Y0-ARF-161

PLATELET ACTIVATING FACTOR RECEPTOR

Signal Mechanisms and Molecular Biology

Edited by

Shivendra D. Shukla

Department of Pharmacology
School of Medicine
University of Missouri-Columbia

CRC Press
Boca Raton   Ann Arbor   London   Tokyo

Library of Congress Cataloging-in-Publication Data

Platelet activating factor receptor: signal mechanisms and molecular
  biology / editor, Shivendra D. Shukla.
      p.   cm.
   Includes bibliographical references and index.
   ISBN 0-8493-7299-2
   1. Platelet activating factor--Receptors.   2. Cellular signal
transduction.   I. Shukla, Shivendra D.   II. Series: Pharmacology &
toxicology (Boca Raton, Fla.)
QP752.P62P58   1992
612'.01577--dc20   92-17515
                                                                              CIP

This book represents information obtained from authentic and highly regarded sources. Reprinted material is quoted with permission, and sources are indicated. A wide variety of references are listed. Every reasonable effort has been made to give reliable data and information, but the author and the publisher cannot assume responsibility for the validity of all materials or for the consequences of their use.

Neither this book nor any part may be reproduced or transmitted in any form or by any means, electronic or mechanical, including photocopying, microfilming, and recording, or by any information storage and retrieval system, without permission in writing from the publisher.

Direct all inquiries to CRC Press, Inc., 2000 Corporate Blvd., N.W., Boca Raton, Florida, 33431.

© 1993 by CRC Press, Inc.

International Standard Book Number 0-8493-7299-2

Library of Congress Card Number 92-17515

Printed in Mexico   1 2 3 4 5 6 7 8 9 0

Printed on acid-free paper

FOREWORD

Three decades ago, the biological activity of platelet activating factor (PAF) was described. In 1979 its structure was identified as 1-*O*-alkyl-2-acetyl-*sn*-glycero-3-phosphocholine. Since then, the progress made on PAF research has established this phospholipid as a novel biological mediator active at nanomolar concentrations. Role(s) of PAF in mammalian cells/systems, e.g., platelets, neutrophils, lymphocytes, macrophages, basophils, eosinophils, heart, lung, liver, kidney, eye, brain, skin, and intestine, have been identified. It is also viewed as important in lower animals and microorganisms. An additional uniqueness is the fact that PAF, being a phospholipid, can be synthesized in almost any cell because membrane phospholipids are its precursor.

Developments in the pathophysiology and pharmacology of PAF have been overwhelming. Especially noteworthy is the research on PAF antagonists. However, research on the PAF receptor, its characterization, and its signal transduction mechanisms was begun only recently. Several signal transduction pathways are activated by PAF, and these developments have highlighted the complexities of PAF receptor functions. PAF is the most potent phospholipid agonist known to date and is the first phospholipid for which a receptor has been cloned. This progress has paved the way for investigations into the molecular mechanism of PAF receptor signaling and its regulation. This is the first book that offers a comprehensive account of these developments on the PAF receptor, its characterization, its multiple signaling pathways, and cloning of the receptor. It is my expectation that the book will be an important source for comprehending progress in this field and will serve as a basis for future research investigations.

I would like to thank my parents and family members, especially my wife, Asha, and children Roshni (Bobby), Sundeep (Sunny), and Bivek (Bimmy) for their love, understanding, and support. Thanks also are due to all the contributors whose excellent chapters in this book will undoubtedly serve as a milestone in PAF research for years to come. Finally, I am grateful to Ms. Judy Richey for her prompt and splendid secretarial assistance in the editing of the book.

Shivendra D. Shukla

THE EDITOR

Shivendra D. Shukla, Ph.D., is Associate Professor and Director of Graduate Studies in the Department of Pharmacology, School of Medicine, University of Missouri at Columbia, Missouri.

Dr. Shukla graduated in 1968 from Banaras Hindu University (BHU), Varanasi, India, with a B.Sc. degree and was awarded the M.Sc. degree (Biochemistry) from the same institution in 1970. Subsequently, he served as lecturer in Biochemistry at BHU. He obtained his Ph.D. degree in Biochemistry in 1977 from the University of Liverpool, England. Dr. Shukla conducted postdoctoral research work in the Department of Biochemistry, University of Birmingham, England (1977–1980), and in the Department of Biochemistry, University of Texas Health Sciences Center at San Antonio, Texas (1980–1983). He was appointed Research Assistant Professor at UTHSC-SA in 1983 before moving to the University of Missouri-Columbia as Assistant Professor of Pharmacology in 1984.

Dr. Shukla is a member of the American Society for Biochemistry and Molecular Biology, American Society for Pharmacology and Experimental Therapeutics, American Association for the Advancement of Science, American Heart Association, Physiological Society of India, Indian Science Congress Association, New York Academy of Sciences, and Sigma Xi Society of North America.

Dr. Shukla was awarded the Atomic Energy Commission Scholarship and the University Gold Medal at Banaras Hindu University. He has also received the National Institutes of Health Research Career Development Award. He has published over 60 research papers. His research work has been supported by research grants from the American Heart Association and the National Institutes of Health. His current research interests include the involvement of phospholipases in cell signaling, and platelet activating factor receptor signal transduction and its molecular biology.

SERIES PREFACE

The series, *Pharmacology and Toxicology: Basic and Clinical Aspects,* has been created in recognition of the fact that, from time to time, a new area of interest within a discipline matures to a critical mass that merits organization and integration of the respective observations into a free-standing monograph. In order for such an undertaking to be successful, each editor and/or author must be qualified to identify and select sources best suited to communicate essential aspects of that subject. Such is the case with *Platelet Activating Factor Receptors: Signal Mechanisms and Molecular Biology.* Dr. Shukla has assembled a list of international contributors whose expertise in their respective areas is well known.

Mannfred A. Hollinger, Ph.D.
Series Editor
Professor
Department of Medical Pharmacology and Toxicology
University of California, Davis
Davis, California

Pharmacology & Toxicology: Basic and Clinical Aspects

Mannfred A. Hollinger, Series Editor
University of California, Davis

Published Titles
Pharmacology of the Skin, 1991, Hasan Mukhtar
Inflammatory Cells and Mediators in Bronchial Asthma, 1990, Devendra K.
   Agrawal and Robert G. Townley
In Vitro *Methods of Toxicity*, 1992, Ronald R. Watson
Basis of Toxicity Testing, 1992, Donald J. Ecobichon
Human Drug Metabolism from Molecular Biology to Man, 1992, Elizabeth Jeffery
Platelet Activating Factor Receptor: Signal Mechanisms and Molecular Biology,
   1992, Shivendra D. Shukla

Forthcoming Titles
Neural Control of Airways, Peter J. Barnes
Alcohol Consumption, Cancer and Birth Defects: Mechanisms Involved in
   Increased Risk Associated with Drinking, Anthony J. Garro
Preclinical & Clinical Modulation of Anticancer Drug Toxicity, Kenneth D. Tew
Rational Drug Design, David B. Weiner and William V. Williams
Receptor Characterization and Their Regulations, Devendra K. Agrawal and
   William V. Williams
Biopharmaceutics of Ocular Drug Delivery, Peter Edman
Beneficial and Toxic Effects of Aspirin, Susan E. Feinman
Placental Pharmacology, B. B. Rama Sastry
Placental Toxicology, B. B. Rama Sastry
Classical Receptor Theory, Terry P. Kenakin
Pharmacology of Intestinal Secretion, Timothy S. Gaginella
Animal Models of Mucosal Inflammation, Timothy S. Gaginella

CONTRIBUTORS

Nicolas G. Bazan
Professor of Ophthalmology,
 Biochemistry and Molecular
 Biology, and
Director, Department of
 Ophthalmology and the
 Neuroscience Center
Louisiana State University
 Medical Center
New Orleans, Louisiana

Lee-Young Chau
Associate Researcher
Institute of Biomedical Sciences
Academia Sinica
Taipei, Taiwan

Neng-neng Cheng
Faculty of Pharmaceutical
 Sciences
Teikyo University, Sagamiko
Kanagawa, Japan

Leanne M. Delbridge
Senior Research Assistant
Department of Physiology
University of Melbourne
Parkville, Victoria, Australia

Animesh Dhar
Research Assistant Professor
Department of Pharmacology
University of Missouri at
 Columbia
Columbia, Missouri

John Philip Doucet
Research Fellow
Department of Ophthalmology and
 the Neuroscience Center
Louisiana State University
 Medical Center
New Orleans, Louisiana

Sagrario Fernandez-Gallardo
Research Fellow
Green Center for Reproductive
 Biology
The University of Texas
Dallas, Texas

Giora Feuerstein
Director of Cardiovascular
 Pharmacology
Department of Pharmaceuticals
Smithkline Beecham
 Pharmaceuticals
King of Prussia, Pennsylvania

Eitan Friedman
Director
Division of Neurochemistry
Professor of Psychiatry and
 Pharmacology
Medical College of Pennsylvania
Philadelphia, Pennsylvania

Teruo Fukuda
Graduate Student
Department of Pharmaceutical
 Sciences
Teikyo University, Sagamiko
Kanagawa, Japan

Carolina Garcia
Becaria MEC-FPI
Laboratorio de Nefrologia
Fundacion Jimenez Diaz
Madrid, Spain

Maria Del Carmen Garcia
Becaria MEC-FPI
Departmento de Bioquimica y
 Fisiologia
Universidad de Valladolid
Valladolid, Spain

Miguel Angel Gijon
Becario pre-Doctoral
Departmento de Bioquimica y
  Fisiologia
Universidad de Valladolid
Valladolid, Spain

Donald J. Hanahan
Professor
Department of Biochemistry
University of Texas Health
  Sciences Center
San Antonio, Texas

Shuntaro Hara
Research Associate
Faculty of Pharmaceutical
  Sciences
University of Tokyo
Tokyo, Japan

Yu-Shen Hsu
Research Assistant
Institute of Biomedical Sciences
Academia Sinica
Taipei, Taiwan

San-Bao Hwang
Director of Biochemistry
CytoMed Inc.
Cambridge, Massachusetts

Keizo Inoue
Professor
Faculty of Pharmaceutical
  Sciences
University of Tokyo
Tokyo, Japan

Yueh-Jin Jii
Research Assistant
Institute of Biomedical Sciences
Academia Sinica
Taipei, Taiwan

Ichiro Kudo
Associate Professor
Faculty of Pharmaceutical
  Sciences
University of Tokyo
Tokyo, Japan

Paul G. Lysko
Associate Senior Investigator
Department of Pharmacology
Smithkline Beecham
  Pharmaceuticals
King of Prussia, Pennsylvania

Tatsuya Miyamoto
Graduate Student
Department of Pharmaceutical
  Sciences
Teikyo University, Sagamiko
Kanagawa, Japan

Faustino Mollinedo
Investigador Cientifico del CSIC
Centro de Investigaciones
  Biologicas
Consejo Superior de
  Investigaciones Cientificas
Madrid, Spain

Joseph T. O'Flaherty
Professor of Medicine
Department of Medicine
Wake Forest University School of
  Medicine
Winston-Salem, North Carolina

Merle S. Olson
Professor and Chairman
Department of Biochemistry
The University of Texas Health
  Science Center
San Antonio, Texas

Mariano Sanchez-Crespo
Professor de Investigacion del
  CSIC
Departmento de Bioquimica y
  Fisiologia
Universidad de Valladolid
Valladolid, Spain

Takao Shimizu
Professor
Department of Biochemistry
The University of Tokyo
Tokyo, Japan

Shivendra D. Shukla
Associate Professor and Director
  of Graduate Studies
Department of Pharmacology
University of Missouri at
  Columbia
Columbia, Missouri

Alastair G. Stewart
Chief Scientist/NH & MRC
  Research Fellow
Microsurgery Research Center
St. Vincent's Hospital
Melbourne, Australia

Takayuki Sugiura
Lecturer
Department of Pharmaceutical
  Sciences
Teikyo University, Sagamiko
Kanagawa, Japan

Archi W. Thurston, Jr.
Graduate Research Associate
Department of Pharmacology
University of Missouri at
  Columbia
Columbia, Missouri

Yamini B. Tripathi
Senior Lecturer
Department of Medicinal
  Chemistry
Banaras Hindu University
Varanasi, India

Keizo Waku
Professor
Department of Pharmaceutical
  Sciences
Teikyo University, Sagamiko
Kanagawa, Japan

Tian-Li Yue
Associate Senior Investigator
Department of Pharmacology
Smithkline Beecham
  Pharmaceuticals
King of Prussia, Pennsylvania

Yuexin C. Zhu
Research Specialist
Department of Pharmacology
University of Missouri at
  Columbia
Columbia, Missouri

CONTENTS

PLATELET ACTIVATING FACTOR RECEPTOR
Signal Mechanisms and Molecular Biology

Chapter 1

PLATELET ACTIVATING FACTOR — PAST, PRESENT, AND FUTURE

Donald J. Hanahan

TABLE OF CONTENTS

ISBN 0-8493-7299-2
© 1993 by CRC Press, Inc.

I. INTRODUCTION

It was announced in 1979 that the component apparently responsible for most of the biological responses noted in systemic anaphylaxis (as one example) was best represented by a phosphoglyceride with the following structure:

$$
\begin{array}{c}
\qquad\qquad CH_2O(CH_2)_x CH_3 \\
\qquad O \quad | \\
\qquad \| \quad | \\
CH_3\ C\ O\ CH \\
\qquad\qquad | \qquad O \\
\qquad\qquad\qquad \| \\
\qquad CH_2O\ \overset{|}{\underset{|}{P}}\ OCH_2\ CH_2\ \overset{+}{N(CH_3)_3} \\
\qquad\qquad O-
\end{array}
$$

where X = 15:0, 17:0 or 17:1

It is interesting to note that three papers[1-3] are considered, in this field, as providing proof of the structure of the naturally occurring mediator. Actually, these publications reported only on the semisynthesis of the above phosphoglyceride, which had thin layer chromatographic (TLC) and biological characteristics similar to the naturally occurring material. The first proof of the structure of platelet activating factor (PAF) isolated from stimulated rabbit basophils was reported[4] nearly 9 months subsequent to these publications. In any event these findings certainly stimulated the field of phospholipid chemistry and biochemistry. To the hardcore lipid chemist, however, it was difficult to accept the fact that an acetate group could be one of the acyl groups on a phosphoglyceride present in cellular membranes. Usually these contained two long chain fatty acyl groups on the *sn*-1 and *sn*-2 position.

It is interesting to note that in neutrophils the fatty acyl group on the *sn*-1 position is replaced by an alkyl ether group and forms part of a cycle in which fatty acyl group on the *sn*-2 position (arachidonic acid) can be released during stimulation of these cells and an acetate group can be inserted. As shall be discussed below, strong evidence also exists for the presence of an 1-O-acyl-2 acetyl-*sn*-glycerophosphocholine in stimulated cells and that it has biological activity. The field of PAF chemistry, biochemistry, and biology has expanded in an almost explosive manner, covering areas from the basic research on its mode of action on a cell to an understanding of its pathophysiologic behavior, to investigations on its positive effects on embryo implantation, fetal development, and termination of pregnancy. A number of reviews have been published on these topics,[5-7] and coupled with the presentations given in this book will show that the field covers a very broad area. An important point, however, is where does the field go now? What questions need to be answered? It is, of course, possible to discuss several areas in need of further study or explanation, but only a few are cited below.

II. ROLE OF ENDOGENOUS PLATELET ACTIVATING FACTOR IN CELLS

Is the only reason for the formation of PAF to participate in the arachidonate cycle mentioned above, or does it have some specific site of action? One example of a "specific" site of action would be in the PAF-mediated glycogenolysis in the perfused rat liver.[8] The exact mode of action of PAF in this instance is unclear, but it does illustrate the fact that PAF has some normophysiologic activity. A similar phenomena has been shown to occur in the fetal lung[9] and can be related to the ensuing formation of long-chain saturated fatty acids required for surfactant formation. Obviously, then, further study needs to be undertaken to elucidate the behavior of intracellularly produced PAF. Of particular importance is the observation that stimulated cells, such as neutrophils, can produce large quantities of PAF without any evident alteration of the behavior of the cell. The identical amount of PAF, however, would considerably alter neutrophils or platelets, if added extracellularly to the cell. Thus, a case for some type of endogenous regulators of PAF must be invoked and is discussed below.

III. A CASE OF INTRACELLULAR INHIBITORS

It has been evident to those interested in assaying for cellular formation of PAF, that one first must extract the total lipids to recover the PAF, and that this total lipid extract, although derived from a stimulated cell, will not give a positive assay for PAF. The second point is that the total lipid extract must be separated by TLC to recover the PAF fraction. This has been a repeated observation and certainly supports the presence of intracellular inhibitors. This proposal has been strengthened by the recent findings that such an inhibitor could be isolated from perfused rat liver. It was identified as a long-chain, unsaturated fatty acid[10] which appears to inhibit the PAF-induced activation of platelets at the polyphosphoinositide synthesis step. Undoubtedly other endogenous regulators of PAF remain to be discovered.

IV. DOES EVIDENCE EXIST FOR SUBCELLULAR RECEPTORS FOR PLATELET ACTIVATING FACTOR?

Pursuant to the discussion above, the metabolic action of PAF, one must address the high potential for an intracellular receptor. To date, none has been detected or fully identified, but it seems very likely that it is only a matter of time until such receptors are found. The problems attendant on defining the intracellular receptors, however, could be significant. At least at present one would have to fragment the cell and isolate subcellular components of the cell and examine whether binding of labeled PAF does occur and whether a specific binding occurs. In such situations, it is always possible that the fractionation procedure has led to artifact production. Then, given a putative receptor(s) is indicated, the next questions are what is the function of the binding site(s), is a signal developed, or is a particular reaction influenced? If so, what are they and how important are they to the normal function of cells? This presents provocative possibilities, but the proper experiments would be difficult to design.

V. EXTRACELLULAR PLATELET ACTIVATING FACTOR RECEPTOR CHARACTERIZATION

This is an exciting area for exploration now that cloning of the gene encoding the cell surface receptor for PAF has been achieved.[11] This breakthrough should allow insight into the structural nature of the receptor and how it binds PAF with such a high specificity, whereas simple removal of the acetate moiety leads to an inactive product and no binding to the specific receptor for PAF. As has been well documented in the literature, the most prevalent substituent on the sn-2 position is an acetyl group. Interestingly, both the C-2 and C-3 derivatives have similar EC_{50} values on platelets, while the synthetic C-4 or longer-chain derivatives have little or no biological activity. Obviously, the structural configuration of the PAF molecule possesses some uniqueness and one hypothetical structure could be viewed as in Figure 1. Such a quasi-cyclical structure does have some validity given the observation that the phosphorothioate derivatives of PAF do have significant differences in biological activity, depending on the stereoconfiguration of the phosphate.[12] Consequently,

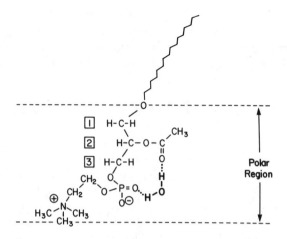

FIGURE 1.

the conformation about the phosphate also contributes to the activity of the particular derivative. These parameters should be an important part of any detailed study of the interaction of PAF with its receptor.

Finally, as regards the receptor, two other questions should be asked: (1) are all PAF receptors created equal?, and (2) if more than one class of receptors exist on a cell do they have similar or different specificities? Pursuant to the latter question, simple removal of the choline moiety from PAF leads to the phosphoric acid derivative, which has significant biological activity. While PAF is inhibited by the PAF receptor inhibitor, CV 3988, the phosphoric acid derivative is not inhibited by this reagent. Even more interesting is the finding that cells can be desensitized to the phosphoric acid derivative and not to the PAF molecule. The reverse situation also is found.

VI. NATURALLY OCCURRING ANALOGUES OF PLATELET ACTIVATING FACTOR

Several years ago the occurrence of the 1-acyl analogue of PAF was announced.[13] Though it has much lower biological activity than the 1-O-alkyl compound, it appears to interact with the same receptor as PAF. Other reports substantiating this early observation have been made. The 1-O-acyl analogue is normally found in much lower amounts than the 1-O-alkyl analogue. Recently, however, a very provocative finding[14] demonstrated that the 1-O-alkyl form is the major component in vascular endothelial cells. Other shorter-chain length substituents have been found in brain.[15]

Thus, the question to be raised is whether the 1-O-acyl derivative has a different mode of action than the 1-O-alkyl, and hence, influences quite different reaction pathways. This puzzle remains to be solved.

In closing, it seems that the field of PAF is very active, but still provides the challenge of understanding how a quite simple phosphoglyceride structure can exert such a potent and diverse biological activity.

REFERENCES

1. **Benveniste, J., Tence, M., Varenne, P., Bidault, J., Boullet, C., and Polonsky, J.,** Semi-synthese et structure purposee du facteur activant les plaquettesPAF: PAF-acether, un alkyl ether analogue de la lysophosphatidylcholine, *C. R. Acad. Sci. Paris,* 28, 1037, 1979.

2. **Demopoulos, C. A., Pinckard, R. N., and Hanahan, D. J.,** Platelet activating factor. Evidence for 1-O-alkyl-2-acetyl-*sn*-glycero-3-phosphorylcholine as the active component. A new class of lipid chemical mediators, *J. Biol. Chem.,* 254, 355, 1979.

3. **Blank, M. L., Snyder, F., Byers, L. W., Brooks, B., and Muirhead, E. E.,** Antihypertensive activity of an alkyl ether analog of phosphatidylcholine, *Biochem. Biophys. Res. Commun.,* 90, 1194, 1979.

4. **Hanahan, D. J., Demopoulos, C. A., Liehr, J., and Pinckard, R. N.,** Identification of platelet activating isolated from rabbit platelets as acetylglycerlether phosphorylcholine, *J. Biol. Chem.,* 255, 5514, 1980.

5. **Hanahan, D. J.,** Platelet activating factor: a biologically active phosphoglyceride, *Annu. Rev. Biochem.,* 55, 483, 1986.

6. **Snyder, F.,** Platelet activating factor and related acetylated lipids as potent biologically active cellular mediators, *Am. J. Physiol.,* 259, C697, 1990.

7. **Prescott, S. M., Zimmerman, G. A., and McIntyre, T. M.,** Platelet activating factor, *J. Biol. Chem.,* 265, 17381, 1990.

8. **Shukla, S. D., Buxton, D. B., Olson, M. S., and Hanahan, D. J.,** Acetylglyceryl ether phosphorylcholine. A potent activator of hepatic phosphoinositide metabolism and glycogenolysis, *J. Biol. Chem.,* 258, 10212, 1983.

9. **Johnston, J. M.,** The function of PAF in the communication between the fetal and maternal compartments during parturition, in *Platelet-Activating Factor and Diseases,* Saito, K. and Hanahan, D. J., Eds., International Medical Publishers, Tokyo, 1989, 129.

10. **Nunez, D., Randon, J., Gandhi, C., Siafaka-Kapadai, A., Olson, M. S., and Hanahan, D. J.,** The inhibition of platelet activating factor-induced platelet activation by oleic acid is associated with a decrease in polyphosphoinositide metabolism, *J. Biol. Chem.,* 265, 18330, 1990.

11. **Honda, Z. I., Nakamura, M., Miki, I., Minami, M., Watanabe, T., Seyama, Y., Okado, H., Toh, H., Ito, K., Miyamoto, T., and Shimizu, T.,** Cloning by functional expression of platelet-activating factor receptor from guinea pig lung, *Nature,* 349, 342, 1991.

12. **Rosario-Jansen, T., Jiang, R.-T., Tsai, M.-D., and Hanahan, D. J.,** Phospholipids chiral at phosphorus. Synthesis and sterospecificity of phosphorothioate analogues of platelet-activating factor, *Biochemistry,* 27, 4619, 1988.

13. **Mueller, H. W., O'Flaherty, J. T., and Wykle, R. L.,** The molecular species distribution of platelet-activating factor synthesized by rabbit and human neutrophils, *J. Biol. Chem.,* 259, 14554, 1984.

14. **Mueller, H. W., Nollert, M. U., and Eskin, S. G.,** Synthesis of 1-acyl-2-[³H] acetyl-*sn*-glycero-3-phosphocholine. A structural analog of platelet activating factor by vascular endothelial cells, *Biochem. Biophys. Res. Commun.,* 176, 1557, 1991.

15. **Tokumura, A., Takauchi, K., Asai, T., Kamiyasu, K., Ogawa, T., and Tsukatani, H.,** Novel molecular analogues of phosphatidylcholine in a lipid extract from bovine brain: 1-long chain acyl-2-short chain acyl-*sn*-glycero-3-phosphocholines, *J. Lipid Res.,* 30, 219, 1989.

Chapter 2

CHARACTERIZATION OF PLATELET ACTIVATING FACTOR RECEPTORS USING RADIOLIGAND BINDING STUDIES

San-Bao Hwang

TABLE OF CONTENTS

ISBN 0-8493-7299-2
© 1993 by CRC Press, Inc.

I. INTRODUCTION

Platelet activating factor (PAF; 1-*O*-alkyl-2-acetyl-*sn*-glycero-3-phosphocholine) is a phospholipid mediator that is synthesized by different cell types and exerts a wide range of pathophysiological effects.[1] Activation of cellular responses by PAF is mediated by interaction with specific receptors that can be labeled with [³H]PAF.[2] The binding of [³H]PAF to high-affinity binding sites is endothermic and largely entropy driven.[3] Specific PAF receptors are present in cell and tissue preparations from many animal species including human platelets,[4-8] neutrophils,[9-12] eosinophils,[13] mononuclear leukocytes,[14,15] macrophages,[16,17] human lung,[18] rat liver tissues,[19,20] rat brain,[21,22] and rabbit eyes.[23]

With the assay development of either PAF receptor binding or PAF-induced aggregation of platelets, PAF receptor antagonists with novel structures were then identified.[2,24] Figure 1 lists several selected PAF receptor antagonists. All of these PAF receptor antagonists are able to block cellular responses induced by PAF and have been demonstrated to be valuable in the characterization of PAF receptors and the evaluation of the role of PAF in several human diseases. We used these PAF receptor antagonists to demonstrate differences in PAF receptors between species and PAF receptor heterogeneity within the same species. These included the PAF-like PAF antagonists, CV-6209 and Ono-6240; natural products; kadsurenone and Fusijawa compound FR 72112 derived from the fermentation product, FR 900452; and other synthetic compounds, benzodiazepine analogue WEB 2086, the indene analogue L-651,142, Rhone Poulenc compounds, 52770 RP, and tetrahydrofuran analogues developed at Merck such as L-652,731, L-653,150, L-659,989, L-670,241 and MK 287 (Figure 1).

II. SOLUBILIZATION OF PLATELET ACTIVATING FACTOR RECEPTORS

The PAF receptor is a membrane-bound protein.[5] It can only be solubilized with detergent. A specific binding protein for PAF with a molecular weight of 160 to 180 kDa has been solubilized and isolated;[25,26] however, no additional data were provided to unambiguously demonstrate that the isolated PAF binding protein was a specific PAF receptor with binding characteristics comparable to those of intact platelets. A digitonin-solubilized PAF receptor protein complex with an Mw of 220 kDa was also reported.[27] The solubilized receptor complex bound specifically to [³H]PAF. This binding can be blocked by either unlabeled PAF or the PAF receptor antagonist, L-652,731. Dissociation of [³H]PAF from the receptor complex was facilitated by Na^+ and Li^+. K^+ and Cs^+ showed no effects on the binding of [³H]PAF to the solubilized receptor complex. GTP synergized the effect of Na^+-induced dissociation of [³H]PAF from the receptor complex. The solubilized PAF receptor from rabbit platelets had a molecular weight of 52,000.[28] Solubilization and partial purification of PAF binding protein was also reported from the membrane of human platelets, and mononuclear leukocytes.[29] The solubilized PAF receptor from human showed a molecular weight of 65 kDa in polyacrylamide gels; however, no binding parameters for [³H]PAF to the solubilized receptor are yet available. We have recently reported that PAF receptors from human platelets can be solubilized with lauryldimethylamine oxide (LDAO).[30] The solubilized receptors retained roughly the same affinity to [³H]PAF as the receptors in the membranes (Figure 2). From several repeated experiments, PAF receptors from human platelet membranes solubilized with LDAO showed an equilibrium dissociation constant (K_d) of 2.02 ± 0.48 nM, which is not significantly different from the K_d value of PAF receptor in human platelet membranes ($K_d = 2.32 \pm 0.27$ nM). Therefore, the solubilized PAF receptor in LDAO retained roughly the same conformation as that in isolated membranes. This is the first step for the purification of PAF receptors.

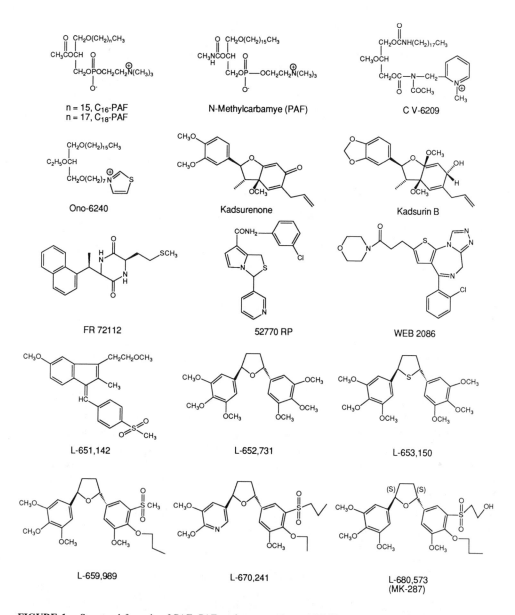

FIGURE 1. Structural formula of PAF, PAF analogues, and several PAF receptor antagonists described in the text.

III. G-PROTEIN INVOLVEMENT

PAF receptors belong to a superfamily of G-protein coupled receptors. GTP specifically inhibited the binding of [³H]PAF to isolated rabbit platelet membranes[31] at either 37° or at 0°C. Other nucleotides at similar concentrations showed no inhibitory effects. Further evidence to support the coupling of PAF receptors to G-protein arises from the measurement of PAF-stimulated GTPase activity (hydrolysis of [γ-³²P]GTP into ³²Pᵢ and GDP). PAF stimulated GTPase activity in a highly dose-dependent fashion.[11,31] The concentration required to stimulate half-maximal effects was at 0.7 nM, which was roughly the same as the K_d value of [³H]PAF binding to rabbit platelet membranes.[31] It reached a maximal effect at

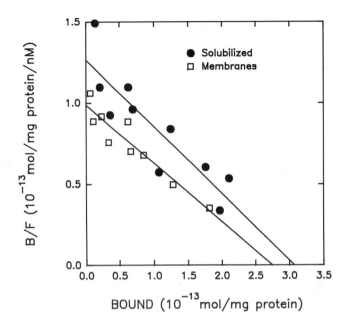

FIGURE 2. Scatchard plots of [³H]C₁₈-PAF binding to isolated human platelet membranes and solubilized PAF receptors from human platelets. The detergent used for solubilization was LDAO with a final concentration of 4 mM.

20 nM. The stimulation of GTPase activity is PAF specific. The biological inactive enantiomer of PAF showed no GTPase activity even at 0.1 µM concentration. The activated GTPase activity can be specifically inhibited by the PAF receptor antagonist, kadsurenone. However, the inactive analogue, kadsurin B, showed no inhibitory effect at the concentrations at which kadsurenone showed significant inhibition. These results suggest that PAF-induced GTPase activity is a receptor-mediated process and the PAF receptor is coupled to G-protein. The PAF receptor has recently been cloned and functionally expressed in *Xenopus* oocytes.[32] The cloned PAF receptor contained 342 amino acids. The hydropathy analysis of this 342 amino acid sequence showed seven transmembrane segments, a specific feature for those receptors coupled to G-protein.

IV. SPECIES DIFFERENCES

PAF receptors showed differences between species. Species differences between PAF receptors were first reported by Hwang and Lam[6] in 1986. L-652,731 and the thiophene analogue, L-653,150, showed differences in potency in inhibiting the binding of [³H]PAF between human platelet and rabbit platelet membranes. L-659,989, a more potent tetrahydrofuran analogue than L-652,731 and L-653,150, showed differences in potency in inhibiting the tritium-labeled PAF between humans and rabbits.[33] In the human, L-659,989 showed identical potency in either human platelet, human polymorphonuclear membrane (PMN), or human lung membranes. However, in rabbit platelet and rabbit PMN membranes, L-659,989 is about ten times more potent than in humans. PAF receptors also showed differences between humans and rats.[12] The indene analogue, L-651,142 showed differences in potency in inhibiting the binding of [³H]PAF to either human PMNs or rat peritoneal PMNs. L-651,142 was about six times more potent in humans than in rats.

V. MULTIPLE CONFORMATIONAL STATES OF PLATELET ACTIVATING FACTOR RECEPTORS

In rabbit platelets, sodium and lithium specifically inhibited the binding of tritium-labeled PAF.[31] Lithium is about 10 to 30 times less potent than sodium in inhibiting [^{3}H]PAF binding. Potassium, cesium, rubidium, magnesium, calcium, and manganese potentiated the binding. The inhibition by sodium appears to be due to the decrease in the affinity of PAF to the receptor, whereas the potentiation by magnesium is mainly due to the increase in the detected receptor number.[31] The detectable receptor number for PAF in the presence of 10 mM MgCl$_2$ is about twice that found either in the presence of 150 mM NaCl or in the absence of cations. On the other hand, the ionic effects on the binding of [^{3}H]L-659,989 are quite different than those for [^{3}H]PAF. Sodium and lithium as well as potassium, magnesium, and calcium potentiated the binding of [^{3}H]L-659,989 to rabbit platelet membranes.[34] The detectable receptor number for [^{3}H]L-659,989 in the presence of 150 mM NaCl was about the same as that detected in 10 mM MgCl$_2$. Because both PAF and L-659,989 bind to the same receptor and share a common binding site,[33,34] the difference in the detectable receptor number under different ionic conditions suggests the coexistence of several conformational states of the receptor and that PAF and L-659,989 bind differently to those states.

The existence of multiple conformational states of the PAF receptor can be further confirmed by the competitive binding studies of [^{3}H]L-659,989 by PAF under different ionic conditions and either in the presence or absence of GTP.[34] The K$_d$ of [^{3}H]L-659,989 binding to rabbit platelet membranes is the same in 10 mM MgCl$_2$ as in 150 mM NaCl, and is not altered by the presence of GTP.[34] In the presence of 10 mM MgCl$_2$, the effective dose of PAF to inhibit 50% of specific [^{3}H]L-659,989 binding (ED$_{50}$) is 1.4 nM, whereas in the presence of 150 mM NaCl, the ED$_{50}$ value of PAF is shifted to about 1 μM, which is about 1000-fold higher than that in 10 mM MgCl$_2$. GTP at 1 mM also effectively shifted the PAF competition curve to the right, from an ED$_{50}$ value of 1.4 to 10 nM in the presence of 10 mM MgCl$_2$ and from 1 to 2 μM in the presence of 150 mM NaCl. The competitive curves of [^{3}H]L-659,989 binding to rabbit platelet membranes by PAF under the assay conditions of 10 mM MgCl$_2$, 10 mM MgCl$_2$ and 1 mM GTP, or 150 mM NaCl can be best fitted with two sites rather than with one site.[34,35] The competition curve of PAF in the presence of both 150 mM NaCl and 1 mM GTP can be best fitted with one site.[34,35] The equilibrium dissociation constant (K$_B$) for PAF binding to rabbit platelet membranes in the presence of 150 mM NaCl and 1 mM GTP can thus be determined indirectly from the Schild plot of the inhibition of [^{3}H]L-659,989 binding by PAF, and is found to be 0.93 μM.[34,35] This is probably the lowest K$_d$ value of PAF receptors for PAF. Multiple conformational states of a single type of PAF receptors are therefore confirmed. However, the biological significance of these multiple conformational states of PAF receptors needs to be further elucidated.

VI. RECEPTOR HETEROGENEITY

Considerable variation exists between different cell types in their sensitivity to PAF. Femtomolar concentrations are normally required to significantly enhance interleukin-1 (IL-1) production in lymphocytes,[36] whereas stimulation of eosinophil or neutrophil superoxide generation required micromolar concentrations.[37,38] Differences in sensitivity in the same cell type were also noticed. Activation of acetyltransferase and PAF synthesis in neutrophils was 10 to 30 times more sensitive to activation by PAF than was degranulation.[38] Multiple molecular species of PAF are produced as a result of inflammatory processes.[39,40] PAF species produced vary with both cell of origin and stimulus.[39,40] Moreover, identical cells

TABLE 1
Equilibrium Dissociation Constants (K_d) of
[^{3}H]C$_{16}$-PAF and [^{3}H]C$_{18}$-PAF to
Isolated Membranes

Source of membranes	K_d (nM)	
	[^{3}H]C$_{16}$-PAF	[^{3}H]C$_{18}$-PAF
Rabbit platelets	0.53 ($\pm$ 0.06)	ND
Human platelets	0.40 ($\pm$ 0.10)	2.05 ($\pm$ 0.32)
Human PMNs	0.47 ($\pm$ 0.14)	3.15 ($\pm$ 0.24)
Human monocytes	ND	2.32 ($\pm$ 0.17)
Rat peritoneal PMNs	0.61 ($\pm$ 0.10)	ND
Human lung tissue	0.51 ($\pm$ 0.17)	ND
Rat liver tissue	0.51 ($\pm$ 0.14)	ND

Note: ND, not determined.

from different animal species produced different spectra of PAF molecules.[39,40] Differences in rank orders of potency of PAF and PAF structural analogues in different cell types from the same species have also been reported.[41,42] These results suggest the presence of PAF receptor heterogeneity.

With the isolated membranes, we have looked at the binding of tritium-labeled PAF ([^{3}H]C$_{16}$-PAF or [^{3}H]C$_{18}$-PAF) to rabbit platelets, human platelets, human PMNs, human mononuclear leukocytes, rat peritoneal PMNs, and human lung and rat liver tissues. PAF receptors in these isolated membrane fragments all showed identical affinity to C$_{16}$-PAF and C$_{18}$-PAF with equilibrium dissociation constants of about 0.5 and 2 nM, respectively (Table 1). These receptor binding data showed no differences between receptors from different species or from different cells and tissues within the same species. However, differences in PAF receptors between cells isolated from the same species have been demonstrated from radioligand binding studies with other tritium-labeled agonists or from the competitive binding studies by receptor antagonists with different chemical structures.[2,43] The K_d values for the nonmetabolizable PAF analogue, *N*-methylcarbamyl-PAF in human platelets and PMNs are different. In human platelet membranes, the K_d value for tritium-labeled *N*-methylcarbamyl-PAF is 2.18 $\pm$ 0.48 nM (mean $\pm$ standard deviation, n = 8), which is significantly different from the K_d value in human PMNs (5.18 $\pm$ 0.54 nM, n = 8).

In rabbit platelets, sodium specifically inhibited the binding of tritium-labeled PAF.[31] Lithium is about 10 to 20 times less potent than sodium in inhibition. The inhibitory effects of sodium have been attributed to a direct linkage between receptors and adenylate cyclase through an inhibitory G-protein.[2] The sodium binding site is located on the cytoplasmic side of plasma membranes and is probably not on the PAF receptor itself, but on a nearby regulatory protein.[35] A membrane component different than G-proteins with a molecular weight of 168 kDa[44] has been identified in the opioid receptor complex to act as an allosteric inhibitor that mediates the effect of sodium on the receptor. The mechanism of the inhibitory effect by Li$^+$ on specific [^{3}H]PAF binding is not well characterized; however, the inhibitory effect by Li$^+$ may be related to the coupling of PAF receptor to the specific G-protein. Li$^+$ has been shown to attenuate the ADP ribosylation of the G$_i$-protein of the cell membranes,[45] and Haslam and Vanderwel[46] reported that PAF inhibited basal, prostaglandin E$_1$-stimulated, and fluoride-stimulated adenylate cyclase activities in human platelets. Potassium, magnesium, calcium, and manganese potentiated the binding. The mechanism for these potentiation effects is not known, but it may also be attributed to the interaction between PAF receptors and other closely coupled regulatory proteins. Therefore, differences in the ionic modulation of [³H]PAF binding to different membrane systems may indicate the differences in the signal transduction mechanism of PAF receptors from different sources.

Similar ionic effects on the tritium-labeled PAF binding in rabbit platelet membranes were also observed in human platelet membranes.[11] Sodium and lithium inhibited the binding. Sodium is ten times more potent than lithium in inhibiting the specific PAF binding. Potassium, magnesium, and calcium potentiated the binding. In human PMN membranes, potassium, magnesium, and calcium again potentiated the binding, whereas sodium and lithium showed no effects on the specific tritium-labeled PAF binding even up to 300 mM concentrations.[11] In human monocyte membranes, as in human platelet membranes, both sodium and lithium showed inhibitory effects on the binding of PAF, but unlike those in human platelet membranes, sodium and lithium showed roughly the same potency in inhibiting the binding of [³H]PAF to human monocyte membranes.[15] Even though potassium or divalent cations, when applied alone, showed an increase in the specific PAF binding in the above three cell types, the potentiation effects of potassium and magnesium are not additive. In the presence of both potassium and magnesium, potassium showed no effect on the magnesium-potentiated PAF binding in human platelet membranes.[11] However, in human PMN membranes, potassium inhibited the magnesium-potentiated PAF binding.[11] In human monocyte membranes, potassium showed no effect on the magnesium-potentiated PAF binding, but sodium and lithium inhibited the magnesium-potentiated specific binding at an identical potency.[15] ZnCl$_2$ has also been demonstrated to specifically inhibit the specific [³H]PAF binding to human platelets and the PAF-induced aggregation in human platelets.[47] However, it showed no significant inhibition of the binding of [³H]PAF to human PMN membranes and human monocyte membranes at ZnCl$_2$ concentrations, which gave a significant inhibition in human platelet membranes.[15,43] These results suggest that the signal transduction mechanism of PAF receptors and possibly the PAF receptor itself are different among the three cell types. Indeed, in the competition of tritium-labeled binding, we found differences in potency in two PAF receptor antagonists between human platelet and human PMN membranes.[2,11,43] In isolated membranes, Ono-6240 is found to be about ten times more potent in human platelet membranes than in human PMN membranes in inhibiting the specific binding of PAF as well as the PAF-induced GTPase activity.[11] At the cellular level, Ono-6240 is again ten times more potent in inhibiting the PAF-induced human platelet aggregation than in inhibiting the PAF-induced human PMN aggregation.[11] On the other hand, FR 72112 is found to be three times more potent in human PMNs in inhibiting the PAF binding than in human platelets.[2,43] We also found two compounds showing similar potencies in human platelet and human PMN membranes, but had different potencies in human monocyte membranes.[15] CV-6209 showed similar potency in competing with the tritium-labeled PAF binding to either human platelet or human PMN membranes, but was less potent in inhibiting the binding of [³H]PAF to human monocyte membranes. On the other hand, 52770 RP showed similar potency in human platelet and human PMN membranes, but was more potent in human monocyte membranes in inhibiting PAF receptor binding. These results further confirmed the difference of PAF receptors within these three cell types. Therefore, PAF receptors as well as signal transduction mechanisms within three types of cells isolated from circulating blood are different.

VII. EXISTENCE OF INTRACELULLAR RECEPTORS

In the preparation of human platelet membranes, we separated the membrane fragments further into two fractions with a discontinuous sucrose density gradient.[6] One membrane fraction was collected from the interface banding at 0.25 and 1.03 M sucrose, and was called membrane fraction A. The other was collected from the interface between 1.03 and 1.5 M

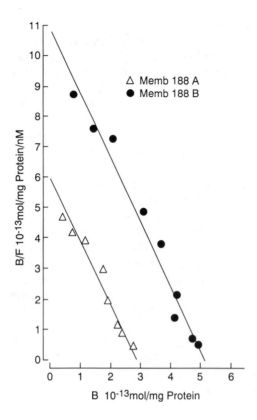

FIGURE 3. Scatchard plots of [^{3}H]C$_{16}$-PAF binding to human platelet membranes: membrane fraction A (extracellular membranes) and membrane fraction B (intracellular membranes). Membrane protein, 100 μg, was added to tubes containing [^{3}H]C$_{16}$-PAF ranging from 0.6 to 5 n*M* in medium containing 10 m*M* MgCl$_2$, 10 m*M* Tris, and 0.25% bovine serum albumin, pH 7.0.

sucrose, and was called membrane fraction B. As demonstrated by several enzyme and receptor markers,[48] membrane fraction A has more alkaline phosphatase than membrane fraction B.[49] Wheat germ agglutinin (WGA) potentiates the binding of PAF to membrane fraction A but not to membrane fraction B.[50] These results suggest that membrane fraction A is a membrane fraction enriched with plasma membranes. On the other hand, membrane fraction B contains more inositol-(1,4,5)-trisphosphate receptors[51] and higher activity of antimycin-insensitive NADH-cytochrome *c* reductase.[49] Therefore, membrane fraction B is likely to be enriched with intracellular membranes. However, as shown in Figure 3, these intracellular membranes have PAF receptors with identical K$_d$ value to [^{3}H]C$_{16}$-PAF as those in plasma membranes, but the maximal detectable receptor sites in membrane fraction B are about twice those in membrane fraction A. Because the intracellular membrane fraction (membrane fraction B) contains consistently more PAF receptor sites than the plasma membrane-enriched fraction (membrane fraction A), the intracellular membrane also contains PAF receptors.[6,50] Thus far, no difference has been found between intra- and extracellular PAF receptors in human platelets. Several PAF analogues and PAF receptor antagonists including C$_{16}$-PAF, C$_{18}$-PAF, *N*-methylcarbamyl-PAF, two of the tetrahydrofuran analogues, L-670,241 and MK 287, and 52770 RP, showed identical K$_d$ values in both intracellular and extracellular membranes.[52] These intracellular receptors may mediate the function of PAF produced and retained inside the cells.

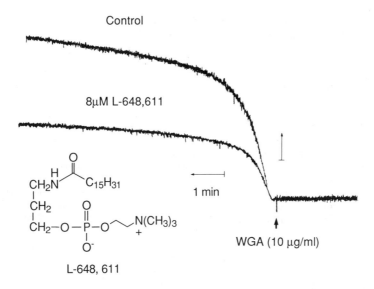

FIGURE 4. Inhibition of WGA-induced aggregation of human platelets by L-648,611. L-648,611 in dimethylsulfoxide or the same volume of dimethylsulfoxide (1.5 µl) was added to a 0.5-ml platelet suspension and incubated for 15 min before the addition of WGA to induce the aggregation of human platelets.

VIII. POSSIBLE FUNCTIONS OF INTRACELLULAR PAF RECEPTORS

WGA induced platelet aggregation even in the presence of both cyclooxygenase inhibitor (aspirin) and ADP scavenger (creatine phosphate/creatine phosphokinase).[50] This WGA-induced human platelet aggregation can be blocked by a PAF acetyltransferase inhibitor, L-648,611 (Figure 4). CV-6209, a PAF receptor antagonist, also inhibited the WGA-induced aggregation of human platelets.[50] These results suggest that WGA may stimulate PAF synthesis and the synthesized PAF may be involved in WGA-induced platelet aggregation. Indeed, activation of acetyltransferase can be observed even at concentrations of WGA below those for the induction of platelet aggregation.[50] WGA-induced PAF synthesis in intact platelets was further confirmed by the measurement of the incorporation of tritium-labeled acetate into PAF either in the presence or absence of the PAF acetylhydrolase inhibitor, phenylmethylsulfonyl fluoride.[50] Synthesis of PAF preceded platelet aggregation.[50] Most importantly, this PAF synthesis can be blocked by the PAF synthesis inhibitor, L-648,611.[50] These results suggest that PAF synthesized and retained inside the cell may act as an intracellular mediator and the intracellular PAF receptors may mediate the function of the intracellular PAF.

REFERENCES

1. **Braquet, P., Touqui, L., Shen, T. Y., and Vargaftig, B. B.,** Perspectives in platelet-activating factor research, *Pharmacol. Rev.,* 39, 97, 1987.
2. **Hwang, S.-B.,** Specific receptors of platelet-activating factor, receptor heterogeneity, and signal transduction mechanisms, *J. Lipid Mediators,* 2, 123, 1990.
3. **Borea, P. A., Montesi, L., Muzzolini, A., and Fantozzi, R.,** Temperature dependence of [³H]PAF binding to washed human platelets, *Biochem. Pharmacol.,* 41, 629, 1991.

4. **Valone, F. H., Cole, E., Reinhold, V. R., and Goetz, E. J.,** Specific binding of phospholipid platelet-activating factor by human platelets, *J. Immunol.,* 129, 1637, 1982.

5. **Hwang, S.-B., Lee, C. S. C., Cheah, M. J., and Shen, T. Y.,** Specific receptor sites for 1-O-alkyl-2-O-acetyl-*sn*-glycero-3-phosphocholine (platelet activating factor) on rabbit platelet and guinea pig smooth muscle membranes, *Biochemistry,* 22, 4756, 1983.

6. **Hwang, S.-B. and Lam, M.-H.,** Species difference in the specific receptor of platelet activating factor, *Biochem. Pharmacol.,* 35, 4511, 1986.

7. **Homma, H., Tokumura, A., and Hanahan, D. J.,** Binding and internalization of platelet-activating factor 1-O-alkyl-2-acetyl-*sn*-glycero-3-phosphocholine in washed rabbit platelets, *J. Biol. Chem.,* 262, 10582, 1987.

8. **Tahraoui, L., Floch, A., Mondot, S., and Cavero, I.,** High affinity specific binding sites for tritiated platelet-activating factor in canine platelet membranes: counterparts of platelet-activating factor receptors mediating platelet aggregation, *Mol. Pharmacol.,* 34, 145, 1988.

9. **Valone, F. H. and Goetzl, E. J.,** Specific binding by human polymorphonuclear leukocytes of the immunological mediator 1-O-alkyl-2-acetyl-*sn*-glycero-3-phosphocholine, *Immunology,* 48, 141, 1983.

10. **O'Flaherty, J. T., Surles, J. R., Redman, J., Jacobson, D., Piantadosi, C., and Wykle, R. L.,** Binding and metabolism of platelet-activating factor by human neutrophils, *J. Clin. Invest.,* 78, 381, 1986.

11. **Hwang, S.-B.,** Identification of a second putative receptor of platelet-activating factor from human polymorphonuclear leukocytes, *J. Biol. Chem.,* 263, 3225, 1988.

12. **Hwang, S.-B.,** High affinity receptor binding of platelet-activating factor in rat peritoneal polymorphonuclear leukocytes, *Eur. J. Pharmacol.,* 196, 169, 1991.

13. **Ukena, D., Krogel, C., Dent, G., Yukawa, T., Sybrecht, G., and Barnes, P. J.,** PAF-receptors on eosinophils: identification with a novel ligand, [³H]WEB-2086, *Biochem. Pharmacol.,* 38, 1702, 1989.

14. **Ng, D. S. and Wong, K.,** Specific binding of platelet-activating factor (PAF) by human peripheral blood mononuclear leukocytes, *Biochem. Biophys. Res. Commun.,* 155, 311, 1988.

15. **Hwang, S.-B., Lam, M.-H., and Wu, K.,** Specific binding of tritium-labeled platelet-activating factor to human mononuclear leukocyte membranes: a third putative receptor of platelet-activating factor, in *Prostaglandins, Leukotrienes, Lipoxins, and PAF,* Bailey, J. M., Ed., Plenum Press, New York, 1991, 281.

16. **Prpic, V., Uhing, R. J., Weiel, J. E., Jakoi, L., Gawdi, G., Herman, B., and Adams, D. O.,** Biochemical and functional responses stimulated by platelet-activating factor in murine peritoneal macrophages, *J. Cell Biol.,* 107, 363, 1988.

17. **Valone, F. H.,** Identification of platelet-activating factor receptor in P388D₁ murine macrophages, *J. Immunol.,* 140, 2389, 1988.

18. **Hwang, S.-B., Lam, M.-H., and Shen, T. Y.,** Specific binding sites for platelet activating in human lung tissues, *Biochem. Biophys. Res. Commun.,* 128, 972, 1985.

19. **Hwang, S.-B.,** Specific receptor sites for platelet activating factor on rat liver plasma membranes, *Arch. Biochem. Biophys.,* 257, 339, 1987.

20. **Chao, W., Liu, H., DeBuysere, M., Hanahan, D. J., and Olson, M. S.,** Identification of receptors for platelet-activating factor in rat Kupffer cells, *J. Biol. Chem.,* 264, 13591, 1989.

21. **Domingo, M. T., Spinnewyn, B., Chabrier, P. E., and Braquet, P.,** Presence of specific binding sites for platelet-activating factor (PAF) in the brain, *Biochem. Biophys. Res. Commun.,* 151, 730, 1988.

22. **Marcheselli, V. L., Rossowska, M. J., Domingo, M.-T., Braquet, P., and Bazan, N. G.,** Distinct platelet-activating factor binding sites in synaptic endings and in intracellular membranes of rat cerebral cortex, *J. Biol. Chem.,* 265, 9140, 1990.

23. **Domingo, M. T., Chabrier, D. E., Van Delft, J. L., Verbeij, N. L., Van Haeringen, N. J., and Braquet, P.,** Characterization of specific binding sites for PAF in the iris and ciliary body of rabbit, *Biochem. Biophys. Res. Commun.,* 160, 250, 1989.

24. **Shen, T. Y., Hwang, S.-B., Doebber, T. W., and Robbins, J. C.,** The chemical and biological properties of PAF agonists, antagonists and biosynthetic inhibitors, in *Platelet-Activating Factor and Related Lipid Mediators,* Synder, F., Ed., Plenum Press, New York, 1987, 153.

25. **Valone, F. H.,** Isolation of a platelet membrane protein which binds the platelet-activating factor 1-O-hexadecyl-2-acetyl-*sn*-glycero-3-phosphorylcholine, *Immunology,* 52, 169, 1984.

26. **Nishihira, J., Ishibashi, T., Imai, Y., and Muramatsu, T.,** Purification and characterization of the specific binding protein for platelet activating factor (1-O-alkyl-2-acetyl-*sn*-glycero-3-phosphocholine) from human platelets, *Tohoku J. Exp. Med.,* 147, 145, 1985.

27. **Chau, L.-Y. and Jii, Y.-J.,** Characterization of ³H-labelled platelet-activating factor receptor complex solubilized from rabbit platelet membranes, *Biochim. Biophys. Acta,* 970, 103, 1988.

28. **Chau, L.-Y., Tsai, Y.-M., and Cheng, J.-R.,** Photoaffinity labeling of platelet-activating factor binding sites in rabbit platelet membranes, *Biochem. Biophys. Res. Commun.,* 161, 1070, 1989.

29. **Shen, T. Y., Hussaini, I., Hwang, S.-B., and Chang, M. N.,** Recent development of platelet-activating factor antagonists, *Adv. Prostaglandin Thromboxane Leukotriene Res.,* 19, 359, 1989.

30. **Hwang, S.-B.,** Receptor heterogeneity and function of intracellular receptors of platelet-activating factor, in *Prostaglandins, Leukotrienes, Lipoxins and PAF,* 11th Spring Symposium of The George Washington University, Bailey, J. M., Ed., 1991, 20 (Abstract).

31. **Hwang, S.-B., Lam, M.-H., and Pong, S. S.,** Ionic and GTP regulation of binding of platelet-activating factor to receptors and platelet-activating factor-induced activation of GTPase in rabbit platelet membranes, *J. Biol. Chem.,* 261, 532, 1986.

32. **Honda, Z.-i., Nakamura, M., Miki, I., Minami, M., Watanabe, T., Seyama, Y., Okado, H., Toh, H., Ito, K., Miyamoto, T., and Shimizu, T.,** Cloning by functional expression of platelet-activating factor receptor from guinea-pig lung, *Nature,* 349, 342, 1991.

33. **Hwang, S.-B., Lam, M.-H., Alberts, A. W., Bugianesi, R. L., Chabala, J. C., and Ponpipom, M. M.,** Biochemical and pharmacological characterization of L-659,989: an extremely potent, selective and competitive receptor antagonist of platelet-activating factor, *J. Pharmacol. Exp. Ther.,* 246, 534, 1988.

34. **Hwang, S.-B., Lam, M.-H., and Hsu, A. H.-M.,** Characterization of platelet-activating factor (PAF) receptor by specific binding of [^{3}H]L-659,989, a PAF receptor antagonist, to rabbit platelet membranes: possible multiple conformational states of a single type of PAF receptors, *Mol. Pharmacol.,* 35, 48, 1989.

35. **Hwang, S.-B. and Lam, M.-H.,** L-659,989: a useful probe for the detection of multiple conformational states of PAF receptors, *Lipids,* 26, 1148, 1991.

36. **Braquet, P. and Rola-Pleszczynski, M.,** The role of PAF in immunological responses: a review, *Prostaglandins,* 34, 143, 1987.

37. **Kroegel, C., Yukawa, T., Westwick, J., and Barnes, P. J.,** Evidence for two platelet activating factor receptors on eosinophils: dissociation between PAF-induced intracellular calcium mobilization and degranulation and superoxides anion generation in eosinophils, *Biochem. Biophys. Res. Commun.,* 162, 511, 1989.

38. **Doebber, T. W. and Wu, M. S.,** Platelet-activating factor (PAF) stimulates the PAF-synthesizing enzyme acetyl-CoA: 1-alkyl-*sn*-glycero-3-phosphocholine O^2-acetyltransferase and PAF synthesis in neutrophils, *Proc. Natl. Acad. Sci. U.S.A.,* 84, 7557, 1987.

39. **Pinckard, R. N., Ludwig, J. C., and McManus, L. M.,** Platelet-activating factor, in *Inflammation: Basic Principles and Clinical Correlates,* Gallins, J. I., Goldstein, I. M., and Snyderman, R., Eds., Raven Press, New York, 1988, 139.

40. **Ramesha, C. S. and Pickett, W. C.,** Species-specific variations in the molecular heterogeneity of platelet-activating factor, *J. Immunol.,* 138, 1559, 1987.

41. **Hayashi, H., Kudo, I., Inoue, K., Onozaki, K., Tsushima, S., Nomura, H., and Nojima, S.,** Activation of guinea pig peritoneal macrophages by platelet-activating factor (PAF) and its agonists, *J. Biochem.,* 97, 1737, 1985.

42. **Levi, R., Genovese, A., and Pinckard, R. N.,** Alkyl chain homologs of platelet-activating factor and their effects on the mammalian heart, *Biochem. Biophys. Res. Commun.,* 161, 1341, 1989.

43. **Hwang, S.-B. and Wang, S.,** Receptor heterogeneity and the existence of intracellular receptors of platelet-activating factor, in *Platelet-Activating Factor Antagonists: New Developments and Clinical Application,* O'Flaherty, J. T. and Ramwell, P. W., Eds., Portfolio Publishing, The Woodlands, TX, 1990, 13.

44. **Ott, S., Costa, T., and Herz, A.,** Sodium modulates opioid receptors through a membrane component different from G-proteins. Demonstration by target size analysis, *J. Biol. Chem.,* 263, 10524, 1988.

45. **Kawamoto, H., Watanabe, Y., Imaizumi, T., Iwasaki, T., and Yoshida, H.,** Effects of lithium ion on ADP ribosylation of inhibitory GTP-binding protein by pertussis toxin, islet-activating protein, *Eur. J. Pharmacol. Mol. Pharmacol.,* 206, 33, 1991.

46. **Haslam, R. J. and Vanderwel, M.,** Inhibition of platelet adenylate cyclase by 1-O-alkyl-2-O-acetyl-*sn*-glyceryl-3-phosphorylcholine (platelet activating factor), *J. Biol. Chem.,* 257, 6879, 1982.

47. **Nunez, D., Kumar, R., and Hanahan, D. J.,** Inhibition of [^{3}H]platelet activating factor (PAF) by Zn^{2+}: a possible explanation for its specific PAF antiaggregating effects in human platelets, *Arch. Biochem. Biophys.,* 272, 466, 1989.

48. **Hwang, S.-B. and Wang, S.,** Wheat germ agglutinin-potentiated specific binding of platelet-activating factor (PAF) to human platelet membranes: possible existence of endogeneous modulator of PAF receptor and intracellular PAF receptor, in *Platelet-Activating Factor in Immune Responses and Renal Diseases,* Braquet, P., Hsieh, K. H., Pirotzky, E., and Mencia-Huerta, J. M., Eds., Excerpta Medica Asia, Hong Kong, 1989, 9.

49. **Hwang, S.-B., Lam, M.-H., and Chang, M. N.,** Specific binding of [^{3}H]dihydrokadsurenone to rabbit platelet membranes and its inhibition by the receptor agonists and antagonists of platelet-activating factor, *J. Biol. Chem.,* 261, 13720, 1986.

50. **Hwang, S.-B. and Wang, S.,** Wheat germ agglutinin potentiates specific binding of platelet-activating factor to human platelet membranes and induces platelet-activating factor synthesis in intact platelets, *Mol. Pharmacol.,* 39, 788, 1991.

51. **Hwang, S.-B.,** Specific binding of tritium-labeled inositol 1,4,5-trisphosphate to human platelet membranes: ionic and GTP regulation, *Biochim. Biophys. Acta,* 1064, 351, 1991.

52. **Hwang, S.-B.,** Function and regulation of extracellular and intracellular receptors of platelet-activating factor, *Ann. N.Y. Acad. Sci.,* 629, 217, 1991.

Chapter 3

SOLUBILIZATION OF FUNCTIONAL PLATELET ACTIVATING FACTOR RECEPTOR FROM RABBIT PLATELETS

Lee-Young Chau, Yueh-Jin Jii, and Yu-Shen Hsu

TABLE OF CONTENTS

ISBN 0-8493-7299-2
© 1993 by CRC Press, Inc.

I. INTRODUCTION

The participation of specific receptors on the surface of target cells to mediate the biological functions of platelet activating factor (PAF) is well documented. Specific [³H]PAF binding activity assessed by radioligand binding assay was demonstrated in a variety of cells and tissue membrane preparations.[1-7] Pharmacological studies with several PAF antagonists showed differences in the rank order of potency in various cells, suggesting the existence of the subtypes of PAF receptor.[8-12] Nonetheless, activation of the PAF receptor in a number of cells has been shown to lead primarily to the membrane polyphosphoinositide breakdown,[13-19] as well as the calcium influx,[20-25] and it has been suggested that the PAF receptor belongs to the G-protein-coupled receptor superfamilies. Disclosure of the structural characteristics of the putative PAF receptor proteins and their interactions with the regulatory G-proteins is fundamentally important for the understanding of the molecular mechanisms underlying the initiation of the intracellular events following PAF stimulation on target cells. In order to isolate the receptor proteins for further characterization, one must first solubilize the membrane-bound receptor in an active form before any purification step is undertaken. Several receptors for peptide hormones and neurotransmitters were successfully solubilized by mild detergent treatment and purified to homogeneity.[26-31] In the case of the PAF receptor, it appeared to be a more elaborative work because of the complication caused by the lipid nature of the ligand. When the ligand-receptor binding assay is conducted with intact cells or the membrane preparations, bovine serum albumin (BSA) is routinely added to the binding assay buffer to assist the solubility of PAF in the aqueous solution. The separation of cell- or membrane-bound [³H]PAF from BSA-bound [³H]PAF can be easily achieved via a filtration or a centrifugation procedure. Once the receptor is solubilized in the aqueous solution, the separation of receptor-bound [³H]PAF from BSA-bound [³H]PAF becomes a difficult task. Although the increase of the detergent concentration in the binding buffer helps the solubility of PAF, it is also possible that the PAF molecule would incorporate into the detergent micelles. To deal with these problems, an alternative approach can be undertaken to solubilize the receptor proteins which are prebound with ligands. Through this method, there is no need to carry out the receptor-binding assay after the solubilization step. In this chapter, the authors describe the successful solubilization of a [³H]PAF receptor complex from rabbit platelet membranes via a nonionic detergent, digitonin. Further characterization of this receptor complex revealed that it retained the sensitivity to the specific modulation by sodium ion and GTP,[35] suggesting that this functional PAF-receptor complex is composed of the PAF binding unit and other regulatory components, such as the G-protein. The dissociation of the PAF binding unit from other components was further demonstrated by treating the receptor complex with the zwitterionic detergent, 3-[3-chloamidopropyl)dimethylammonio]-1-propanesulfonate (CHAPS), which converted the large [³H]PAF binding complex into a smaller [³H]PAF binding species. When the [³H]PAF prelabeled platelet membranes were solubilized by CHAPS, a specific [³H]PAF labeled species similar in size as that obtained from the CHAPS-treated large complex was observed, again supporting that the ligand-binding site of the PAF receptor resides in the CHAPS-solubilized small species.

II. METHODS

A. PREPARATION OF PLATELET MEMBRANES

Rabbit platelets were isolated as described previously.[32] After washing twice by ice-cold buffer containing 25 mM Tris-HCl pH 7.4, 150 mM NaCl and 2 mM EDTA, the platelets were spun down and resuspended in 10 mM Tris-HCl pH 7.4 containing 5 mM

EDTA and 0.1 mM PMSF at 1 × 10⁹ platelets per milliliter. The platelets were sonicated at 4°C for 8 × 15 s followed by centrifugation at 30,000 × g for 30 min at 4°C. The pellets were resuspended in the same buffer and stored at −70°C until use.

B. SOLUBILIZATION OF [³H]PAF PRELABELED PLATELET MEMBRANES

Platelet membrane proteins (1.25 mg) were incubated with [³H]PAF (100,000 to 200,000 cpm) in 2 ml of 25 mM Tris-HCl pH 7.4 containing 0.1 M KCl, 10 mM MgCl₂, and 0.25% BSA in the presence or absence of unlabeled PAF at 4°C for 1 h. The membranes were then collected by centrifugation at 30,000 × g for 30 min at 4°C. The pellets were washed once with binding buffer without BSA and spun down again at 4°C. The [³H]PAF prelabeled membranes were incubated with 2% digitonin or 1% CHAPS in 0.25 ml of 25 mM Tris-HCl pH 7.4 containing 0.5 M KCl, 10 mM MgCl₂, 2 mM EDTA, and 0.1 mM PMSF at 4°C for 30 min. The detergent-solubilized proteins were separated from insoluble residues by centrifugation at 100,000 × g for 1 h at 4°C.

C. SUCROSE-DENSITY GRADIENT ULTRACENTRIFUGATION OF SOLUBILIZED [³H]PAF RECEPTOR COMPLEX

Detergent-solubilized extracts were layered on the top of 4 ml of 5 to 20% sucrose gradient in 25 mM Tris-HCl pH 7.4 containing 10 mM MgCl₂, 0.5 M KCl, 2 mM EGTA, 0.1 mM PMSF, and indicated percentage of detergent. The centrifugation was conducted in a Beckman SW60Ti rotor at 200,000 × g for 16 h at 4°C. At the end of centrifugation, fractions were collected from the top of the gradients and the radioactivities were determined by liquid scintillation counting. The sedimentation coefficient of the radiolabeled components was deduced from the calibration curve constructed by the following markers: cytochrome c (1.71S), carbonic anhydrase (2.75S), BSA (4.6S), bovine r-globulin (7.2S), and catalase (11.4S).

III. RESULTS

The binding of [³H]PAF to rabbit platelet membranes was carried out at 4°C for 1 h to reach equilibrium. At the end of the incubation, the membrane-bound [³H]PAF was separated from the free [³H]PAF by centrifugation. After a wash by ice-cold buffer, the prelabeled membranes were spun down again and solubilized with 2% digitonin. Analysis of the detergent-solubilized extracts by 5 to 20% sucrose gradient ultracentrifugation revealed two radiolabeled peaks (Figure 1). The major peak, which represents over 85% of the radio-activity, was a large species with a sedimentation coefficient of 10.5S. The minor peak was a much smaller species with a sedimentation coefficient of 7.5S. When unlabeled PAF, at concentration of 0.5 and 5 nM, was present in the preincubation medium, the labeling to the 10.5S peak was reduced by 20 and 70%, respectively, whereas the 7.5S peak was virtually unaffected, suggesting that the 10.5S species is a specific PAF-binding macro-molecule. The specificity was further demonstrated by the experiment with lysoPAF, which is the inactive metabolite of PAF. As shown in the same figure, lysoPAF at a concentration of 1 μM did not significantly alter the labeling to both species. The specificity of the 10.5S component was further confirmed by the competition experiments with specific PAF antag-onists, L652731[33] and SRI-63441.[34] Both compounds substantially attenuated the labeling of [³H]PAF to the 10.5S peak but not the 7.5S peak (Figure 2). Taken together, these results strongly suggested that the 10.5S species is a specific [³H]PAF receptor complex. The binding of [³H]PAF to the receptor complex appeared to be very stable, because incubation of the complex with 1 μM of unlabeled PAF at 37°C for 2 h did not affect the binding of [³H]PAF to the 10.5S component as shown in Figure 3B. This high affinity, however, was reduced

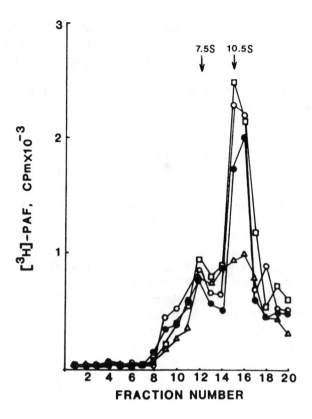

FIGURE 1. Identification of the specific [³H]PAF receptor complex solubilized by digitonin. Platelet membranes preincubated with [³H]PAF alone (○) or in the presence of 0.5 nM unlabeled PAF (●), 5 nM unlabeled PAF (△), and 1 μM unlabeled lysoPAF (□) were solubilized with 2% digitonin. After sedimentation at 100,000 × g for 30 min, the supernatants were centrifuged separately through 5 to 20% sucrose-density gradients for 16 h at 200,000 × g. (From Chau, L.-Y. and Jii, Y.-J., *Biochim. Biophys. Acta,* 970, 103, 1988. With permission.)

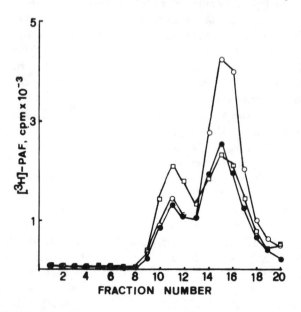

FIGURE 2. Effect of PAF antagonists on the formation of [³H]PAF receptor complex. Platelet membranes preincubated with [³H]PAF in the absence (○) or presence of 1 μM L-652731 (●) and 1 μM SRI-63441 (□) were solubilized by digitonin and then centrifuged on sucrose-density gradients.

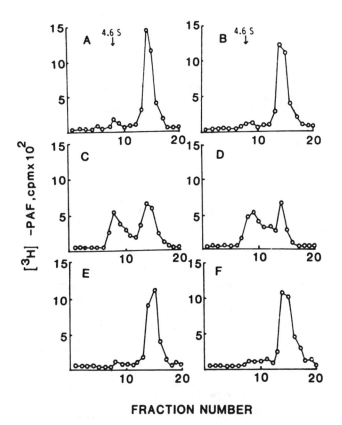

FRACTION NUMBER

FIGURE 3. The differential effects of monovalent cations on the digitonin-solubilized [³H]PAF receptor complex. Isolated [³H]PAF receptor complex was incubated with 0.1% BSA alone (A), or 0.1% BSA, 1 μM PAF in the absence (B) or presence of 150 mM of LiCl (C), NaCl (D), KCl (E), and CsCl (F) at 37°C for 2 h followed by sucrose-density gradient ultracentrifugation. The position of the BSA (4.6S) peak is indicated by arrow. (From Chau, L.-Y. and Jii, Y.-J., *Biochim. Biophys. Acta,* 970, 103, 1988. With permission.)

in the presence of Li⁺ and Na⁺, as reflected by the shift of the radioactivity from the 10.5S peak to a peak corresponding to BSA (4.6S) (Figures 3C and D). Other monovalent ions, K⁺ and Cs⁺, were not effective at the same concentration (Figures 3E and F). The specific effect of Na⁺ and Li⁺ ions apparently was similar to that observed in the membrane-bound PAF receptor of platelets.[35] Because it is known that the receptors coupled to G-proteins are subjected to the modulation by guanosine triphosphate (GTP),[36] the effect of GTP on the stability of the 10.5S complex was also examined. As shown in Figure 4, GTP facilitated the dissociation of [³H]PAF from the receptor complex in a time-dependent fashion. Furthermore, the effects of Na⁺ ion and GTP appeared to be additive. Experiments with different nucleotides demonstrated that the effect of GTP is specific, since other nucleotides at the same concentrations were ineffective (Table 1). These results suggested that the 10.5S complex is composed of PAF receptor binding unit and other regulatory components. To clarify this issue, the [³H]PAF labeled 10.5S macromolecule recovered from the sucrose-density gradient ultracentrifugation was further treated with 1% CHAPS at 4°C for 30 min. At the end of the incubation, the sample was analyzed again by the 5 to 20% sucrose-density gradient sedimentation in the presence of 0.2% CHAPS. As demonstrated in Figure 5, the radioactivity was shifted from the 10.5S macromolecule to a peak with a lower sedimentation rate. Very likely this small species (4.0S) is the binding unit of the PAF receptor complex. When the [³H]PAF prelabeled platelet membranes were subjected to the solubilization by

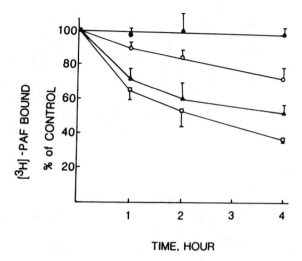

FIGURE 4. Effects of GTP and Na$^+$ ion on the dissociation kinetics of [^{3}H]PAF from the digitonin-solubilized receptor complex. The [^{3}H]PAF-receptor complex was incubated with 0.1% BSA and 1 μM PAF in the absence (●) or presence of 1 mM GTP (○), 50 mM NaCl (▲), mM GTP, and 50 mM NaCl (□) at 37°C for the indicated time. After sedimentation on a sucrose-density gradient, the percent radioactivity remaining bound to the peak corresponding to the [^{3}H]PAF receptor complex was determined. The data shown here are the mean of three separate experiments. (From Chau, L.-Y. and Jii, Y.-J., *Biochim. Biophys. Acta,* 970, 103, 1988. With permission.)

TABLE 1
Effect of Different Nucleotides on the Dissociation of [^{3}H]PAF from the Radioligand-Receptor Complex

Nucleotide (mM)	%[^{3}H]PAF receptor complex remaining
None	99.3 ± 2.7
Guanosine triphosphate (0.5)	91.7 ± 0.3
(1.0)	77.5 ± 2.1
(2.5)	76.0 ± 1.6
ATP (1.0)	96.1 ± 1.4
UTP (1.0)	97.4 ± 1.7

[^{3}H]PAF receptor complex isolated from sucrose density gradient was incubated with 1 μM unlabeled PAF, 0.1% BSA, in the absence or presence of the indicated concentrations of nucleotides at 37°C for 4 h, followed by centrifugation on sucrose-density gradients. The percent of radioactivity remaining bound to the [^{3}H]PAF receptor complex was determined. Data shown are the mean of three separate experiments.

From Chau, L.-Y. and Jii, Y.-J., *Biochim. Biophys. Acta,* 970, 103, 1988. With permission.

1% CHAPS, sucrose-density gradient ultracentrifugation also revealed a [^{3}H]PAF labeled peak with sedimentation coefficient of around 4.0S (Figure 6). The presence of 1 μM unlabeled PAF in the preincubation medium caused the reduction in the labeling of [^{3}H]PAF to this 4.0S species, again indicating that the CHAPS-solubilized species is a specific PAF binding unit which is the likely candidate of PAF receptor.

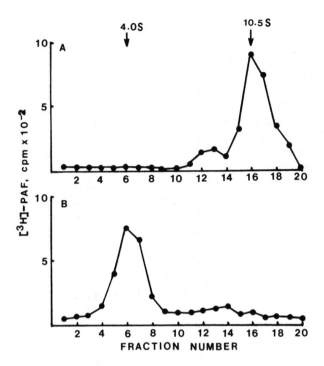

FIGURE 5. Effect of CHAPS on the digitonin-solubilized receptor complex. Isolated digitonin-solubilized [³H]PAF receptor complex (A) was incubated with 1% CHAPS at 4°C for 30 min followed by 5 to 20% sucrose-density gradient sedimentation in the presence of 0.2% CHAPS (B).

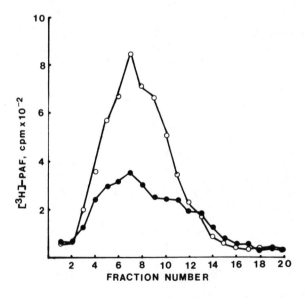

FIGURE 6. Sucrose-density gradient ultracentrifugation of CHAPS-solubilized [³H]PAF binding activity. Platelet membranes preincubated with [³H]PAF alone (○) or in the presence of 1 μ*M* unlabeled PAF (●) were solubilized by 1% CHAPS. The detergent-solubilized membrane proteins were subjected to 5 to 20% sucrose-density gradient ultracentrifugation in the presence of 0.2% CHAPS.

IV. SUMMARY AND CONCLUSION

These results clearly demonstrated that the PAF receptor, after preoccupation with the ligand, can survive the solubilization by CHAPS and digitonin. The observation that the digitonin-solubilized receptor complex was sensitive to the modulation by GTP suggested that the G-protein is likely to be a part of the large complex. Solubilization of the ternary complex of ligand receptor-G-protein has also been demonstrated in a variety of receptors.[37-40] It seems to be consistent with the notion that the binding of ligand to the receptor leads to the formation of the receptor-G-protein complex, which subsequently mediates the transduction of the signal through activation of the effector enzymes or the opening of ion channels.[36] As demonstrated by the conversion of the 10.5S species to the smaller 4.0S species, the interaction between the PAF receptor binding unit and the regulatory component(s) apparently can be interrupted by CHAPS treatment. Because PAF receptor subtypes may exist and couple to different G-proteins in various cell types, it will be relevant to see whether heterogeneous species of the PAF receptor complex can be solubilized from different cells and tissues by using the same approaches.

ACKNOWLEDGMENTS

This work was supported by Grants NSC-76-0412-B001-03 and NSC-77-0412-B001-01 from the National Science Council of Taiwan.

REFERENCES

1. **Inarrea, P., Gomez-Cambronero, J., Nieto, M., and Sanchez Crespo, M.,** Characteristics of the binding of platelet-activating factor to platelets of different animal species, *Eur. J. Pharmacol.*, 105, 309, 1984.
2. **Valone, F. H., Cole, S. E., Reinhold, V. R., and Goetzl, E. J.,** Specific binding of phospholipid platelet-activating factor by human platelets, *J. Immunol.*, 129, 1637, 1982.
3. **Hwang, S.-B., Lee, C. S. C., Cheah, M. J., and Shen, T. Y.,** Specific receptor sites for 1-O-alkyl-2-O-acetyl-*sn*-glycero-3-phosphocholine (platelet activating factor) on rabbit platelet and guinea pig smooth muscle membranes, *Biochemistry,* 22, 4756, 1983.
4. **Hwang, S.-B., Lam, M.-H., and Shen, T. Y.,** Specific binding sites for platelet activating factor in human lung tissues, *Biochem. Biophys. Res. Commun.*, 128, 972, 1985.
5. **Domingo, M. T., Chabrier, P. E., Van Delft, T. L., Venbeij, N. L., Van Haeringen, N. J., and Braquet, P.,** Characterization of specific binding sites for PAF in the iris and ciliary body of rabbit, *Biochem. Biophys. Res. Commun.*, 160, 250, 1989.
6. **Domingo, M. T., Spinnewyn, B., Chabrier, P. E., and Braquet, P.,** Presence of specific binding sites for platelet-activating factor (PAF) in brain, *Biochem. Biophys. Res. Commun.*, 151, 730, 1988.
7. **Marcheselli, V. L., Rossowska, M. J., Domingo, T., Braquet, P., and Bazan, N. G.,** Distinct platelet-activating factor binding sites in synaptic endings and in intracellular membranes of rat cerebral cortex, *J. Biol. Chem.*, 265, 9140, 1990.
8. **Lambrecht, G. and Parnham, M. J.,** Kadsurenone distinguishes between different platelet activating factor receptor subtypes on macrophages and polymorphonuclear leukocytes, *Br. J. Pharmacol.*, 87, 287, 1986.
9. **Hwang, S.-B.,** Identification of a second putative receptor of platelet-activating factor from human polymorphonuclear leukocytes, *J. Biol. Chem.*, 263, 3225, 1988.
10. **Hwang, S.-B. and Lam, M.-H.,** Species difference in the specific receptor of platelet activating factor, *Biochem. Pharmacol.*, 35, 4511, 1986.
11. **Stewart, A. G. and Dusting, G. J.,** Characterization of receptors for platelet-activating factor on platelets, polymorphonuclear leukocytes and macrophages, *Br. J. Pharmacol.*, 94, 1225, 1988.
12. **Kroegel, C., Yukawa, T., Westwick, J., and Barnes, P. J.,** Evidence for two platelet activating factor receptors on eosinophils: dissociation between PAF-induced intracellular calcium mobilization, degranulation and superoxides anion generation in eosinophils, *Biochem. Biophys. Res. Commun.*, 162, 511, 1989.

13. **Shukla, S. D.,** Platelet-activating factor-stimulated formation of inositol trisphosphate in platelets and its regulation by various agents including Ca^{2+}, indomethacin, CV-3988 and forskolin, *Arch. Biochem. Biophys.,* 240, 674, 1985.

14. **Morrison, W. J. and Shukla, S. D.,** Desensitization of receptor-coupled activation of phosphoinositide-specific phospholipase C in platelets: evidence for distinct mechanisms for platelet-activating factor and thrombin, *Mol. Pharmacol.,* 33, 58, 1988.

15. **Verghese, M. W., Charles, L., Jakoi, L., Dillon, S. B., and Synderman, R.,** Role of a guanine nucleotide regulatory protein in the activation of phospholipase C by different chemoattractants, *J. Immunol.,* 138, 4374, 1987.

16. **Fisher, R. A., Shukla, S. D., Debuysere, M. S., Hanahan, D. J., and Olson, M. S.,** The effect of acetylglyceryl ether phosphorylcholine on glycogenolysis and phosphatidylinositol 4,5-bisphosphate metabolism in rat hepatocytes, *J. Biol. Chem.,* 259, 8685, 1984.

17. **Grandison, L.,** Platelet activating factor induces inositol phosphate accumulation in cultures of rat and bovine anterior pituitary cells, *Endocrinology,* 127, 1786, 1990.

18. **Murphy, S. and Welk, G.,** Hydrolysis of polyphoinositides in astrocytes by platelet-activating factor, *Eur. J. Pharmacol.,* 188, 399, 1990.

19. **Prpic, V., Uhing, R. J., Weiel, J. E., Jakoi, L., Gawdi, G., Herman, B., and Adams, D. O.,** Biochemical and functional responses stimulated by platelet-activating factor in murine peritoneal macrophages, *J. Cell Biol.,* 107, 363, 1988.

20. **Naccache, P. H., Molski, M. M., Volpi, M., Becker, E. L., and Sha'afi, R. I.,** Unique inhibitory profile of platelet activating factor induced calcium mobilization, polyphosphoinositide turnover and granule enzyme secretion in rabbit neutrophils towards pertussis toxin and phorbol ester, *Biochem. Biophys. Res. Commun.,* 130, 677, 1985.

21. **Valone, F. H. and Johnson, B.,** Modulation of platelet-activating factor-induced calcium influx and intracellular calcium release in platelets by phorbol esters, *Biochem. J.,* 247, 669, 1987.

22. **Kornecki, E. and Ehrlich, Y. H.,** Neuroregulatory and neuropathological actions of the ether-phospholipid platelet-activating factor, *Science,* 240, 1792, 1988.

23. **Schwertschlag, U. S. and Whorton, A. R.,** Platelet-activating factor-induced homologous and heterologous desensitization in cultured vascular smooth muscle cells, *J. Biol. Chem.,* 263, 13791, 1988.

24. **Bussolino, F., Aglietta, M., Sanavio, F., Stacchini, A., Lauri, D., and Camussi, G.,** Alkyl-ether phosphoglycerides influence calcium fluxes into human endothelial cells, *J. Immunol.,* 135, 2748, 1985.

25. **Kester, M., Men'e, P., Dubyak, G. R., and Dumm, M. J.,** Elevation of cytosolic free calcium by platelet-activating factor in cultured rat mesangial cells, *FASEB J.,* 1, 215, 1987.

26. **Cohen, S., Carpenter, G., and King, L.,** Epidermal growth factor receptor-protein kinase interactions, *J. Biol. Chem.,* 255, 4834, 1980.

27. **Regan, J. W., Nakata, H., DeMarinis, R. M., Caron, M. G., and Lefkowitz, R. J.,** Purification and characterization of the human platelet α_2-adrenergic receptor, *J. Biol. Chem.,* 261, 3894, 1986.

28. **Shorr, R. L., Lefkowitz, R. J., and Caron, M. G.,** Purification of the β-adrenergic receptor, *J. Biol. Chem.,* 256, 5820, 1981.

29. **Mesikkö, K. and Rajaniemi, H.,** Purification of luteinizing hormone receptor and its subunit structure, *Biochem. Biophys. Res. Commun.,* 95, 1730, 1980.

30. **Hazum, E., Schvartz, I., Waksman, Y., and Keinan, D.,** Solubilization and purification of rat pituitary gonadotropin-releasing hormone receptor, *J. Biol. Chem.,* 261, 13043, 1986.

31. **Takayanagi, R., Inagami, T., Snajdar, R. M., Imada, T., Tamura, M., and Misono, K. S.,** Two distinct forms of receptors for atrial natriuretic factor in bovine adrenocortical cells. Purification, ligand binding, and peptide mapping, *J. Biol. Chem.,* 262, 12104, 1987.

32. **Chau, L.-Y. and Jii, Y.-J.,** Characterization of ^{3}H-labelled platelet activating factor receptor complex solubilized from rabbit platelet membranes, *Biochim. Biophys. Acta,* 970, 103, 1988.

33. **Hwang, S.-B., Lam, M.-H., Biftu, T., Beattie, T. R., and Shen, T. Y.,** trans-2,5-Bis(3,4,5-trimethoxyphenyl)tetrahydrofuran. An orally active specific and competitive receptor antagonist of platelet activating factor, *J. Biol. Chem.,* 260, 15639, 1985.

34. **Saunders, R. N. and Handley, D. A.,** Platelet-activating factor antagonists, *Annu. Rev. Pharmacol. Toxicol.,* 27, 237, 1987.

35. **Hwang, S.-B., Lam, M.-H., and Pong, S. S.,** Ionic and GTP regulation of binding of platelet-activating factor to receptors and platelet-activating factor-induced activation of GTPase in rabbit platelet membranes, *J. Biol. Chem.,* 261, 532, 1986.

36. **Gilman, A. G.,** G proteins: transducers of receptor-generated signals, *Annu. Rev. Biochem.,* 56, 615, 1987.

37. **Fitzgerald, T. J., Uhing, R. J., and Exton, J. H.,** Solubilization of the vasopression receptor from rat liver plasma membranes. Evidence for a receptor GTP-binding protein complex, *J. Biol. Chem.,* 261, 16871, 1986.

38. **Couvineau, A., Amiranoff, B., and Laburthe, M.,** Solubilization of the liver vasoactive intestinal peptide receptor. Hydrodynamic characterization and evidence for an association with a functional GTP regulatory protein, *J. Biol. Chem.,* 261, 14482, 1986.
39. **Watanabe, T., Umegaki, K., and Smith, W. L.,** Association of a solubilized prostaglandin E_2 receptor from renal medulla with a pertussis toxin-reactive guanine nucleotide regulatory protein, *J. Biol. Chem.,* 261, 13430, 1986.
40. **Mong, S., Wu, H.-L., Stadel, J. M., Clark, M. A., and Crooke, S. T.,** Solubilization of [^{3}H]leukotriene D_4 receptor complex from guinea pig lung membranes, *Mol. Pharmacol.,* 29, 235, 1986.

Chapter 4

MOLECULAR CLONING OF PLATELET ACTIVATING FACTOR RECEPTORS

Takao Shimizu

TABLE OF CONTENTS

ISBN 0-8493-7299-2
© 1993 by CRC Press, Inc.

I. INTRODUCTION

A. EVIDENCE OF THE CELL SURFACE RECEPTOR FOR PLATELET ACTIVATING FACTOR

Since the discovery and structural identification of platelet activating factor (PAF; PAF-acether; 1-O-alkyl-2-acetyl-*sn*-glycero-3-phosphocholine; AGEPC; acetyl glycerol ether phosphorylcholine),[1-5] the presence of the specific receptor for PAF has been postulated. The following observations suggest the existence of the specific PAF receptor:

1. *Strict structural requirement and stereospecificity for PAF action.* Alkyl-ether bond at C-1 is needed for activity, while addition of the ester bond causes loss of activity. At the C-2 position, the acetyl moiety shows the highest biological activity; the longer the acyl chain, the less the biological activity. The naturally occurring R chirality at C-2 is active, whereas the S-form is totally inactive. Phosphocholine, but not phosphoethanolamine, at the C-3 position is required for the biological activity. Such structure-activity relation is well studied and readers are recommended to refer to the intensive review article by Braquet et al.[6]

2. *Development of specific antagonists.* Essentially three classes of PAF antagonists are reported, including phospholipid PAF analogues, natural products (especially those isolated from herbal plants), and the synthetic compounds from *in vitro* screening efforts. The structure and potencies of each antagonist are described in References 6 and 7.

3. *Specific and saturable bindings of [³H]PAF and [³H]WEB 2086 to membrane fraction.* More direct evidence was presented by ligand-binding experiments. High affinity binding sites for [³H]PAF were found in human,[8,9] rabbit platelets,[10,11] and human leukocyte membrane.[12] The development of the tritium-labeled PAF antagonist, [³H]WEB 2086, proved to be the best tool for this experiment because it is metabolically stable and the nonspecific binding is relatively low[13,14] (see below). Rat platelets do not aggregate with PAF,[15] and it is in accordance with the finding that they do not possess the bindings sites for PAF.

4. *Elucidation of the second messenger system.* Following receptor activation, at least three types of signal transducing systems (hence, second messenger generating systems) are activated: phospholipase C,[16-23] which breaks down phosphatidylinositol-4,5-bis-phosphate (PIP_2); phospholipase A_2,[24-26] which releases arachidonic acid and other unsaturated fatty acids; and the decrease of cyclic AMP (cAMP),[24,27] either by inhibiting the adenylate cyclase or stimulating the cAMP phosphodiesterase. These results strongly indicate that PAF binds to the membrane surface receptor.

B. INOSITOL LIPID TURNOVER, CA^{2+} ENTRY, AND TYROSINE PHOSPHORYLATION

As presented above, evidence is growing that PAF stimulates breakdown of polyphosphoinositides (for a review, see Reference 28). Thus, generated products inositol 1,4,5-trisphosphate (IP_3) and diacylglycerol (DG) serve as second messengers and play roles in intracellular Ca^{2+} mobilization and in the activation of protein kinase C, respectively. The role of protein kinase C in the PAF response remains to be clarified.[29,30] Although some reports show that the Ca^{2+} channel opening is required for the PAF action,[31,32] most of the PAF bioactivity is attributable to the intracellular mobilization of Ca^{2+} by IP_3 formation. Ca^{2+} influx may be a consequence of IP_3 production since the microinjection of IP_3 to *Xenopus laevis* oocytes[33] and mouse lacrimal acinar cells[34] caused the Ca^{2+} influx. Recently, two groups reported the tyrosine phosphorylation induced by PAF in rabbit platelets[35] and human polymorphonuclear leukocytes.[36] Dhar et al.[35] described that IP_3 formation, as well as platelet aggregation, were inhibited by genistein, a tyrosine kinase inhibitor. Furthermore, they showed that pp60[c-src] is one of the major phosphorylated proteins at *tyr* residue in the blood platelets, as evidenced by immunoprecipitation with anti-*c-src* and anti-phosphotyrosine antibodies.[37]

The cross-talk between phosphatidylinositol (PI) turnover and tyrosine phosphorylation is observed with various ligands including certain growth factors (platelet-derived growth factor, PDGF; epidermal growth factor, EGF) and other ligands (bradykinin, thrombin, fMLP, etc.).[38] The receptors for these growth factors were isolated, and the mechanism of the cross-talk has been intensively studied.[39-42] The receptors for these growth factors have a single polypeptide chain with one transmembrane domain. The cytosolic domain contains both the tyrosine kinase activity and autophosphorylation sites. Thus, phosphorylated receptors can physically associate with a protein family possessing SH2 (*src* homology) domain.[43] This family includes various proteins (GAP, GTPase activating protein; *src*; and *crk*) including phospholipase Cγ. It remains unclear, though, how phosphorylated phospholipase C initiates the PI turnover.[44] It has been challenging to determine the primary structure of PAF receptor(s) and to elucidate a seemingly complicated signal transduction mechanism involving the cross-talk between PI turnover and tyrosine phosphorylation.

II. MOLECULAR CLONING OF PLATELET ACTIVATING FACTOR RECEPTORS

A. EXPRESSION CLONING OF PLATELET ACTIVATING FACTOR RECEPTOR FROM GUINEA PIG LUNG[45]

Xenopus laevis oocytes are a good model for cloning various proteins, receptors, and channels. The oocyte has a highly efficient translation machinery.[46] They effectively translate exogenous mRNA, carry out the post-translational modifications, and transport exogenous protein to an appropriate cellular component. Thus, the functional membrane receptor appears in the cell surface membrane 48 to 72 h after mRNA injection, when the microinjected mRNA encodes a functional receptor. The oocyte system offers another advantage in that the receptor that links to G-protein coupled PI turnover can be detected. Intracellular increase in the Ca^{2+} concentration is determined by the inward current through the Ca^{2+}-dependent Cl^- channel. By using this system, receptors for substance K[47] and serotonin[48] have actually been characterized. We decided to employ this method. No data were available on PAF receptor(s) at the protein level, although the intensive efforts were made to purify and characterize the PAF receptor (binding protein).[49-52] According to these results, the estimated M_r of PAF receptor is between 50 and 180 kDa.[53] Because no lipid autacoid receptor had been cloned, any approach using homology was not feasible.

Cloning strategy of guinea pig lung PAF receptor. When mRNA prepared from guinea pig lung was injected into oocytes and incubated at 22°C for 3 d, a prominent inward current (>50 nA) was observed with 10^{-7} M PAF (Figure 1). Via sucrose-density gradient centrifugation, we further purified the mRNA according to the amplitude of the inward current. Several fractions with approximately 3 kb-size mRNA were combined and used for cDNA synthesis (Pharmacia). Using the cDNA, a λZap II (Stratagene) library was constructed. Phage DNA was prepared via the alkali-sodium dodecyl sulfate (SDS) method from each 6 × 10^4 phage aliquot, digested at Not I site, downstream to T7 promoter, and the template was transcribed *in vitro* using T7 RNA polymerase. The transcript, rather than the tissue mRNA, was injected into oocytes, and the positive fraction was divided by sibling by monitoring the PAF-induced Cl^- current electrophysiologically. Finally, a single clone was

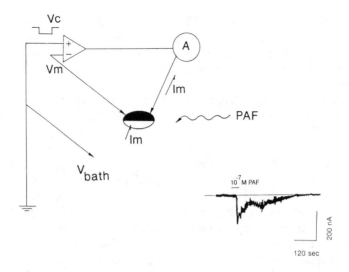

FIGURE 1. Electrophysiological determination of PAF receptor expression on oocytes. Membrane potential (Vm) was held below the reversal potential of Cl^- in oocytes (Vc) in modified Ringer's solution (115 mM NaCl/2 m M KCl/1.8 mM CaCl$_2$/5 mM HEPES, pH 7.4), and PAF-induced inward current (Im) was recorded. A typical trace of the biphasic inward current with 10^{-7} M PAF is illustrated in the inset.

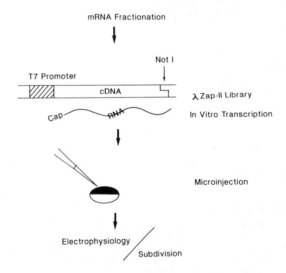

FIGURE 2. Cloning strategy of PAF receptor. After sucrose-density gradient, positive fractions were combined and subjected to cDNA synthesis. The cDNA was ligated with phage vector, λZAP II. *In vitro* transcribed mRNA was injected to oocytes for the electrophysiological detection.

isolated and subjected to DNA sequence analysis.[45] The cloning strategy is summarized in Figure 2.

B. CLONING OF PLATELET ACTIVATING FACTOR RECEPTOR FROM HUMAN LEUKOCYTES

We isolated human homologue of PAF receptor from leukocytes (>90% neutrophils) by the homology-probing approach.[54] A 0.8-kb Sma I fragment of the guinea pig receptor cDNA was radiolabeled by the multiprimer labeling system (Amersham) and was used as a probe. From 3 × 10⁴ clones, a single clone (1.8 kb) coding for PAF receptor was isolated which was functionally full-length.[54]

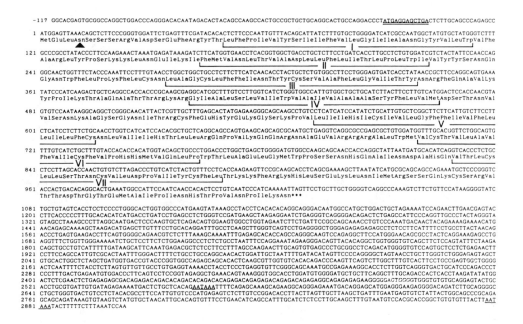

FIGURE 3. Nucleotide and deduced amino acid sequences of guinea pig lung PAF receptor. Designations I to VII beneath the amino acid sequences are putative transmembrane domains.[45]

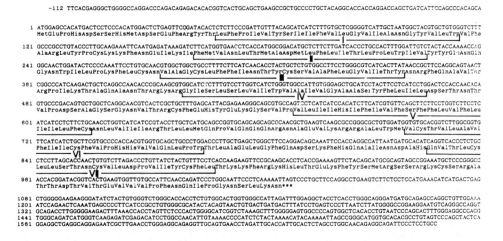

FIGURE 4. Nucleotide and deduced amino acid sequences of human leukocyte PAF receptor.[54] Solid bars indicate the putative transmembrane segments.

III. PRIMARY STRUCTURE AND PROPERTIES OF PLATELET ACTIVATING FACTOR RECEPTORS

A. PRIMARY STRUCTURE OF PLATELET ACTIVATING FACTOR RECEPTORS

The nucleotide sequences and deduced amino acid sequences of thus cloned receptors are shown in Figures 3 and 4. Both guinea pig lung and human leukocyte receptors are composed of 342 amino acids.[45,54] Overall identity was 83%, whereas >90% homology was observed in the transmembrane domains. Conserved amino acids between two species are illustrated in a single letter in Figure 5. Hydropathy analysis revealed that these receptors

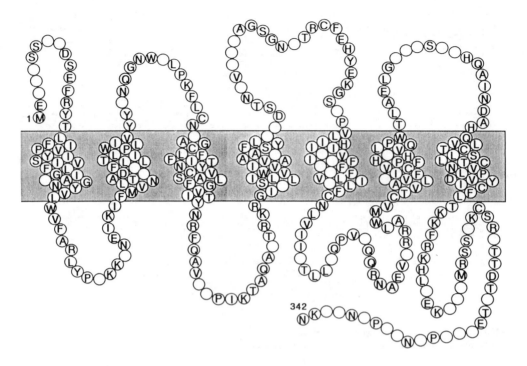

FIGURE 5. Homology between guinea pig lung and human leukocyte receptors. Conserved amino acids are illustrated in a single letter. Overall homology is 83%, while that in the transmembrane domains is 91%.

have seven putative transmembrane segments, characteristic of the G-protein coupled receptor superfamily. As shown in Figure 5, two cysteines in the second and third extracellular loops, three prolines in the sixth and seventh transmembrane domains, and eight residues of serine and threonine and one cysteine in the C terminal cytoplasmic loop, were all conserved. In contrast to the guinea pig lung receptor and other G-protein coupled receptors so far sequenced, the *N*-glycosylation site in the N terminal extracellular domain is absent in the human leukocyte receptor.

B. PHARMACOLOGIC PROPERTIES OF PLATELET ACTIVATING FACTOR RECEPTORS

To elucidate the pharmacologic properties of PAF receptors, the cloned cDNA was expressed in both oocytes and COS-7 cells. As shown in Figure 6, addition of PAF elicited dose-dependent increases in the Cl^- current amplitude. The ED_{50} value was around 10 nM under the assay conditions. Partial agonist, 1-*O*-octadecyl-2-acetoamide-2-deoxyglycero-3-phosphocholine is less potent by two orders of magnitude. The Ca^{2+} increase by PAF was almost completely inhibited by equimolar concentrations of PAF antagonists, CV-6209 and Y-24180.[45] It is difficult to carry out the binding experiment using oocytes, because only small amounts of expressed receptors show large electrophysiological responses. Therefore, we subcloned a PAF receptor cDNA to a mammalian expression vector, pEUKC1, to transfect into COS-7 cells. Binding assays were performed with [³H]WEB 2086 as a ligand. B_{max} values and corresponding K_d values are 6.9 pmol/mg of protein and 6.4 nM for guinea pig lung receptor,[45] and 9.2 pmol/mg of protein, and 1.3 nM for human leukocyte receptor.[54] COS-7 cells overexpress PAF receptor on their surface at a density of 10^6 sites per cell. Scatchard plot analysis using both human and guinea pig clones shows a single entity of the binding sites. These K_d values are practically identical with those reported in the liter-

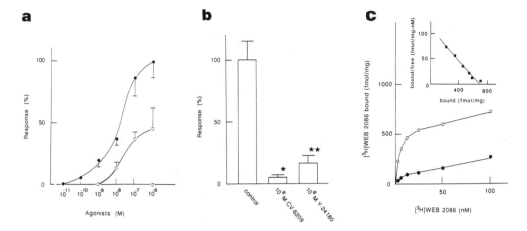

FIGURE 6. Pharmacological properties of PAF receptor. (a) Dose-response relation of PAF (●), 1-O-octadecyl-2-acetamido-2-deoxy-glycero-3-phosphocholine (○) and lyso-PAF (□). The mean amplitude of the inward current induced by 10^{-6} M PAF was defined as 100%. (b) Inhibition of PAF-induced current by specific antagonists, CV-6209 and Y-24180. Both concentrations of PAF and antagonists were 10^{-8} M. (c) Saturation isotherm and derived Scatchard plot of [^{3}H]WEB2086 to COS-7 cell membrane. (○) and (●) represent specific and nonspecific bindings, respectively.

ature.[53] The receptor activation is susceptible to desensitization with PAF application (Figure 7). Because IP$_3$ response did not change before or after PAF application, this decreased response is not due to depletion of Ca^{2+} store.

C. DISTRIBUTION OF PLATELET ACTIVATING FACTOR RECEPTOR mRNA

In the guinea pig tissues, PAF receptor mRNA (band 2 in Figure 8) is most abundant in leukocytes, followed by lung, spleen, and kidney.[45] Although it is not detectable in the RNA blotting method, other organs such as brain have a functional PAF receptor;[55] this agrees well with the finding by Marchesselli et al.,[56] who showed the specific binding of PAF in the rat cerebral cortex. In the guinea pig kidney, the mRNA was most abundant in the cortex, followed by the outer and inner medulla.[57] Structures and their relations to the PAF receptor of two other bands (bands 1 and 3) in Figure 8 remain to be clarified. Because the washing procedures are stringent, they may represent some homologous mRNAs in those tissues. In humans cells, PAF receptor is predominant in peripheral granulocytes. When EoL-1 cells (eosinophilic leukemia cells) are stimulated with IL-5 and granulocyte macrophage colony stimulating factor (CSF), they expressed a fairly large amount of PAF receptor mRNA. In contrast, human erythroleukemic (HEL) cells show a faint band, either nonstimulated or stimulated with phorbol 12-tetradecanoyl 13-acetate. More precise elucidation of localization of PAF receptor by *in situ* hybridization with anti-mRNA probe or histochemistry with antireceptor antibody is ongoing in our laboratory.

D. SIGNAL TRANSDUCTION THROUGH G-PROTEIN(S) AND PHOSPHOINOSITIDE TURNOVER

The involvement of G-protein(s) following receptor activation was demonstrated by the injection of the inactive analogue of GTP, GDPβS in the oocytes. More than 70% of the response was inhibited by the GDPβS pretreatment. In transfected COS-7 cells and oocytes injected with *in vitro* transcribed receptor mRNA, PAF at 10^{-8} M rapidly increased IP$_3$ formation. All these results suggest that PAF stimulates PI turnover through G-protein(s). The type of G-protein(s) involved in the PAF response can differ from cell to cell. In fact,

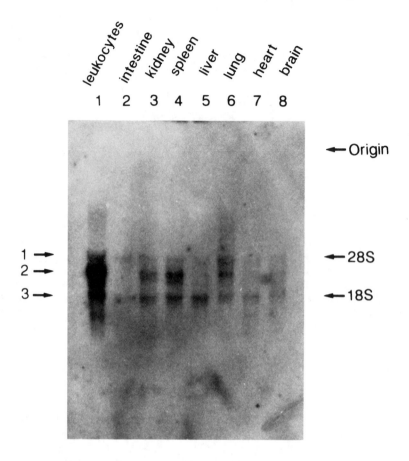

FIGURE 7. RNA blot analysis of PAF receptor in various tissues of guinea pig.[45]

it was reported by several investigators that the PAF response in rabbit platelets[21] and the human monocytic cell line U937[23] was resistant to the islet-activating peptide (IAP) treatment, while responses in rabbit neutrophils,[21] human macrophages,[58] and human platelets[44] were sensitive to IAP treatment. Thus, both IAP-sensitive (G_i) and IAP-insensitive (possibly G_q) G proteins are involved in the signaling pathway of PAF, depending on cell type and the nature of responses. It remains unclear whether tyrosine phosphorylation is a consequence of the cloned receptor activation, or whether there is another type of PAF receptor that belongs to a growth factor receptor family.

IV. CONCLUSIONS AND PERSPECTIVES

In this chapter, I described our recent work on a molecular cloning of PAF receptors from guinea pig lung and human leukocytes. These represent the first successful examples of receptor cloning of lipid mediators. Soon after our work, a thromboxane A_2/prostaglandin H_2 receptor was also cloned from human placental and megakaryocytic leukemia cell libraries.[59] Between the two kinds of lipid mediator receptors, overall homology is around 40%, which is not more than an average value among a G-protein coupled receptor superfamily. Some small domains or peptide sequences may be common and characteristic for lipid mediators. We must wait for such conclusions until receptors for prostaglandins and leukotrienes are cloned (for a review, see Reference 60). The following are problems for the future which should be investigated: (1) Do subtype(s) of the PAF receptor exist in

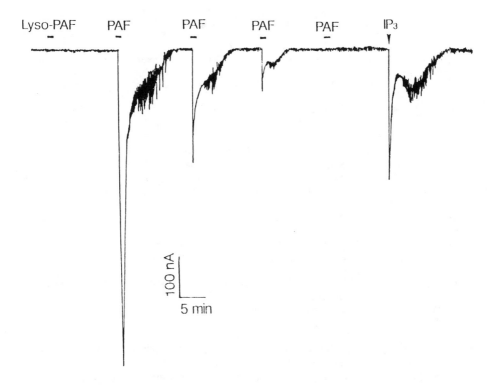

FIGURE 8. Desensitization of the inward current by repeated application of PAF. Microinjection of IP_3 evoked Cl^- current in the desensitized oocytes, suggesting the phenomenon is not due to the Ca^{2+} depletion.

different tissues? (2) What are the roles of intracellular PAF and are intracellular PAF receptors present? (3) How does tyrosine phosphorylation occur through G-protein coupled receptor? Alternatively, is there another growth factor-type receptor present for PAF? (4) What type of G-protein(s) and effector(s) couple with each PAF receptor? (5) What is the mechanism of the PAF receptor desensitization? Is it due to the *ser/thr* phosphorylation; are other types of protein kinases involved? (6) Which peptide sequence of the PAF receptor is required in the ligand binding, and which domains are involved in transducing signals through G-protein(s)? (7) How are messages transmitted to the nucleus to induce early oncogene expression, and cellular proliferation? Structural information on PAF receptor described in this chapter will help to elucidate the mechanism of PAF actions as well as the rational design of more specific PAF antagonists for various inflammatory and allergic disorders. This review has covered the cloning and structure of the PAF receptors. Readers are recommended to refer to the excellent review articles contained in References 6, 28, 61 to 63 which deal with other related areas of PAF research.

ACKNOWLEDGMENTS

This series of work has been done in collaboration with Z. Honda, M. Nakamura, T. Izumi, H. Bito, T. Takano, M. Minami, C. Sakanaka, H. Mutoh, and T. Kishimoto in our laboratory. The secretarial assistance of N. Ooigawa is greatly acknowledged. The work was supported by a Grant-in-Aid from the Ministry of Education, Science and Culture and the Ministry of Health and Welfare of Japan, and the Toray Science Foundation.

REFERENCES

1. **Benveniste, J., Henson, P. M., and Cochrane, C. G.,** Leukocyte-dependent histamine release from rabbit platelets. The role of IgE, basophils, and a platelet-activating factor, *J. Exp. Med.,* 136, 1356, 1972.
2. **Benveniste, J., LeCouedic, J. P., Polonsky, J., and Tence, M.,** Structural analysis of purified platelet-activating factor by lipases, *Nature,* 269, 170, 1977.
3. **Demopoulos, C. A., Pinckard, R. N., and Hanahan, D. J.,** Platelet-activating factor. Evidence for 1-*O*-alkyl-2-acetyl-*sn*-glyceryl-3-phosphorylcholine as the active component (a new class of lipid chemical mediators), *J. Biol. Chem.,* 254(19), 9355, 1979.
4. **Blank, M. L., Snyder, F., Byers, L. W., Brooks, B., and Muirhead, E. E.,** Antihypertensive activity of an alkylether analog of phosphatidylcholine, *Biochem. Biophys. Res. Commun.,* 90, 1194, 1979.
5. **Vargaftig, B. B., Lefort, J., Chignard, M., and Benveniste, J.,** Platelet-activating factor induces a platelet-dependent bronchoconstriction unrelated to the formation of prostaglandin derivatives, *Eur. J. Pharmacol.,* 65, 185, 1980.
6. **Braquet, P., Touqui, L., Shen, T. Y., and Vargaftig, B. B.,** Perspectives in platelet-activating factor research, *Pharmacol. Rev.,* 39, 97, 1987.
7. **Meade, C. J., Heuer, H., and Kempe, R.,** Biochemical pharmacology of platelet-activating factor (and PAF antagonists) in relation to clinical and experimental thrombocytopenia, *Biochem. Pharmacol.,* 41, 657, 1991.
8. **Valone, F. H., Coles, E., Reinhold, V. R., and Goetzl, E. J.,** Specific binding of phospholipid platelet-activating factor by human platelets, *J. Immunol.,* 129, 1637, 1982.
9. **Korth, R., Hirafuji, H., Keraly, C. L., Delautier, D., Bidault, J., and Benveniste, J.,** Interaction of the PAF antagonist WEB 2086 and its hetrazepine analogues with human platelets and endothelial cells, *Br. J. Pharmacol.,* 98, 653, 1989.
10. **Terashita, Z., Imura, Y., and Nishikawa, K.,** Inhibition by CV-3988 of the binding of [^{3}H]-platelet activating factor (PAF) to the platelet, *Biochem. Pharmacol.,* 34, 1491, 1985.
11. **Hwang, S.-B., Lam, M.-H., and Pong, S.-S.,** Ionic and GTP regulation of binding of platelet-activating factor to receptors and platelet-activating factor-induced activation of GTPase in rabbit platelet membrane, *J. Biol. Chem.,* 261, 532, 1986.
12. **Hwang, S. B.,** Identification of a second putative receptor of platelet-activating factor from human polymorphonuclear leukocytes, *J. Biol. Chem.,* 263, 3225, 1988.
13. **Ukena, D., Dent, G., Birke, F. W., Robaut, C., Sybrecht, G. W., and Barnes, P. J.,** Radioligand binding of antagonists of platelet-activating factor to intact human platelets, *FEBS Lett.,* 228, 285, 1988.
14. **Dent, G., Ukena, D., Sybrecht, G. W., and Barnes, P. J.,** [^{3}H]WEB 2086 labels platelet activating factor receptors in guinea pig and human lung, *Eur. J. Pharmacol.,* 169, 313, 1989.
15. **Inarrea, P., Gomez-Cambronero, J., Nieto, M., and Sanchez-Crespo, M.,** Characteristics of the binding of platelet-activating factor to platelets of different animal species, *Eur. J. Pharmacol.,* 105, 309, 1984.
16. **Shukla, S. D. and Hanahan, D. J.,** AGEPC (platelet activating factor) induced stimulation of rabbit platelets: Effects on phosphatidylinositol, di- and triphosphoinositides and phosphatidic acid metabolism, *Biochem. Biophys. Res. Commun.,* 106, 697, 1982.
17. **Shukla, S. D. and Hanahan, D. J.,** An early transient decrease in phosphatidylinositol 4,5-bisphosphate upon stimulation of rabbit platelets with acetylglycerylether phosphorylcholine (platelet activating factor), *Arch. Biochem. Biophys.,* 227, 626, 1983.
18. **Mauco, G., Chap, H., and Douste-Blazy, L.,** Platelet activating factor (PAF-acether) promotes an early degradation of phosphatidylinositol-4,5-bisphosphate in rabbit platelets, *FEBS Lett.,* 153, 361, 1983.
19. **MacIntyre, D. E. and Pollack, W. K.,** Platelet-activating factor stimulates phosphatidylinositol turnover in human platelets, *Biochem. J.,* 212, 433, 1983.
20. **Shukla, S. D.,** Platelet activating factor-stimulated formation of inositol trisphosphate in platelets and its regulation by various agents including Ca^{2+}, indomethacin, CV-2988, and forskolin, *Arch. Biochem. Biophys.,* 240, 674, 1985.
21. **Naccache, P. H., Molski, M. M., Volpi, M., Becker, E. L., and Sha'afi, R. I.,** Unique inhibitory profile of platelet activating factor induced calcium mobilization, polyphosphoinositide turnover and gradual enzyme secretion in rabbit neutrophils towards pertussis toxin and phorbol ester, *Biochem. Biophys. Res. Commun.,* 130, 677, 1985.
22. **Brass, L. F., Woolkalis, M. J., and Manning, D. R.,** Interaction in platelets between G proteins and the agonists that stimulate phospholipase C and inhibit adenylyl cyclase, *J. Biol. Chem.,* 263, 5348, 1988.
23. **Barzaghi, G., Sarau, H. M., and Mong, S.,** Platelet-activating factor-induced phosphoinositide metabolism in differentited U937 cells in culture, *J. Pharm. Exp. Ther.,* 248, 559, 1989.
24. **Murayama, T. and Ui, M.,** Receptor-mediated inhibition of adenylate cyclase and stimulation of arachidonic acid release in 3T3 fibroblasts. Selective susceptibility to islet-activating protein, pertussis toxin, *J. Biol. Chem.,* 260, 7226, 1985.

25. **Levine, L.,** Platelet-activating factor stimulates arachidonic acid metabolism in rat liver cells (C-9 cell line) by a receptor-mediated mechanism, *Mol. Pharmacol.,* 34, 791, 1988.

26. **Nakashima, S., Suganuma, A., Sato, M., Tohmatsu, T., and Nozawa, Y.,** Mechanism of arachidonic acid liberation in platelet-activating factor-stimulated human polymorphonuclear neutrophils, *J. Immunol.,* 143, 1295, 1989.

27. **Houselay, M. D., Bojanic, D., Gawler, D., O'Hagen, S., and Wilson, A.,** Thrombin, unlike vasopressin, appears to stimulate two distinct guanine nucleotide regulatory proteins in human platelets, *Biochem. J.,* 238, 109, 1986.

28. **Shukla, S. D.,** Inositol phospholipid turnover in PAF transmembrane signalling, *Lipids,* 26, 1028, 1991.

29. **O'Flaherty, J. T. and Nishihara, J.,** Arachidonic metabolites, platelet-activating factor, and the mobilization of protein kinase C in human polymorphonuclear neutrophils, *J. Immunol.,* 138, 1889, 1987.

30. **Uhing, R. J., Prpic, V., Hollenbach, P. W., and Adams, D. O.,** Involvement of protein kinase C in platelet-activating factor-stimulated diacylglycerol accumulation in murine peritoneal macrophages, *J. Biol. Chem.,* 264, 9224, 1989.

31. **Naccache, P. H., Molski, M. M., Volpi, M., Becker, E. L., and Sha'afi, R. I.,** Unique inhibitory profile of platelet-activating factor induced calcium mobilization, phosphophoinositide turnover and granule enzyme secretion in rabbit neutrophils towards pertussis toxin and phorbol ester, *Biochem. Biophys. Res. Commun.,* 130, 677, 1985.

32. **Avdonin, P. V., Cheglakov, I. B., Boogry, E. M., Svitina-Ulitina, I. V., Mazaev, A. B., and Tkachuk, V. A.,** Evidence for the receptor-operated calcium channels in human platelet plasma membrane, *Thromb. Res.,* 46, 29, 1987.

33. **Sugiyama, H., Ito, I., and Hirono, C.,** A new type of glutamate receptor linked to inositol phospholipid metabolism, *Nature,* 325, 531, 1987.

34. **Bird, G. St. J., Rossier, M. F., Hughes, A. R., Shears, S. B., Armstrong, D. J., and Putney, J. W. Jr.,** Activation of Ca^{2+} entry into acinar cells by a non-phosphorylatable inositol trisphosphate, *Nature,* 352, 162, 1991.

35. **Dhar, A., Paul, A. K., and Shukla, S. D.,** Platelet activating factor stimulation of tyrosine kinase and its relationship to phospholipase C in rabbit platelets: studies with genistein and monoclonal antibody to phosphotyrosine, *Mol. Pharmacol.,* 37, 519, 1990.

36. **Gomez-Cambronero, J., Wang, E., Johnson, G., Huang, C. K., and Sha'afi, R. I.,** Platelet-activating factor induces tyrosine phosphorylation in human neutrophils, *J. Biol. Chem.,* 266, 6240, 1991.

37. **Dhar, A. and Shukla, S. D.,** Involvement of pp60[c-src] in platelet activating factor-stimulated platelets: evidence for translocation from cytosol to membrane, *J. Biol. Chem.,* 266, 18797, 1991.

38. **Cantley, L. C., Auger, K. R., Carpenter, C., Duckworth, B., Graziani, A., Kapeller, R., and Soltoff, S.,** Oncogenes and signal transduction, *Cell,* 64, 281, 1991.

39. **Anderson, D., Koch, C. A., Grey, L., Ellis, C., Moran, M. F., and Pawson, T.,** Binding of SH2 domains of phospholipase Cγ1, GAP and Src to activated growth factor receptors, *Science,* 250, 979, 1990.

40. **Kim, H. K., Kim, J. W., Zilberstein, A., Margolis, B., Kim, J. G., Schlessinger, J., and Rhee, S. G.,** PDGF stimulation of inositol phospholipid hydrolysis requires PLCγ1 phosphorylation on tyrosine residues 783 and 1254, *Cell,* 65, 435, 1991.

41. **Kim, J. W., Sim, S. S., Kim, U.-H., Nishibe, S., Wahl, M. I., Carpenter, G., and Rhee, S. G.,** Tyrosine residues in bovine phospholipase Cγphosphorylated by the epidermal growth factor receptor *in vitro, J. Biol. Chem.,* 265, 3940, 1990.

42. **Margolis, B., Rhee, S. G., Felder, S., Mervic, M., Lyall, R., Levitzki, A., Ullrich, A., Zilberstein, A., and Schlessinger, J.,** EGF induces tyrosine phosphorylation of phospholipase C-II: a potential mechanism for EGF receptor signalling, *Cell,* 57, 1101, 1989.

43. **Meisenhelder, J., Suh, P.-G., Rhee, S. G., and Hunter, T.,** Phospholipase C-γ is a substrate for the PDGF and EGF receptor protein-tyrosine kinases *in vivo* and *in vitro, Cell,* 57, 1109, 1989.

44. **Goldschmidt-Clermont, P., Kim, J. W., Machesky, L. M., Rhee, S. G., and Pollard, T. D.,** Regulation of phospholipase C-γ1 by profilin and tyrosine phosphorylation, *Science,* 251, 1231, 1991.

45. **Honda, Z., Nakamura, M., Miki, I., Minami, M., Wantanabe, T., Seyama, Y., Okado, H., Toh, H., Ito, K., Miyamoto, T., and Shimizu, T.,** Cloning by functional expression of platelet-activating factor receptor from guinea-pig lung, *Nature,* 349, 342, 1991.

46. **Colman, A.,** Translation of eukaryotic messenger RNA in *Xenopus* oocytes, in *Transcription and Translation,* Hames, B. D. and Higgins, S. J., Eds., IRL Press, Oxford, 1984, 271.

47. **Masu, Y., Nakayama, K., Tamaki, H., Harada, Y., Kuno, M., and Nakanishi, S.,** cDNA cloning of bovine substance-K receptor through oocyte expression system, *Nature,* 329, 836, 1987.

48. **Julius, D., MacDermott, A. B., Axel, R., and Jessells, T. M.,** Molecular characterization of a functional cDNA encoding the serotonin 1c receptor, *Science,* 241, 558, 1988.

49. **Valone, F. H.,** Isolation of a platelet membrane protein which binds the platelet-activating factor, 1-O-hexadecyl-2-acetyl-*sn*-glycero-3-phosphorylcholine, *Immunology,* 52, 169, 1984.

50. **Nishihara, J., Ishibashi, T., Imai, Y., and Muramatsu, T.**, Purification and characterization of the specific binding protein for platelet activating factor (1-O-alkyl-2-acetyl-*sn*-glycero-3-phosphocholine) from human platelets, *Tohoku J. Exp. Med.*, 147, 145, 1985.

51. **Chau, L. Y. and Jii, Y. J.**, Characterization of ^{3}H-labeled platelet activating factor receptor complex solubilized from rabbit platelet membranes, *Biochim. Biophys. Acta*, 970, 103, 1988.

52. **Chau, L. Y., Tsai, Y. M., and Cheng, J. R.**, Photoaffinity labeling of platelet activating factor binding sites in rabbit platelet membranes, *Biochem. Biophys. Res. Commun.*, 161, 1070, 1989.

53. **Valone, F. H.**, Platelet-activating factor binding to specific cell membrane receptors, in *Platelet-Activating Factor and Related Lipid Mediators*, Snyder, F., Ed., Plenum Press, New York, 1987, 137.

54. **Nakamura, M., Honda, Z., Izumi, T., Sakanaka, C., Mutoh, H., Minami, M., Bito, H., Seyama, Y., Matsumoto, T., Noma, M., and Shimizu, T.**, Molecular cloning and expression of platelet-activating factor receptor from human leukocytes, *J. Biol. Chem.*, 266, 20400, 1991.

55. **Bito, H., Honda, Z., Nakamura, M., Shimizu, T., Kudo, Y., and Seyama, Y.**, Platelet-activating factor receptor in the rat brain, in *Abstract of the 3rd IBRO World Cong. Neurosc.*, Montreal, August 4 to 9, 1991, 368.

56. **Marchesselli, V. L., Rossowska, M. J., Domingo, M.-T., Braquet, P., and Bazan, N. G.**, Distinct platelet-activating factor binding sites in synaptic endings and in intracellular membranes of rat cerebral cortex, *J. Biol. Chem.*, 265, 9140, 1990.

57. **Takano, T., Honda, Z., Watanabe, T., Uchida, S., Shimizu, T., and Kurokawa, K.**, Demonstration of platelet activating factor receptor in guinea pig kidney, *Biochem. Biophys. Res. Commun.*, 177, 54, 1991.

58. **Huang, S. J., Monk, P. N., Downes, C. P., and Whetton, A. D.**, Platelet-activating factor-induced hydrolysis of phosphatidyl-inositol-4,5-bisphosphate stimulates the production of reactive oxygen intermediates in macrophages, *Biochem. J.*, 249, 839, 1988.

59. **Hirata, M., Hayashi, Y., Ushikubi, F., Yokota, Y., Kageyama, R., Nakanishi, S., and Narumiya, S.**, Cloning and expression of cDNA for a human thromboxane A_2 receptor, *Nature*, 349, 617, 1991.

60. **Shimizu, T. and Wolfe, L. S.**, Arachidonic acid cascade and signal transduction, *J. Neurochem.*, 55, 1, 1990.

61. **Hanahan, D. J.**, Platelet activating factor: a biologically active phosphoglyceride, *Annu. Rev. Biochem.*, 55, 483, 1986.

62. **Snyder, F.**, Ed., *Platelet-Activating Factor and Related Lipid Mediators*, Plenum Press, New York, 1987.

63. **Prescott, S. M., Zimmerman, G. A., and McIntyre, T. M.**, Platelet activating factor, *J. Biol. Chem.*, 265, 17381, 1990.

Chapter 5

PLATELET ACTIVATING FACTOR RECEPTOR FUNCTIONS VIA PHOSPHOINOSITIDE TURNOVER AND TYROSINE KINASE

Shivendra D. Shukla, Archie W. Thurston, Jr., Cindy Y. Zhu, and Animesh Dhar

TABLE OF CONTENTS

ISBN 0-8493-7299-2
© 1993 by CRC Press, Inc.

I. INTRODUCTION

Elucidation of the structure of platelet activating factor (PAF) as 1-O-alkyl-2-acetyl-*sn*-glycero-3-phosphocholine in 1979[1-3] led to intense research activity into its receptors and signal transduction mechanisms.[4-6] Thus, issues such as characterization of PAF receptor binding, isolation of receptors, and identification of second messengers were targeted in many laboratories. With these investigations, it became apparent that PAF modulated multiple signaling pathways.[7,8] The importance of second messengers, e.g., Ca^{2+}, inositol trisphosphate (IP$_3$), diglyceride (DG), cAMP, etc., in relation to PAF receptor function began to emerge. Differences in the binding properties of the receptor to [^{3}H]PAF or to radiolabeled antagonists have provided evidence for the heterogeneity in PAF receptors.[9] The PAF receptor has been cloned and its molecular features are also now being explored.[10,11] In this chapter, the developments related to PAF receptor coupled phosphoinositide (PPI) turnover and tyrosine kinase is reviewed extensively. The interrelationships between phosphoinositide-specific phospholipase C (PLC) mediated pathway and other signaling routes affected by PAF are also discussed.

The past two decades have also witnessed a surge in investigations on phosphoinositide turnover and tyrosine kinase as important pathways for the cell signal transduction.[12] Since its discovery by Hokins,[13] followed by the historical proposals of Michell[14] and Berridge and Irvine,[15] it is now well recognized that PPI turnover is an important pathway for intracellular cell signaling. Several diverse stimuli activate PLC, which primarily hydrolyzes phosphatidylinositol-4,5-bisphosphate (PIP$_2$).[15] Inositol-1,4,5-trisphosphate (IP$_3$) and DG are products of PIP$_2$. IP$_3$ initiates the release of Ca^{2+} from intracellular stores,[16] while DG activates protein kinase C (PKC).[17] However, the entire cascade of PI turnover is gaining complexity. A family of water-soluble inositol polyphosphates, including IP$_4$, IP$_5$, IP$_6$, and cyclic inositol phosphates have been identified.[18] Similarly, at least seven isozymes of PKC have been documented and their sensitivity to Ca^{2+} and/or phospholipids exhibits a diversity in their function.[17]

Agonist coupled activation of PLC has been widely documented to be mediated via GTP binsing protein(s).[19,20] A family of G-proteins of high and low molecular weight, which could be both membrane bound or cytosolic, have been identified.[19,20] Of this family, G$_i$, G$_q$, G$_o$, G$_p$, G$_z$, and G? have been proposed to activate PLC. A further interesting dimension arises with the observations that at least four (perhaps more) types of physicochemically and immunologically different phospholipases C, e.g., PLC$_\alpha$, PLC$_\gamma$, PLC$_\beta$, and PLC$_\delta$, exist.[21,22] At present, a unified mechanism for PLC activation has not been perceived.

Tyrosine kinase(s) have also emerged as key players involved in cell responses and in growth and differentiation[23] after its discovery by Hunter and Cooper.[24] Significant advances have been made in establishing the role of tyrosine kinase activity in PLC$_\gamma$ activation. In particular, tyrosine kinases which are receptors for epidermal growth factor (EGF) and platelet-derived growth factor (PDGF) have been shown to cause phosphorylation of tyrosine residues in PLC$_\gamma$. This phosphorylation is responsible for its translocation from cytosol to membrane.[25] *In vivo* phosphorylation of PLC$_{\gamma 1}$ at tyrosine residues by EGF resulted in an increase in the catalytic activity.[26] However, phosphorylation of purified bovine PLC$_{\gamma 1}$ did not cause any significant increase in the catalytic activity. It has been suggested that a modulating protein may be necessary for PLC catalytic activity *in vivo*.[22] Other components in receptor signaling and PI turnover, e.g., phosphatidylinositol kinase or GTPase activating protein (GAP), are also substrates for cellular tyrosine kinases.[27]

II. PLATELET ACTIVATING FACTOR-STIMULATED PHOSPHOINOSITIDE TURNOVER

PAF-stimulated turnover of PPI was first reported in rabbit platelets. In these studies, a rapid incorporation of carrier-free ^{32}P into PI, PIP, and PIP_2 was stimulated by PAF.[28,29] This reflected activation of the PI cycle, and the ^{32}P incorporation was a result of a synthesis of PPI.[13] When rabbit platelets prelabeled with [^3H]inositol were challenged with PAF, a rapid (5 to 10 s) and transient decrease in [^3H]PIP_2[35] and a concomitant increase in water-soluble [^3H]IP_3 was demonstrated.[30] This established the activation of PI-specific PLC by PAF. Studies with platelets from horse,[31] human,[32] and pig,[33] have further documented and characterized this response. In the past decade, numerous groups have shown that PAF activates inositol lipid turnover in a wide spectrum of cells originating from blood, kidney, liver, lung, intestine, epithelium, etc. (Table 1). In most cases, this response is rapid, transient, and occurs at a PAF concentration range of 10^{-9} to 10^{-7} M. However, it is of interest to mention that in astrocytes, IP_3 production by PAF occurred at concentrations below 1 nM PAF, but not with concentrations above it.[74]

A. CHARACTERISTICS OF PHOSPHOLIPASE C ACTIVATION AND DESENSITIZATION

In general, PAF activation of PLC is independent of extracellular Ca^{2+};[7] however, in the absence of extracellular Ca^{2+}, functional responses of cells to PAF (e.g., aggregation of platelets or degranulation of neutrophils) may not occur. This indicates that external Ca^{2+} serves as an important link between receptor activation and cell response. In platelets, the relationship between binding of [^3H]PAF to the activation of PLC (i.e., IP_3 production) was explored. Interestingly, it became apparent that fractional occupancy of the receptor is sufficient to activate the PLC maximally.[78] Such studies led to the suggestion that not all PAF receptors are coupled to PLC activation.

In several cells or systems the biochemical and physiological responses of PAF are prone to the process of desensitization. For example, pretreatment of platelets with PAF renders them insensitive (or desensitized) to any subsequent challenge by PAF.[79] The phenomenon of desensitization has also been addressed in relation to PLC activation. It was noted that [^3H]inositol-labeled rabbit platelets that were incubated with increasing concentrations of PAF and subsequently challenged by the same concentration of PAF had greatly diminished [^3H]IP_3 production (i.e., PLC activity).[80] Platelets incubated with fixed concentrations of PAF and then challenged with increasing concentrations of PAF had log-dose response curves of [^3H]IP_3 production progressively shifted to the right, i.e., to higher concentrations. Pretreatment of platelets with 10 nM PAF rendered their PLC completely unresponsive to PAF. These studies demonstrated that PPI turnover was desensitized in platelets preexposed to PAF, i.e., homologous desensitization. Interestingly, platelets desensitized to PAF exhibited full PLC activation by thrombin. On the contrary, pretreatment with thrombin desensitized platlets to both PAF and thrombin, thus indicating heterologous desensitization. These observations clearly identify distinct mechanisms for PAF and thrombin receptor signaling pathways and also demonstrate that PLC activation is an early step in the mechanism underlying desensitization.[80] Besides platelets, similar desensitization of the PLC response also occurred in other cells, e.g., U937 cells,[70] and anterior pituitary cells.[68] It is noteworthy that other PAF responses, e.g., Ca^{2+} mobilization[81] and protein phosphorylations[82] are also desensitized. The mechanism of PAF receptor coupled PLC desensitization is not defined. It is not due to depletion of (1) the PIP_2 pool[83] or (2) due to PKC, because staurosporine (a PKC inhibitor) had no effect on the desensitization.[84] In desensitized rabbit platelets, the [^3H] PAF binding was little affected, suggesting that the down-regulation of the receptor

TABLE 1
List of Cells/Tissues in Which PAF Stimulates Inositol Lipid Turnover

Cells or tissues	Response Monitored	Ref.
Platelets		
Rabbit	[^{32}P] incorporation in PPI	29
	PA production	29, 34
	PIP$_2$ breakdown	35, 36
	IP$_3$ production	30
Porcine	IP$_3$ production	33
Horse	PA production, decrease in PIP$_2$	31, 37
Human	PA production, decrease in PIP$_2$	32, 38–43
Macrophages		
Alveolar	Decrease in PIP$_2$	75
Peritoneal (murine)	IP$_3$ production	44, 45
Bone marrow derived	IP$_3$ production	46
Neutrophils		
Rabbit	Decrease in [^{32}P] PIP$_2$	47
Human	IP$_3$ production	48, 49 (see also 50)
Peripheral blood mononuclear leukocytes (human)	IP$_3$ production	51
B cell line SKW6.4 (human)	^{32}P-labeling of PI	52, 77
B-lymphoblastoid cells (HSCE or LA350)	IP$_3$ production	53
Eosinophils (guinea pig)	IP$_3$ production	54
Kidney		
Epithelial cells (LLC-PK-1)	Decrease in PI, increase in DG	55
Mesengial cells	IP$_3$ production	56
Juxtaglomerular cells	Decrease in [^{32}P] PIP$_2$	57
Liver		
Hepatocytes	Decrease in [^{32}P]PIP$_2$	58 (see also 59)
Kupffer cells	IP (total)	60
	IP$_3$ production	61
Bovine pulmonary artery endothelial cells	IP$_3$ production	62
Aortic smooth muscle cells	Decrease in PI, increase in DG	55
Aortic cultured vascular smooth muscle cells	IP$_3$ production	63
Ileal plasmalemmal vesicles	Decrease in [^{32}P] PIP$_2$	64
Rat myometrium (uterus)	IP$_1$ production	65
Guinea pig pancreatic lobule	IP$_3$ production	66
Porcine thyroid cells (cultured)	^{32}P-labeling of PI	67
Anterior pituitary cells (rat and bovine)	IP$_3$ production	68
Skin cells (human keratinocytes)	IP$_3$ production	69
Monocytic leukemic U937 cells (human)	IP$_3$ production	70
Human erythroleukemia cells (HEL cells)	IP$_3$ production	71
Epidermoid carcinoma cells (A-431 cells)	IP$_3$ production	72
Swiss mouse 3T3 fibroblasts	Decrease in PI, increase in DG	73
Astrocytes	IP$_3$ production	74
Oocytes (transfected with PAF receptor cDNA)	IP$_3$ production	11
COS-7 cells (transfected with PAF receptor cDNA)	IP$_3$ production	11
Neurohybrid NG108-15 cells	IP$_3$ production	76

may not be the explanation.[100,169] However, prior treatment of human platelets with unlabeled PAF rendered the platelets incapable of binding [^{3}H]PAF, presumably through the loss of available binding sites.[39] In yet another study, there was no loss of the binding sites, but the affinity of [^{3}H]PAF was proposed to be altered in desensitized platelets.[85] The mechanism for desensitization thus remains open. The involvement of G-proteins, tyrosine kinase, or protein phosphorylation in this desensitization process has yet to be explored.

PAF-stimulated PPI hydrolysis was primarily due to PLC activation, as discussed in the preceding section; however, such is not always the case. There are several examples in which PAF receptor activation has been demonstrated to deacylate PI and other lipids to produce arachidonic acid via phospholipase A_2-mediated pathway. The existence of this mechanism has been documented in eye smooth muscle,[86] vascular smooth muscle cells,[55,87] hepatocytes,[59,88,89] Kupffer cells,[61,90] macrophages,[91-93] neutrophils,[94,95] brain cells,[96] B cells,[52] 3T3 fibroblasts,[73] and endothelial cells.[97] The arachidonic acid thus produced can be metabolized to a variety of prostaglandins.

B. MECHANISM OF PHOSPHOLIPASE C ACTIVATION: ROLE OF G-PROTEINS AND TYROSINE KINASE

Several stimuli cause PI turnover mediated by PLC. Two separate mechanisms for agonist stimulation of PLC activity have been proposed thus far. In one case, G-proteins act as transducers of PLC activity, e.g., in α_1 or M_1 receptors, etc.[18,19] In the other case, tyrosine kinase plays the role of transducer, e.g., with EGF or PDGF receptors.[22] A further complexity lies in the fact that several high and low molecular weight G-proteins exist in mammalian cells[98,99] and that their specific roles are unknown.

Interestingly, both G-proteins and tyrosine kinase have been suggested to be involved in the PAF activation of PLC.[8] While strong arguments have been presented for both mechanisms, the identity of these components and evidence for their direct involvement in PAF signaling is not well established. In several cells in which GTPγs has been observed to activate PLC, PAF also activated PLC. As is now well known, the α subunit of the trimeric G-protein (α, β, γ subunits) possesses GTPase activity and hydrolysis of GTP bound to the α subunit renders this subunit inactive and favors its association with the β-γ subunit.[19,20] In platelets,[100,101] neutrophils,[102] and A431 cells,[103] PAF stimulates GTPase and therefore an involvement of G-proteins can be implied in PAF receptor function. Several studies have also used pertussis toxin (PT) as a tool to monitor the involvement of G-proteins in PLC activation. PT causes ADP-ribosylation of the α subunit of G_i and inactivates it.[19,20] Observations obtained using PT do not allow us to draw any firm conclusions about the functional involvement of G-proteins in PAF signaling mechanisms. In studies with platelets[114] and A431 cells,[103] PAF-stimulated PPI turnover was only partially sensitive to PT treatment. In macrophage[46] and neutrophils,[47,49] the PPI turnover by PAF was sensitive to the toxin while U937 cells[70] and peripheral blood mononuclear leukocytes (PBML)[51] were insensitive. Further, in neutrophils, PT does block functional changes induced by PAF,[50] but does not block Ca^{2+} rise.[47] PT had no effect on PAF-induced Ca^{2+} increase in PBML cells[162] or in polymorphonuclear leukocytes.[49] PAF-stimulated GTPase activity in human platelet membrane was insensitive to PT,[9,40,102] while it was affected in neutrophil membranes.[102] PT treatment completely inhibited PAF stimulated GTPase in A431 cell membranes.[103] A G-protein that is distinct from G_s or G_i has been implicated in PAF-mediated PI metabolism in platelets.[119] It should be noted that GTP causes a shift to the right in the binding of PAF, one of the characteristics of the ligand binding to G-protein coupled receptors.[9,19] The experimental evidence discussed above illustrates the complexities of G-protein involvement in PAF actions. Most likely, more than one type of G-protein is involved in PAF receptor functions and this could very well differ from cell to cell. Further, as discussed later in the case with A431 cells, the possibility of dual mechanisms of PLC activation involving both G-protein and tyrosine kinase also exists.[103]

Another mechanism for PLCγ activation is via its phosphorylation by tyrosine kinase. It has been shown, particularly with EGF, that phosphorylation of PLCγ by the EGF receptor induces translocation of the PLCγ from cytosol to membrane fraction and also activates this enzyme. Phosphorylation on Tyr 783 is considered essential for PLC-γ1 activation.[22] Whether phosphorylation of PLC by this mechanism causes an increase in PLC activity by PAF is presently unknown. PLCγ activation in hepatocytes is claimed to be coupled to both G-protein and tyrosine kinase.[104,105]

New developments on PAF receptor responses in A431 cells offer interesting insights into the unique features of PLC activation by PAF. In this cell line, PT pretreatment abolished 50% of the PAF-stimulated IP_3 production, while genistein, a tyrosine kinase inhibitor, totally blocked PLC stimulation. Staurosporine (a PKC inhibitor) potentiated PLC activation, while PMA (a PKC activator) abolished PLC activation, as also observed in rabbit platelets.[84] Pretreatment of A431 cells with forskolin, an adenylate cyclase activator, decreased PAF-stimulated PI hydrolysis. Interestingly, PT treatment of A431 cell membranes led to the total abolition of PAF-stimulated GTPase. Thus, the possible involvement of PT insensitive G-proteins in PAF activation of PLC was ruled out in this particular cell line. These studies have led to the proposal of dual mechanisms involved in PLC activation in A431 cells where tyrosine kinase mediates the PLC stimulation and part of this stimulation is dependent upon a PT-sensitive G-protein.[103] In a recent report, PT sensitive G-proteins were proposed to be involved in signal transduction responsible for positive and negative regulation of A431 cell growth, despite the fact that EGF-stimulated PI turnover was not susceptible to PT treatment.[156] This draws a distinction between PAF- and EGF-mediated signal transduction pathways in A431 cells.[155]

A variety of pharmacological agents and PAF antagonists have been used to define the characteristics of PAF-stimulated PPI turnover (Table 2). Several structurally dissimilar PAF antagonists blocked the PPI turnover, indicating the dependency of this phenomenon on PAF receptor occupancy.[107] In addition, PKC activators, tyrosine kinase inhibitors, PLC inhibitors, and adenylate cyclase activators all inhibited PAF stimulation of PLC. On the other hand, PKC inhibitors and Ca^{2+} chelators either potentiated or had no effect on the PLC activation (see Table 2). Staurosporine potentiated PAF stimulated IP_3 production in platelets[84] and up-regulated the PAF stimulation of respiratory burst in neutrophils.[152] Results from these pharmacological manipulations are providing valuable information for establishing the mechanisms involved in PAF receptor signaling (Fig. 1).

C. RELATIONSHIP TO Ca^{2+}

Ca^{2+} mobilization accompanying PPI turnover plays a crucial role in PAF responses. Many investigators have shown that PAF stimulates a rise in cytosolic free Ca^{2+} concentration in a wide variety of cells. This can occur both by release of intracellularly stored Ca^{2+} and by influx of extracellular Ca^{2+}. This aspect has been investigated in detail for platelets. Using Quin-2-loaded human platelets, it was observed that PAF caused a rapid increase in cytosolic free Ca^{2+} concentration to 1 μM.[106,164] With EGTA in the medium, this increase was reduced to only 170 nM, indicating a requirement for external Ca^{2+}.[7,106] Similarly in rabbit platelets (loaded with Fura-2), PAF-stimulated increase in Ca^{2+} occurred via two pathways. In the absence of external Ca^{2+} (i.e., with EGTA) the Ca^{2+} increases were 300 nM, while it rose to 2 μM in the presence of external Ca^{2+}.[81] Of the total increase in cytosolic Ca^{2+} caused by PAF, about 25% is due to release from internal stores, while the remainder can be attributed to the influx. The release of intracellular Ca^{2+} is most likely activated by IP_3 produced by PAF.[7] With EGTA in the medium, PAF fails to aggregate rabbit and human platelets, although IP_3-mediated release of intracellular Ca^{2+} does occur.[7] External Ca^{2+} is thus important for other steps involved in the process leading to aggregation. Ca^{2+} serves as an important link between receptor activation and the physiological response. The PAF-induced increase in Ca^{2+} and the importance of both intracellular Ca^{2+} release and influx has also been documented in human erythroleukemic (HEL) cells (unpublished), U937 cells,[70] neuroblastoma cells,[108] neutrophils,[121] lymphocytes,[153] smooth muscle,[154] and macrophages.[159]

TABLE 2
Effect of Various Chemicals/Treatments on PAF-Stimulated Phospholipase C Pathway

Chemicals	Known property or site of action	Effect	Ref.
Forskolin	Increases cAMP	Inhibition	30, 67, 155
Prostaglandin I_2	Increases cAMP	Inhibition	31
Phorbol myristate acetate	Stimulates PKC	Inhibition	46, 60, 74, 84
Staurosporine	Inhibits PKC	Potentiation	84
Genistein	Inhibits tyrosine kinase	Inhibition	114
2,5-dihydroxycinnamate	Inhibits tyrosine kinase	Inhibition	115
Erbstatin	Inhibits tyrosine kinase	Inhibition	116
Indomethacin	Inhibits cyclooxygenase	No effect	30, 31
		Inhibition	65
Neomycin	Inhibits PLC	Inhibition	42
Manoalide	Inhibits PLC	Inhibition	70
EDTA or EGTA	Cation chelator	No effect	30, 70
		Potentiation (EDTA)	155
Trifluoperazine	Ca^{2+} channel blocker	No effect	31
Verapamil	Ca^{2+} channel blocker	Inhibited Ca^{2+} entry	57
Oleic acid	Fatty acid	Inhibition	117
Zn^{2+}	Cation	Inhibition	118
Pertussis toxin	ADP-ribosylates $G_{\alpha i}$ protein	Inhibition	40, 46, 50, 61
		No inhibition	51, 70, 114, 119
Cholera toxin	ADP-ribosylates $G_{\alpha s}$ protein	No effect	51
CV3988	PAF receptor antagonist	Inhibition	30, 70, 107
CV6209	PAF receptor antagonist	Inhibition	107
SRI-63441	PAF receptor antagonist	Inhibition	107
SRI-63675	PAF receptor antagonist	Inhibition	60, 107
BN50739	PAF receptor antagonist	Inhibition	76
BN52021	PAF receptor antagonist	Inhibition	38, 120
U66985	PAF receptor antagonist	Inhibition	61, 122
U66982	PAF receptor antagonist	Inhibition	122
L659989	PAF receptor antagonist	Inhibition	51
L652731	PAF receptor antagonist	Inhibition	68
WEB 2086	PAF receptor antagonist	Inhibition	53, 54
DNPP	Serine protease inhibitor	Partial inhibition	123
NaTrpEE	Serine protease inhibitor	Partial inhibition	123

PAF-induced increase in Ca^{2+} was also noted in oocytes in which the PAF receptor was specifically expressed.[11] Injection of IP_3 in these cells also caused an increase in cytosolic Ca^{2+} concentration. In another experiment, PAF receptor cDNA was expressed in COS cells.[11] PAF stimulated [^{3}H]IP_3 production in these cells labeled with [^{3}H]inositol.[11] Such direct approaches can help establish the molecular interaction involved between the PAF receptor and the transducer/effector.

In a few studies, the mechanism of PAF stimulated Ca^{2+} increases have been explored. Elevation of cAMP in platelets, e.g., by PGI_2, eliminated the PAF-induced Ca^{2+} increase.[164] Such increases in cAMP also inhibit PAF-stimulated PI turnover (Table 2). This suggested a negative (inhibitory) role of cAMP (and perhaps of cAMP-dependent protein kinase) in the PAF-stimulated PLC activation and Ca^{2+} mobilization. The involvement of PKC in Ca^{2+} hemostasis has also been addressed. Phorbol esters inhibited the PAF-induced increase in Ca^{2+},[164] while staurosporine (a PKC inhibitor) had no effect on the Ca^{2+} mobilization caused

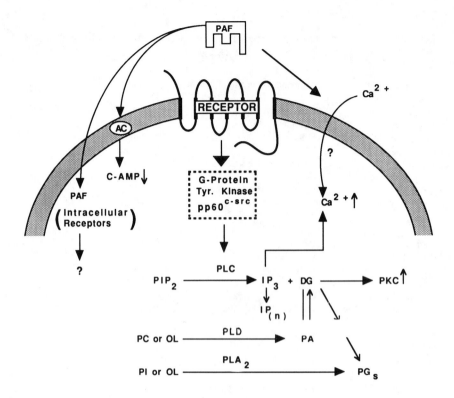

FIGURE 1.   A simplified model of PAF receptor activated signal transduction pathways. The diagram depicts the relationship between PAF receptor and major signaling pathways activated by PAF. The scheme is simplified for clarity. Various phospholipids shown are located in plasma membranes. The dotted box indicates that the interactions among these components are not known. AC, adenylate cyclase; DG, diglyceride; IP_3, inositol 1,4,5 trisphosphate; $IP_{(n)}$, other inositol phosphates; OL, other lipids; PA, phosphatidic acid; PC, phosphatidylcholine; PGs, prostaglandins; PLA_2, phospholipase A_2; PLC, phospholipase C; PLD, phospholipase D; PI, phosphatidyli- nositol; PIP_2, PI-4,5 bisphosphate; PKC, protein kinase C; Tyr kinase, tyrosine kinase.

by PAF.[81] Another PKC inhibitor, K252a, was also without effect on PAF-induced Ca^{2+} rise.[109] These results illustrate that activation of PKC is not a requirement for the Ca^{2+} mobilization.

In rabbit platelets, as low as 10^{-12} M PAF caused an increase in cytosolic Ca^{2+}.[81] At this concentration of PAF, no detectable increase in IP_3 could be observed.[30] This raises the possibility of an IP_3-independent increase in Ca^{2+}. In this regard, PAF stimulates receptor operated Ca^{2+} channels in human platelets[110-112] and eosinophils.[157] In some studies, Ca^{2+} channel blockers inhibited the PAF-stimulated rise in Ca^{2+},[57,112,113] while in other cases these had no effect.[108] It is intriguing to note that in one study, PAF at concentrations as high as 10 to 100 μM were used to cause a rise in Ca^{2+} in GH_4C_1 rat pituitary cells.[113] These concentrations far exceed the critical micellar concentration of PAF (about 1 μM)[158] and would have a detergent-like effect on cells.

The mechanism of PAF-induced Ca^{2+} influx is not known. PAF may directly cause influx or this influx may be mediated by other products generated in membranes by PAF, e.g., phosphatidic acid[163] or lipoxygenase-generated products.[165] Similarly, the importance of the proposed PAF receptor operated Ca^{2+} channel will also be of great interest to investigate.

III. PLATELET ACTIVATING FACTOR STIMULATION OF TYROSINE KINASE

Tyrosine kinases were at first thought to be involved mainly in receptors for growth factors. However, platelets, which are terminally differentiated nonproliferative cells, contain very high levels of protein tyrosine kinase activity in both particulate and cytosolic fractions.[124,125] It was later reported that human and rabbit platelets express high levels of pp60[c-src] tyrosine kinase, which shows homology to the retroviral oncogene product pp60[v-src].[126] Several reports have recently demonstrated that thrombin,[127-129] collagen,[129] and vasopressin[130] also stimulate tyrosine kinase in platelets. These observations indicate that tyrosine-specific protein kinases may regulate the cellular process in platelets (and perhaps in other cells) that are distinct from cell growth.

As stated earlier, PT did not completely inhibit inositol phosphate production in saponin permeabilized rabbit platelets.[114] This observation also suggested the existence of additional mechanisms for PAF stimulation of PLC. In order to assess whether PLC activation and protein phosphorylation stimulated by PAF were mediated by tyrosine kinase, the involvement of this enzyme in the PAF signaling mechanism was investigated using a monoclonal antibody to phosphotyrosine and genistein (a putative inhibitor of tyrosine kinases) as probes.[114] Genistein inhibited PAF-induced platelet aggregation and PLC activation in a dose-dependent manner. These data suggest that tyrosine kinase activity is an important early step in PAF receptor-stimulated IP$_3$ production. To determine if this inhibition of PLC activity by genistein was due to tyrosine kinase inhibition rather than PKC inhibition, experiments involving staurosporine were pursued. Staurosporine, a PKC inhibitor, potentiated PAF stimulation of [^{3}H]inositol trisphosphate production. Interestingly, genistein inhibited the combined stimulation of IP$_3$ production that is observed with staurosporine plus PAF. The possibility of the inhibition of PAF responses due to the blockade of PAF binding by genistein in rabbit platelets was next considered; apparently genistein did not inhibit the specific binding of [^{3}H]PAF to platelets.[114]

Pretreatment of platelets with genistein decreased the PAF-stimulated phosphorylation of several proteins including 20, 40, and 50 kDa proteins.[114] Genistein blocked 20 and 50 kDa protein phosphorylation, whereas 40 kDa protein phosphorylation was partially blocked. It is known that the 40 kDa protein is phosphorylated by PKC. The partial decrease in phosphorylation of PKC substrates by genistein treatment may be best explained by the effect of this inhibitor on PAF-stimulated PLC activity. In this scenario, if PLC is not activated to produce DG or to increase Ca^{2+} transiently (by IP$_3$), then neither Ca^{2+}-dependent myosin light chain kinase nor DG-dependent PKC would be activated. This might also explain why genistein inhibited phosphorylation of a 20 kDa myosin light chain kinase substrate, and a 40 kDa PKC substrate. Phosphorylation of a 50 kDa protein was the most affected by genistein treatment. PMA-mediated phosphorylation of the 40 kDa protein was also partially affected by genistein and the significance of this partial inhibition is not clearly understood. Western blot analysis with phosphotyrosine monoclonal antibody showed that 50 and 60 kDa proteins are the only ones that react predominantly with this antibody in platelets. Phosphoamino acids in the 50 and 60 kDa proteins were analyzed. It was demonstrated that PAF stimulated an increase in [^{32}P] phosphotyrosine levels of both the 50 and 60 kDa proteins and this was inhibited by genistein treatment. Erbstatin, another tyrosine kinase inhibitor, was also shown to inhibit PAF-induced protein tyrosine phosphorylation, PPI hydrolysis, PKC activation, and aggregation of rabbit platelets.[116] In P388D$_1$ cells, a macrophage-like cell line, genistein had a small inhibitory effect on lipopolysaccharide (LPS) priming and a significant inhibitory effect on primed PAF stimulation of arachidonic acid metabolism in these cells. The release of arachidonic acid is mediated mostly by a phospholipase A$_2$ (PLA$_2$)-like enzyme. Therefore, PAF-stimulated PLA$_2$ activation also appears to be mediated through tyrosine kinase. In another study with neutrophils, PAF was demonstrated to cause an increase in tyrosine phosphorylation of 41, 54, 66, 104, and 116 kDa proteins in a dose-dependent manner.[120] Lyso-PAF and other biologically inactive PAF analogues do not stimulate tyrosine phosphorylation in human neutrophils, thus indicating specificity for PAF. The PAF receptor-mediated tyrosine phosphorylation in neutrophils can be blocked by the PAF antagonist BN-52021.[120] The PAF-induced tyrosine phosphorylation of 66, 116, and 104 kDa proteins were selectively inhibited by PT treatment, whereas the 41 kDa protein remained unchanged after PT treatment. The calcium chelator EGTA significantly inhibited tyrosine phosphorylation of the 41 kDa protein, although the intracellular calcium chelator bis(-O-aminophenoxy) ethane-*NN, N'N'*-tetraacetic acid (BAPTA) stimulated the PAF-induced tyrosine phosphorylation of this protein. BAPTA also stimulated the PAF-induced tyrosine phosphorylation of 66, 106, and 116 kDa proteins. This study indicated the complexity of PAF-induced tyrosine phosphorylation in human neutrophils, and suggests that PAF may be able to affect directly or indirectly tyrosine specific kinases or phosphatases.[120] All these observations indicate that PAF stimulates tyrosine kinases in different cells such as platelets, macrophages, and neutrophils and that this kinase activity is involved in PAF receptor coupled signaling mechanism.[8]

The major tyrosine kinase in platelets is pp60^{c-src}. On the basis of the above observations, we therefore investigated the characteristics of PAF-stimulated tyrosine protein kinases and their relationship to pp60^{c-src} using a phosphotyrosine monoclonal antibody and a pp60^{c-src} antibody as probes.[131] It was established that PAF stimulated tyrosine phosphorylation of 50, 60, 71, 82, and 300 kDa proteins using phosphotyrosine monoclonal antibody affinity chromatography. The immunoreactivity of pp60^{c-src} monoclonal antibody to tyrosine phosphorylated proteins was next examined. The immunoprecipitation of ^{32}P-labeled platelets, stimulated by PAF with the monoclonal antibody to pp60^{v-src} (the viral counterpart of pp60^{c-src}), confirmed an increase in the phosphorylation of the 60 kDa protein. This suggested that PAF increased phosphorylation of pp60^{c-src}. It was reported earlier that there is a tendency for the pp60^{c-src} to undergo proteolysis during purification from human platelets.[132,133] Thus, the 50 kDa protein, which is a pp60^{c-src} immunoreactive species, perhaps represents the proteolytic product of the pp60^{c-src} in rabbit platelets, and this protein species was also phosphorylated. It has been observed that PAF-induced pp60^{c-src} phosphorylation is inhibited by the PAF antagonist CV-6209, whereas lyso-PAF (an inactive analogue) had no effect on the phosphorylation. Genistein inhibited PAF-induced ppo60^{c-src} phosphorylation.

To further explore the relationship between PAF receptor coupled signaling and pp60^{c-src} phosphorylation, we conducted experiments to localize pp60^{c-src}. Membrane and cytosolic fractions from control and PAF-treated platelets were isolated, and their immunoreactivity to pp60^{c-src} monoclonal antibody was monitored. It was observed that immunoreactivity to pp60^{c-src} monoclonal antibody in 50 and 60 kDa proteins was increased in the membrane fraction of PAF-treated platelets with concomitant decrease of these proteins in the cytosolic fraction. This clearly indicated that a proportion of pp60^{c-src} protein might be translocated from cytosol to particulate membrane fractions. This protein may interact, in some manner, with the PAF receptor or associated proteins and could cause tyrosine phosphorylation of protein substrates. It is also interesting to note that the members of the pp60^{c-src} family contain two of the protein domains, SH-2 and SH-3,[27] present in PLCγ, ras-GAP (GTPase activating proteins), and the CRK-oncogenic product. The SH-2 domain of pp60^{c-src} interacts with other proteins or receptors and may serve as a binding site for one protein to another.[27] It is possible that the association of the PAF receptor with a protein (analogous to PLCγ or GAP, which is a substrate for tyrosine kinase or pp60^{c-src}) may play a role in the PAF signaling mechanism.

Recently, the PAF receptor was cloned from guinea pig lung and was shown to contain seven membrane spanning domains, which is typical of G-protein coupled receptors.[10] Two other G-protein coupled receptors, thrombin[134] and angiotensin II,[135] have also been recently cloned. Thrombin-induced tyrosine phosphorylation may have a role in platelet aggregation involving membrane glycoprotein IIb/IIIa.[136,137] Another major platelet glycoprotein, GPIV, is physically associated with src-related protein tyrosine kinases, and ligand interaction with GPIV may activate the signal mechanism mediated by tyrosine phosphorylation.[137] The angiotensin II receptor itself contains a tyrosine phosphorylation domain which might regulate the receptor-ligand interactions and signaling mechanism inside the cell.[135] These two G-protein coupled receptors are clearly linked to tyrosine phosphorylation either directly or indirectly. The PAF receptor happens to contain 12 tyrosine residues. Whether these residues are phosphorylated and whether the receptor has intrinsic tyrosine kinase activity is not known. If the PAF receptor has no intrinsic tyrosine kinase activity, then it may directly or indirectly stimulate tyrosine phosphorylation by pp60[c-src] through an as-yet unknown mechanism. It is possible that another type of PAF receptor exists in platelets which might be linked to tyrosine kinase activity. The translocation of pp60[c-src] from cytosol to membrane and the possible interaction of its SH-2 domain to an unknown membrane component may play an important role in the PAF receptor signal mechanism. pp60[c-src] from human platelet membranes has already been purified and characterized by Feder and Bishop[132] and also by Reuter et al.[133] Recently, a 32-kDa protein was identified in a platelet membrane that interacts with the myristylated amino-terminal peptide of pp60[c-src].[138] The identity or role of the 32 kDa protein has yet to be determined.

IV. INTERRELATIONSHIP BETWEEN PHOSPHOLIPASE C AND OTHER SIGNALING PATHWAYS

A. RELATIONSHIP TO CYCLIC AMP

Agents that stimulate adenylate cyclase activity in cells, and thereby increase cAMP levels, are known to inhibit PAF activation of PLC. For example, treatment of rabbit[30] and horse[31] platelets or A431 cells[155] with forskolin[30,155] or PGI$_2$[31] abolished the PLC response by PAF. On the other hand, PAF itself has an inhibitory effect on the adenylate cyclase activation (e.g., by forskolin, PGI$_2$, or PGE$_2$) in platelets,[139,140] pulmonary artery endothelial cells,[62] thyroid cells,[67] and A431 cells (unpublished). Phentolamine, an α-adrenergic antagonist, did not abolish the PAF-induced inhibition of adenylate cyclase.[101] It is therefore likely that cAMP has a negative feedback effect on the PLC activation process. Equally important, inhibition of the adenylate cyclase by PAF could very well impart a positive effect on PLC activation. The mechanism of this interesting crosstalk between the two pathways and any role of cAMP-dependent protein kinase in this process remains to be ascertained.

B. ACTIVATION OF PHOSPHOLIPASE D

Recently phospholipase D (PLD) -mediated metabolism of phospholipids has drawn considerable attention as a transmembrane signaling event.[141-143] Transphosphatidylation reaction is a unique property of PLD, and in the presence of ethanol, this leads to the formation of phosphatidylethanol. Thus, formation of phosphatidylethanol has been used as a parameter to monitor PLD activation in many cells.[143] In human platelets, PAF induced formation of phosphatidylethanol could not be detected (unpublished). In contrast, PAF has been demonstrated to stimulate PLD activity in kidney,[144] macrophage,[145] neutrophils,[146,167] and A431 cells.[147] In neutrophils other agents such as leukotriene B4 and formyl methionyl leucyl peptide also activated PLD.[146] The outcome of PLD activity is the production of phosphatidic acid which is next hydrolyzed by PA-phosphohydrolase to DG.[143] Obviously, DG thus produced can activate PKC. Therefore, in systems in which both PLC and PLD are activated by PAF, both pathways will affect PKC and subsequent protein phosphory-lations. The relative importance of PLC and PLD in PAF receptor responses has yet to be understood. In A431 cells it was observed that PLC is the predominant pathway as compared to PLD.[147]

V. CONCLUDING REMARKS

Multiple sets of signaling pathways are activated by PAF (Figure 1). Among them, the PAF receptor coupled PI metabolism mediated by PLC occurs rapidly and transiently. The molecular mechanism for the stimulation of PLC remains unresolved. G-protein and tyrosine kinases have been implicated in this process.[8] However, the nature and identity of either of these transducing elements is unknown. Further, the cross-talk between PLC and PKC or cAMP pathways appears to impart regulatory constraints on PLC activation by PAF. It is therefore reasonable to speculate that other hormones or mediators that activate PKC or cAMP may influence the response of cells to PAF *in vivo*.

With the availability of PAF receptor cDNA more direct approaches are now feasible to define the molecular interactions between the PAF receptor and other signaling compo-nents. The mechanism of PLC desensitization and the role of protein phosphorylation in response to PAF can also be better evaluated. Due to the apparent heterogeneity of PAF[148] and PAF receptors,[149] the differences in the signaling pathways associated with them will have to be sorted out and this will be a challenge for future investigations. With some degree of certainty it can be expected that different target systems for PAF have differences in the predominant signaling pathways. PAF can be internalized in cells.[5,166] Whether there are intracellular PAF receptors (Figure 1), and if they elicit their functions through yet another set of signal transduction mechanisms via intracellular membranes is a quite provocative concept for future research.[8,9] The emerging complexities of the PAF receptor signaling and the intercommunication among pathways will be an important part of future investigations. The significance of PAF stimulated PI turnover in disease states, e.g., in platelets of asthmatics[160] or diabetics[161] is just beginning to emerge. Identification of PAF receptor signaling mechanisms will also allow a better understanding of PAF actions in clinical and pathophysiological states.[150,151,168]

ACKNOWLEDGMENTS

We are grateful to Dr. Marilyn James-Kracke for her critical reading of this article. Thanks are also due to Ms. Judy Richey for the excellent typing. The work in the author's laboratory was supported by the National Institute of Diabetes, Digestive and Kidney Diseases grant DK35170 and by a Research Career Development Award DK01782 to Dr. Shukla.

REFERENCES

1. **Demopoulos, C. A., Pinckard, R. N., and Hanahan, D. J.,** Platelet activating factor. Evidence for 1-O-alkyl-2-acetyl-*sn*-glyceryl-3-phosphorylcholine as the active component (a new class of lipid chemical mediators), *J. Biol. Chem.,* 254, 9355, 1979.
2. **Blank, M. L., Snyder, F., Byers, L. W., Brooks, B., and Muirhead, E. E.,** Antihypertensive activity of an alkyl ether analogue of phosphatidylcholine, *Biochem. Biophys. Res. Commun.,* 90, 1194, 1979.

3. **Benveniste, J., Tence, M., Varenne, P., Bidault, J., Boullet, C., and Polonsky, J.,** Semisynthese et structur proposee du facteur activant les plaquettes (P.A.F.): PAF-acether, un alkyl ether analogue de la lysophosphatidylcholine, *C. R. Acad. Sci. (Paris),* 289, 1037, 1979.

4. **Snyder, F.,** Chemical and biochemical aspects of platelet activating factor: a novel class of acetylated ether-linked choline phospholipids, *Med. Res. Rev.,* 5, 107, 1985.

5. **Hanahan, D. J.,** Platelet activating factor: a biologically active phosphoglyceride, *Annu. Rev. Biochem.,* 55, 483, 1986.

6. **Braquet, P. L., Touqui, L., Shen, T. Y., and Vargaftig, B. B.,** Perspectives in platelet activating factor research, *Pharmacol. Rev.,* 39, 97, 1987.

7. **Shukla, S. D.,** Inositol phospholipid turnover in PAF transmembrane signalling, *Lipids,* 26, 1028, 1991.

8. **Shukla, S. D.,** Platelet activating factor receptor and signal transduction mechanisms, *FASEB J.* 6, 2296, 1992.

9. **Hwang, S.,** Specific receptors of platelet activating factor, receptor heterogeneity, and signal transduction mechanisms, *J. Lipid Mediators,* 2, 123, 1990.

10. **Honda, Z., Nakamura, M., Miki, I., Minami, M., Wantanabe, T., Seyama, Y., Okado, H., Toh, H., Ito, K., Miyamoto, T., and Shimizu, T.,** Cloning functional expression of platelet activating factor receptor from guinea pig lung, *Nature,* 349, 342, 1991.

11. **Nakamura, M., Honda, Z., Izumi, T., Sakanaka, C., Mutoh, H., Minami, M., Bito, H., Seyama, Y., Matsumoto, T., Noma, M., and Shimizu, T.,** Molecular cloning and expression of platelet activating factor receptor from human leukocytes, *J. Biol. Chem.,* 266, 20400, 1991.

12. **Ullrich, A. and Schlessinger, J.,** Signal transduction by receptors with tyrosine kinase activity, *Cell,* 61, 203, 1990.

13. **Hokin, L. E.,** Receptors and phosphoinositide-generated second messengers, *Annu. Rev. Biochem.,* 54, 205, 1985.

14. **Michell, R. H.,** Inositol phospholipids and cell surface receptor functions, *Biochim. Biophys. Acta,* 415, 81, 1975.

15. **Berridge, M. J. and Irvine, R. F.,** Inositol trisphosphate, a novel second messenger in cellular signal transduction, *Nature,* 312, 315, 1984.

16. **Berridge, M. J. and Galione, A.,** Cytosolic calcium oscillators, *FASEB J.,* 2, 3074, 1988.

17. **Kikkawa, U., Kishimoto, A., and Nishizuka, Y.,** The protein kinase C family: heterogeneity and its implications, *Annu. Rev. Biochem.,* 58, 31, 1989.

18. **Bansal, V. S. and Majerus, P. W.,** Phosphatidylinositol-derived precursors and signals, *Annu. Rev. Cell Biol.,* 6, 41, 1990.

19. **Gilman, A.,** G-proteins, transducers of receptor generated signals, *Annu. Rev. Biochem.,* 56, 615, 1987.

20. **Simon, M. I., Strathmann, M. P., and Gautam, N.,** Diversity of G-proteins in signal transduction, *Science,* 252, 802, 1991.

21. **Rhee, S. G., Suh, P., Ryu, S., and Lee, S. Y.,** Studies of inositol phospholipid C, *Science,* 244, 546, 1989.

22. **Rhee, S. G.,** Inositol phospholipid-specific phospholipase C: interaction of the γ_1 isoform with tyrosine kinase, *Trends Biochem. Sci.,* 16, 297, 1991.

23. **Yarden, Y. and Ullrich, A.,** Growth factor receptor tyrosine kinases, *Annu. Rev. Biochem.,* 57, 443, 1988.

24. **Hunter, T. and Cooper, J. A.,** Protein tyrosine kinases, *Annu. Rev. Biochem.,* 54, 897, 1985.

25. **Todderud, G., Wahl, M. I., Rhee, S. G., and Carpenter, G.,** Stimulation of phospholipase C-γ_1 membrane association by epidermal growth factor, *Science,* 249, 296, 1990.

26. **Nishibe, S., Wahl, M. I., Hernandez-Sotomayor, S. M., Tonks, N. K., Rhee, S. G., and Carpenter, G.,** Increase of the catalytic activity of phospholipase C-γ_1 by tyrosine phosphorylation, *Science,* 250, 1253, 1990.

27. **Cantley, L. C., Auger, K. R., Carpenter, C., Duckworth, B., Graziani, A., Kapeller, R., and Soltoff, S.,** Oncogenes and signal transduction, *Cell,* 64, 281, 1991.

28. **Shukla, S. D. and Hanahan, D. J.,** Changes in phosphatidylinositol and other inositol phospholipids during stimulation of rabbit platelets by AGEPC (platelet activating factor), *Fed. Proc.,* 41, 912, 1982.

29. **Shukla, S. D. and Hanahan, D. J.,** AGEPC (platelet activating factor) induced stimulation of rabbit platelets: effects on phosphatidylinositol, di- and triphosphoinositides and phosphatidic acid metabolism, *Biochem. Biophys. Res. Commun.,* 106, 697, 1982.

30. **Shukla, S. D.,** Platelet activating factor stimulated formation of inositol triphosphate in plates and its modulation by various agents including Ca^{2+}, indomethacin, CV3988 and forskolin, *Arch. Biochem. Biophys.,* 240, 674, 1985.

31. **Lapetina, E. G.,** Platelet activating factor stimulates the phosphatidylinositol cycle. Appearance of PA is associated with the release of serotonin in horse platelets, *J. Biol. Chem.,* 257, 7314, 1982.

32. **MacIntyre, D. E. and Pollack, W. K.,** Platelet activating factor stimulates phosphatidylinositol turnover in human platelets, *Biochem. J.,* 212, 433, 1983.

33. **Duronio, V., Reany, A., Wong, S., Bigras, C., and Salari, H.,** Characterization of platelet-activating factor receptors in porcine platelets, *Can. J. Physiol. Pharm.,* 68, 1514, 1990.

34. **Ieyasu, H., Takai, Y., Kaibuchi, K., Sawamura, M., and Nishizuka, Y.,** A role of calcium-activated, phospholipid-dependent protein kinase in platelet-activating factor induced serotonin release from rabbit platelets, *Biochem. Biophys. Res. Commun.,* 108, 1701, 1982.

35. **Shukla, S. D. and Hanahan, D. J.,** A transient rapid decrease in TPI upon stimulation of rabbit platelets with AGEPC, *Arch. Biochem. Biophys.,* 227, 626, 1983.

36. **Mauco, G., Chap, H., and Douste-Blazy, L.,** Platelet activating factor (PAF-acether) promotes an early degradation of phosphatidylinositol-4,5-bisphosphate in rabbit platelets, *FEBS Lett.,* 153, 361, 1983.

37. **Billah, M. M. and Lapetina, E. G.,** Platelet activating factor stimulates metabolism of phosphoinositides in horse platelets: possible relation to Ca^{2+} mobilization during stimulation, *Proc. Natl. Acad. Sci. U.S.A.,* 80, 965, 1983.

38. **Simon, M. F., Chap, H., Braquet, P., and Douste-Blazy, L.,** Effect of BN 52021, a specific antagonist of platelet activating factor (PAF-acether), on calcium movements and phosphatidic acid production induced by PAF-acether in human platelets, *Thromb. Res.,* 45, 299, 1987.

39. **Kloprogge, E. and Akkerman, J. W.,** Binding kinetics of PAF-acether to intact human platelets, *Biochem. J.,* 223, 901, 1984.

40. **Brass, L. F., Woolkalis, M. J., and Manning, D. R.,** Interactions in platelets between G proteins and the agonists that stimulate phospholipase C and inhibit adenylyl cyclase, *J. Biol. Chem.,* 263, 5348, 1988.

41. **Shukla, S. D., Morrison, W. J., and Klachko, D. M.,** Responses of platelet activating factor in human platelets stored and aged in plasma: decrease in aggregation, phosphoinositide turnover and receptor affinity, *Transfusion,* 29, 528, 1989.

42. **Tysnes, O. B., Verhoeven, A. J., and Holmsen, H.,** Neomycin inhibits agonist-stimulated polyphosphinositide metabolism and responses in human platelets, *Biochem. Biophys. Res. Commun.,* 144, 454, 1987.

43. **Rao, A. K., Willis, J., Hassell, B., Dangelmaier, C., Holmsen, H., and Smith, J. B.,** Platelet-activating factor is a weak platelet agonist: evidence from normal human platelets and platelets with congenital secretion defects, *Am. J. Hematol.,* 17, 153, 1984.

44. **Uhing, R. J., Prpie, V., Hollenbach, P. W., and Adams, D. O.,** Involvement of protein kinase C in platelet activating factor stimulated diacylglycerol accumulation in murine peritoneal macrophages, *J. Biol. Chem.,* 264, 9224, 1989.

45. **Prpic, V., Uhing, R. J., Weiel, J. E., Jakar, L., Gawdi, G., Herman, B., and Adams, D. O.,** Biochemical and functional responses stimulated by platelet-activating factor in murine periotneal macrophages, *J. Cell Biol.,* 107, 363, 1988.

46. **Huang, S. J., Monk, P. N., Downes, C. P., and Whetton, A. D.,** Platelet activating factor induced hydrolysis of phosphatidylinositol-4,5-bisphosphate stimulates the production of reactive oxygen intermediates in macrophages, *Biochem. J.,* 249, 839, 1988.

47. **Naccache, P. M., Molski, M. M., Volpi, M., Becker, E. L., and Sha'afi, R. I.,** Unique inhibitory profile of PAF induced calcium mobilization, polyphosphoinositide turnover and granule enzyme secretion in rabbit neutrophils towards pertussis toxin and phorbol ester, *Biochem. Biophys. Res. Commun.,* 130, 677, 1985.

48. **Rossi, A. G., McMillan, R. M., and MacIntyre, D. E.,** Agonist-induced calcium flux, phosphoinositide metabolism aggregation and enzyme secretion in human neutrophils, *Agents Actions,* 24, 272, 1988.

49. **Verghese, M. W., Charles, L., Jakoi, L., Dillon, S. B., and Snyderman, R.,** Role of a guanine nucleotide regulatory protein in the activation of phospholipase C by different chemoattractants, *J. Immunol.,* 138, 4374, 1987.

50. **Lad, P. M., Olson, C. V., and Grewal, I. S.,** Platelet activating factor mediated effects on human neutrophil function are inhibited by pertussis toxin, *Biochem. Biophys. Res. Commun.,* 129, 623, 1985.

51. **Ng, D. S. and Wong, K.,** Platelet activating factor (PAF) stimulates phosphatidylinositol hydrolysis in human peripheral blood mononuclear leukocytes, *Res. Commun. Chem. Pathol. Pharm.,* 66, 219, 1989.

52. **Schulam, P. G., Kuruvilla, A., Putcha, G., Mangus, L., Franklin-Johnson, J., and Shearer, W. T.,** Platelet activating factor induces phospholipid turnover, calcium flux, arachidonic acid liberation, eicosanoid generation and oncogene expression in a human B cell line, *J. Immunol.,* 146, 1642, 1991.

53. **Mazer, B., Domenico, J., Sawami, H., and Gelfand, E. W.,** Platelet activating factor induces an increase in intracellular calcium and expression of regulatory genes in human B lymphoblastoid cells, *J. Immunol.,* 146, 1914, 1991.

54. **Kroegel, C., Chilvers, E. R., Giembycz, M. A., Challis, R. A. J., and Barnes, P. J.,** Platelet activating factor stimulates a rapid accumulation of inositol (1,4,5)(tris-phosphate in guinea pig eosinophils: relationship to calcium mobilization and degranulation, *J. Allergy Clin. Immunol.,* 88, 114, 1991.

55. **Kawaguchi, H. and Yasuda, H.**, Platelet activating factor stimulates prostaglandin synthesis in cultured cells, *Hypertension*, 8, 192, 1986.

56. **Bonventre, J. V., Weber, P. C., and Gronich, J. H.**, PAF and PDGF increase cytosolic Ca^{2+} and phospholipase activity in mesangial cells, *Am. J. Physiol.*, 254, F87, 1988.

57. **Pfeilschifter, J., Kurtz, A., and Bauer, C.**, Inhibition of renin secretion by PAF in cultured rat renal juxtaglomerular cells, *Biochem. Biophys. Res. Commun.*, 127, 903, 1985.

58. **Shukla, S. D., Buxton, D., Olson, M. S., and Hanahan, D. J.**, AGEPC: a potent activator of hepatic phosphoinositide metabolism and glycogenolysis, *J. Biol. Chem.*, 258, 19212, 1983.

59. **Okayasu, T., Hasegawa, K., and Ishibashi, T.**, Platelet activating factor stimulates metabolism of phosphoinositide via PLA_2 in primary cultured rat hepatocytes, *J. Lipid Res.*, 28, 760, 1987.

60. **Fisher, R. A., Sharma, R. V., and Bhalla, R. C.**, Platelet activating factor increases inositol phosphate production and cytosolic free Ca^{2+} concentrations in cultured rat Kupffer cells, *FEBS Lett.*, 251, 22, 1989.

61. **Gandhi, C. R., Hanahan, D. J., and Olson, M. S.**, Two distinct pathways of platelet-activating factor-induced hydrolysis of phosphoinositides in primary cultures of rat Kuppfer cells, *J. Biol. Chem.*, 265, 18234, 1990.

62. **Grigorian, G. Y. and Ryan, U. S.**, Platelet activating factor effects on bovine pulmonary artery endothelial cells, *Circ. Res.*, 61, 389, 1987.

63. **Schwertschlag, U. S. and Whorton, A. R.**, Platelet activating factor-induced homologous and heterologous desensitization in cultured vascular smooth muscle cells, *J. Biol. Chem.*, 263, 13791, 1988.

64. **Kester, M., Kumar, R., and Hanahan, D. J.**, Alkylacetyl glycerophosphocholine stimulates Na^+-Ca^{2+} exchange, protein phosphorylation, polyphosphoinositide turnover in rat ileal plasmalemmal vesicles, *Biochim. Biophys. Acta*, 888, 306, 1986.

65. **Varol, F. G., Hadjiconstantinou, M., Travers, J. B., and Neff, N. H.**, Platelet activating factor stimulates phosphatidylinositol hydrolysis in the rat myometrium, *Eur. J. Pharm.*, 159, 97, 1989.

66. **Soling, H., Eibl, H., and Fest, W.**, Acetylcholine-like effect of 1-O-alkyl-2-acetyl-*sn*-glycero-3-phosphocholine (platelet activating factor) and its analogues in exocrine secretory glands, *Eur. J. Biochem.*, 144, 65, 1984.

67. **Haye, B., Aublin, J. L., Champion, S., Lambert, B., and Jacquemin, C.**, Interactions between thyreostimulin and PAF acether on thyroid cell metabolism, *Eur. J. Pharm.*, 104, 125, 1984.

68. **Grandison, L.**, Platelet activating factor induces inositol phosphate accumulation in cultures of rat and bovine anterior pituitary cells, *Endocrinology*, 127, 1786, 1990.

69. **Fisher, G. J., Talwar, H. S., Ryder, N. S., and Voorhees, J. J.**, Differential activation of human skin cells by platelet activating factor: stimulation of phosphoinositide turnover and arachidonic acid mobilization in keratinocytes but not in fibroblasts, *Biochem. Biophys. Res. Commun.*, 163, 1344, 1989.

70. **Barzaghi, G., Saran, H. M., and Mong, S.**, Platelet activating factor-induced phosphoinositide metabolism in differentiated U-937 cells in culture, *J. Pharmacol. Exp. Ther.*, 248, 559, 1989.

71. **Lazarowski, E. R., Winegar, D. A., Nolan, R. D., Oberdisse, E., and Lapetina, E. G.**, Effect of protein kinase A on inositide metabolism and rap-1 G-protein in human erythroleukemia cells, *J. Biol. Chem.*, 265, 13118, 1990.

72. **Thurston, A. W., Jr., Kansra, S., and Shukla, S. D.**, Characterization of PAF receptor responses in A431 cells, a human carcinoid cell line, *FASEB J.*, 5, A895, 1991.

73. **Kawaguchi, H. and Yasuda, H.**, Platelet activating factor stimulates phospholipase in quiescent Swiss mouse 3T3 fibroblasts, *FEBS Lett.*, 176, 93, 1984.

74. **Murphy, S. and Welk, G.**, Hydrolysis of polyphosphoinositides in astrocytes by platelet activating factor, *Eur. J. Pharm.*, 188, 399, 1990.

75. **Kumar, R., King, R., and Hanahan, D. J.**, PAF effects on phosphoinositide turnover in alveolar II macrophages, manuscript submitted.

76. **Yue, T., Gleason, M. M., Gu, J., Lysko, P. G., Hallenbeck, J., and Feuerstein, G.**, Platelet-activating factor (PAF) receptor-mediated calcium mobilization and phosphoinositide turnover in neurohybrid NG108-15 cells: studies with BN50739, a new PAF antagonist, *J. Pharm. Exp. Ther.*, 257, 347, 1991.

77. **Schulam, P. G., Putcha, G., Franklin-Johnson, J., and Shearer, W. T.**, Evidence for a PAF receptor on human lymphoblastoid B cells: activation of the PI cycle and induction of calcium mobilization, *Biochem. Biophys. Res. Commun.*, 166, 1047, 1990.

78. **Shukla, S. D. and Morrison, W. J.**, Platelet activating factor receptor occupancy in relation to the activation and desensitization of phosphoinositide specific phospholipase C, in *Platelet Membrane Receptors*, Jamieson, G. A., Ed., Alan R. Liss, New York, 1988, 341.

79. **Henson, P. M.**, Activation and desensitization of platelets by platelet activating factor (PAF) derived from Ig-E sensitized basophils. I. Characterization of the secretory response, *J. Exp. Med.*, 143, 937, 1976.

80. **Morrison, W. J. and Shukla, S. D.**, Desensitization of receptor coupled activation of phosphoinositide specific phospholipase C in platelets: evidence for distinct mechanisms for platelet activating factor and thrombin, *Mol. Pharmacol.*, 33, 58, 1988.

81. **James-Kracke, M. R., Sexe, R., and Shukla, S. D.,** The role of calcium in activation and desensitization of fura-2 loaded platelets to platelet activating factor and thrombin, *Biochim. Biophys. Acta,* manuscript submitted.

82. **Shukla, S. D., Morrison, W. J., and Dhar, A.,** Desensitization of platelet activating factor stimulated protein phosphorylation in platelets, *Mol. Pharmacol.,* 35, 409, 1989.

83. **Shukla, S. D., Franklin, C., and Carter, M.,** Activation of phospholipase C in platelets by platelet activating factor and thrombin causes hydrolysis of a common pool of phosphatidylinositol-4,5-bisphosphate, *Biochim. Biophys. Acta,* 929, 134, 1987.

84. **Morrison, W. J., Dhar, A., and Shukla, S. D.,** Staurosporine potentiates platelet activating factor stimulated phospholipase C activity in rabbit platelets but does not block its desensitization, *Life Sci.,* 45, 333, 1989.

85. **Chesney, C. M., Pifer, D. D., and Huch, K. M.,** Desensitization of human platelets by platelet activating factor, *Biochem. Biophys. Res. Commun.,* 127, 24, 1985.

86. **Yousufzai, S. Y. K. and Abdel-Latif, A. A.,** Effects of platelet activating factor on the release of arachidonic acid and prostaglandins by rabbit iris smooth muscle: inhibition by calcium channel antagonists, *Biochem. J.,* 228, 697, 1985.

87. **Takayasu-Okishio, M., Terashita, Z., and Kondo, K.,** Endothelin-1 and platelet activating factor stimulate thromboxane A_2 biosynthesis in rat vascular smooth muscle cells, *Biochem. Pharmacol.,* 40, 2713, 1990.

88. **Levine, L.,** Platelet activating factor stimulates arachidonic acid metabolism in rat liver cells (C-9 cell line) by a receptor mediated mechanism, *Mol. Pharmacol.,* 34, 793, 1988.

89. **Garcia-Sainz, J. A.,** Intercellular communication within the liver has clinical implications, *TIPS,* 10, 10, 1989.

90. **Kuiper, J., DeRijke, Y. B., Zijlstra, F. J., VanWaas, M. P., and VanBerkel, J. C.,** The induction of glycogenolysis in the perfused liver by platelet activating factor is mediated by prostaglandin D_2 from Kupffer cells, *Biochem. Biophys. Res. Commun.,* 157, 1288, 1988.

91. **Emilsson, A. and Sundler, R.,** Differential activation of phosphatidylinositol deacylation and a pathway via diphosphoinositide in macrophages responding to zymosan and ionophore A23187, *J. Biol. Chem.,* 259, 3111, 1984.

92. **Kadiri, C., Cherqui, G., Masliah, J., Rybkine, T., Etienne, J., and Bereziat, G.,** Mechanism of *N*-formyl-methionyl-leucyl-phenylalanine and platelet activating factor induced arachidonic acid release in guinea pit alveolar macrophages: involvement of a GTP-binding protein and role of protein kinase A and protein kinase C, *Mol. Pharmacol.,* 38, 418, 1990.

93. **Glaser, K. B. and Dennis, E. A.,** Bacterial lipopolysaccharide priming of $P388D_1$ macrophage like cells for enhanced arachidonic acid metabolism platelet activating factor receptor activation and regulation of phospholipase A_2, *J. Biol. Chem.,* 265, 8658, 1990.

94. **Chilton, F. H., O'Flaherty, J. T., Walsh, C. E., Thomas, M. J., Wykle, R. L., DeChetelet, L. R., and Waite, B. M.,** Platelet activating factor stimulation of the lipoxygenase pathway in polymorphonuclear leukocytes by 1-O-alkyl-2-O-acetyl-*sn*-glycero-3-phosphorylcholine, *J. Biol. Chem.,* 257, 5402, 1982.

95. **Tou, J.-S.,** Platelet-activating factor promotes arachidonate incorporation into phosphatidylinositol and phosphatidylcholine in neutrophils, *Biochem. Biophys. Res. Commun.,* 127, 1045, 1985.

96. **Panetta, T., Marcheselli, V. L., Braquet, P., Spinnevyn, B., and Bazan, N. G.,** Effects of a PAF antagonist (BN 52021) on free fatty acids, diglyceride, polyphosphoinositides and blood flow in the gerbil brain: inhibition of ischemia-reperfusion induced cerebral injury, *Biochem. Biophys. Res. Commun.,* 149, 580, 1987.

97. **Stewart, A. G., Dubbin, P. N., Harris, T., and Dusting, G. J.,** Platelet activating factor may act as a second messenger in the release of icosanoids and superoxide anions from leukocytes and endothelial cells, *Proc. Natl. Acad. Sci. U.S.A.,* 87, 3215, 1990.

98. **Manning, D. R. and Brass, L. F.,** The role of GTP-binding proteins in platelet function, *Thromb. Haemost.,* 66, 393, 1991.

99. **Kaziro, Y., Itoh, H., Kozasa, T., Nakafuku, M., and Satoh, T.,** Structure and function of signal transducing GTP-binding protein, *Annu. Rev. Biochem.,* 60, 349, 1991.

100. **Homma, H. and Hanahan, D. J.,** Attenuation of platelet activating factor-induced stimulation of rabbit platelet GTPase by phorbol ester, dibutyryl cAMP, and desensitization: concomitant effects on PAF receptor binding characteristics, *Arch. Biochem. Biophys.,* 262, 32, 1988.

101. **Avdonin, P. V., Svitina-Ultina, I. V., and Kulikov, V. I.,** Stimulation of high-affinity hormone-sensitive GTPase of human platelets by 1-O-alkyl-2-O-acetyl-*sn*-glyceryl-3-phosphocholine (platelet activating factor), *Biochem. Biophys. Res. Commun.,* 131, 307, 1985.

102. **Hwang, S. B.,** Identification of a second putative receptor of platelet-activating factor from human polymorphonuclear leukocytes, *J. Biol. Chem.,* 263, 3225, 1988.

103. **Thurston, A. T. and Shukla, S. D.,** Dual mechanisms for phospholipase C activation by platelet activating factor receptor involving G-proteins and tyrosine kinase in A431 cells, *FASEB J.,* 6, A1921, 1992.

104. **Johnson, R. M. and Garrison, J. C.,** Epidermal growth factor and angiotensin II stimulate formation of inositol 1,4,5- and inositol 1,3,4 tris-phosphate in hepatocytes: differential inhibition by pertussis toxin and phorbol 12-myristate 13-acetate, *J. Biol. Chem.,* 262, 17285, 1987.

105. **Yang, L., Baffy, G., Rhee, S. G., Manning, D., Hansen, C. R., and Williamson, J. R.,** Pertussis toxin sensitive G_i protein involvement in epidermal growth factor-induced activation of phospholipase C-γ in rat hepatocytes, *J. Biol. Chem.,* 266, 22451, 1991.

106. **Rink, T. J. and Sage, S. O.,** Calcium signaling in human platelets, *Annu. Rev. Physiol.,* 52, 431, 1990.

107. **Morrison, W. J. and Shukla, S. D.,** Antagonism of platelet activating factor receptor binding and stimulated phosphoinositide-specific phospholipase C, *J. Pharmacol. Exp. Ther.,* 250, 831, 1989.

108. **Yue, T. L., Gleason, M. M., Hallenbeck, J., and Feurstein, G.,** Characterization of platelet-activating factor-induced elevation of cytosolic-free calcium level in neurohybrid NCB-20 cells, *Neuroscience,* 41, 177, 1991.

109. **Yamada, K., Iwahashi, K., and Kase, H.,** Parallel inhibition of platelet-activating factor induced protein phosphorylation and serotonin release by K-252A, a new inhibitor of protein kinases in rabbit platelets, *Biochem. Pharm.,* 37, 1161, 1988.

110. **Avdonin, P. V., Cheglakov, I. B., Boogry, E. M., Svitina-Ulitina, I. V., Mazaev, A. V., and Tkachuk, V. A.,** Evidence for the receptor-operated calcium channels in human platelet plasma membrane, *Thromb. Res.,* 46, 29, 1987.

111. **Avdonin, P. V., Cheglakob, I. B., and Ikachuk, V. A.,** Stimulation of non-selective cation channels providing Ca^{2+} influx into platelets by platelet-activating factor and other aggregation inducers, *Eur. J. Biochem.,* 198, 267, 1991.

112. **Valone, F. H. and Johnson, B.,** Decay of the activating signal after platelet stimulation with 1-O-alkyl-2-acetyl-*sn*-glycero-3-phosphorylcholine: changes in calcium permeability, *Thromb. Res.,* 40, 385, 1985.

113. **Yang, J. and Tashijian, A. H., Jr.,** Platelet activating factor affects cytosolic free calcium concentration and prolactin secretion in GH_4C_1 rat pituitary cells, *Biochem. Biophys. Res. Commun.,* 174, 424, 1991.

114. **Dhar, A., Paul, A., and Shukla, S. D.,** Involvement of tyrosine kinase in PAF stimulation of phospholipase C in rabbit platelets: studies with genistein and monoclonal antibody of phosphotyrosine, *Mol. Pharmacol.,* 37, 519, 1990.

115. **Zhu, C. Y. and Shukla, S. D.,** Role of tyrosine kinase in PAF responses in human platelets: studies using inhibitors, *FASEB J.,* 5, A896, 1991.

116. **Salari, H., Duronio, V., Howard, S. L., Demos, M., Jones, K., Reany, A., Hudson, A. T., and Pelech, S. L.,** Erbstatin blocks platelet activating factor-induced protein tyrosine phosphorylation, poly-phosphoinositide hydrolysis, protein kinase C activation, serotonin secretion and aggregation of rabbit platelets, *FEBS Lett.,* 263, 104, 1990.

117. **Nunez, D., Randon, J., Gandhi, C., Siafaka-Kapadia, A., Olson, M. S., and Hanahan, D. J.,** The inhibition of platelet-activating factor-induced platelet activation by oleic acid is associated with a decrease in polyphosphoinositide metabolism, *J. Biol. Chem.,* 265, 18330, 1990.

118. **Nunez, D., Kumar, R., and Hanahan, D. J.,** Inhibition of [³H]platelet activating factor (PAF) binding by Zn^{2+}: a possible explanation for its specific PAF antiaggregating effects in human platelets, *Arch. Biochem. Biophys.,* 272, 466, 1989.

119. **Houslay, M. D., Bojanic, B., and Wilson, A.,** Platelet activating factor and U44069 stimulate a GTPase activity in human platelets which is distinct from the guanine nucleotide regulatory proteins, N_s and N_i, *Biochem. J.,* 234, 737, 1986.

120. **Gomez-Cambronero, J., Wang, E., Johnson, G., Huang, C., and Sha'afi, R. I.,** Platelet activating factor induces tyrosine phosphorylation in human neutrophils, *J. Biol. Chem.,* 266, 6240, 1991.

121. **Gomez-Cambronero, J., Drustin, M., Molski, T. F., Naccache, P. H., and Sha'afi, R. I.,** Calcium is necessary but not sufficient for the platelet-activating factor release in human neutrophils stimulated by physiological stimuli. Role of G-proteins, *J. Biol. Chem.,* 264, 2699, 1989.

122. **Tokumura, A., Homma, H., and Hanahan, D. J.,** Structural analogs of alkyl acetylglycerophosphocholine inhibitory behavior on platelet activation, *J. Biol. Chem.,* 260, 12710, 1985.

123. **Sugatani, J., Miwa, M., and Hanahan, D. J.,** Platelet activating factor stimulation of rabbit platelets is blocked by serine protease inhibitor (chymotroptic protease inhibitor), *J. Biol. Chem.,* 262, 5740, 1987.

124. **Tuy, F. P. D., Henry, J., Rosenfield, C., and Kahn A.,** High tyrosine kinase activity in normal non-proliferating cells, *Nature,* 305, 435, 1983.

125. **Nakamura, S., Takenchi, F., Tamizawa, T., Tarasaki, N., Konda, H., and Yamamura, H.,** Two separate tyrosine protein kinases in human platelets, *FEBS Lett.,* 184, 56, 1985.

126. **Golden, A., Nemeth, S. P., and Brugge, J. S.,** Blood platelets express high levels of the pp60[c-src] specific tyrosine kinase activity, *Proc. Natl. Acad. Sci. U.S.A.,* 83, 852, 1986.

127. **Ferrel, J. E., Jr. and Martin, G. S.,** Platelet tyrosine specific protein phosphorylation is regulated by thrombin, *Mol. Cell. Biol.,* 8, 3603, 1988.
128. **Golden, A. and Brugge, J. S.,** Thrombin treatment induces rapid changes in tyrosine phopshorylation in platlets, *Proc. Natl. Acad. Sci. U.S.A.,* 86, 901, 1989.
129. **Nakamura, S. and Yamamura, H.,** Thrombin and collagen induce rapid phosphorylation of a common set of cellular proteins on tyrosine in human platelets, *J. Biol. Chem.,* 264, 7089, 1989.
130. **Cranot (Grazini), Y., Putten, V. V., and Schrier, R. W.,** Vasopressin dependent tyrosine phosphorylation of a 38 KDa protein in human platelets, *Biochem. Biophys. Res. Commun.,* 168, 566, 1990.
131. **Dhar, A. and Shukla, S. D.,** Involvement of pp60$^{c\text{-src}}$ in PAF stimulated platelets: evidence for translocation from cytosol to membranes, *J. Biol. Chem.,* 266, 18797, 1991.
132. **Feder, D. and Bishop, J. M.,** Purification and enzymatic characterization of pp60$^{c\text{-src}}$ from human platelets, *J. Biol. Chem.,* 265, 8205, 1990.
133. **Reuter, C., Findik, D., and Presek, P.,** Characterization of purified pp60$^{c\text{-src}}$ protein tyrosine kinase from human platelets, *Eur. J. Pharmacol.,* 190, 343, 1990.
134. **Thien-Khai, H. V., Hung, D. T., Wheaton, V. I., and Coughlin, S. R.,** Molecular cloning of a functional thrombin receptor reveals a novel proteolytic mechanism of receptor activation, *Cell,* 64, 1057, 1991.
135. **Force, T., Kyriakis, J. M., Avruch, J., and Bonventre, J. V.,** Endothelin, vasopressin, and angiotensin II enhance tyrosine phosphorylation by protein kinase C-dependent and -independent pathways in glomerular mesangial cells, *J. Biol. Chem.,* 266, 6650, 1991.
136. **Golden, A., Brugge, J. S., and Shattil, S. J.,** Role of platelet membrane glycoprotein IIb-IIIa in agonist-induced tyrosine phosphorylation of platelet protein, *J. Cell. Biol.,* 111, 3117, 1990.
137. **Huang, M., Bolen, J. B., Barnwell, J. W., Shattil, S. J., and Brugge, J. S.,** Membrane glycoprotein IV (CD36) is physically associated with the Fyn, Lyn, and Yes protein kinases in human platelets, *Proc. Natl. Acad. Sci. U.S.A.,* 88, 7844, 1991.
138. **Feder, D. and Bishop, J. M.,** Identification of platelet membrane proteins that interact with amino-terminal peptides of pp60$^{c\text{-src}}$, *J. Biol. Chem.,* 266, 19040, 1991.
139. **Haslam, R. J. and Vanderwel, M.,** Inhibition of platelet adenylate cyclase by 1-O-alkyl-2-O-acetyl-*sn*-glyceryl-3-phosphorylcholine (platelet activating factor), *J. Biol. Chem.,* 257, 6879, 1982.
140. **Miller, D. V., Ayer, D. E., and Gorman, R. R.,** Acetyl glyceryl phosphorylcholine inhibition of prostaglandin I$_2$ stimulated adenosine 3′,5′-cyclic monophosphate levels in human platelets: evidence for thromboxane A$_2$ dependence, *Biochim. Biophys. Acta,* 711, 445, 1982.
141. **Exton, J. H.,** Signalling through phosphatidylcholine breakdown, *J. Biol. Chem.,* 265, 1, 1990.
142. **Billah, M. M. and Anthes, J. C.,** The regulation and cellular functions of phosphatidylcholine hydrolysis, *Biochem. J.,* 269, 281, 1990.
143. **Shukla, S. D. and Halenda, S. P.,** Phospholipase D in cell signalling and its relationship to phospholipase C, *Life Sci.,* 48, 851, 1991.
144. **Kester, M. and Dunn, M. J.,** Platelet-activating factor stimulates phospholipase D in cultured rat mesangial cells, *Kidney Int.,* 37, 208, 1990.
145. **Balsinde, J. and Mollinedo, F.,** Platelet activating factor synergizes with phorbol myristate acetate in activating phospholipase D in the human premonocytic cell line U937. Evidence for different mechanisms of activation, *J. Biol. Chem.,* 266, 18726, 1991.
146. **Kanaho, Y., Kanoh, H., Saitoh, K., and Nozawa, Y.,** Phospholipase D activation by platelet activating factor, leukotriene B4, and formyl-methionyl-leucyl-phenylalanine in rabbit neutrophils: phospholipase D activation is involved in enzyme release, *J. Immunol.,* 146, 3536, 1991.
147. **Fernandez-Gallardo, S. and Shukla, S. D.,** Phospholipase D activation by PAF and EGF in A431 cells, *FASEB J.,* A895, 1991.
148. **Pinckard, R. N., Ludwig, J. C., and McManus, L. M.,** Platelet activating factor, in *Inflammation: Basic Principles and Clinical Correlates,* Gallins, J. I., Goldstein, I. M., and Synderman, R., Eds., Raven Press, New York, 1988, 139.
149. **Hwang, S. B.,** Identification of a second putative receptor of platelet activating factor from human polymorphonuclear leukocytes, *J. Biol. Chem.,* 263, 3225, 1988.
150. **Koltai, M., Hosford, D., Guinot, P., Esanu, A., and Braquet, P.,** Platelet activating factor (PAF). A review of its effects, antagonists, and possible future clinical implications. I., *Drugs,* 42, 9, 1991.
151. **Koltai, M., Hosford, D., Guinot, P., Esanu, A., and Braquet, P.,** Platelet activating factor (PAF). A review of its effects, antagonists, and possible future clinical implications. II., *Drugs,* 42, 174, 1991.
152. **Combadiere, C., Hakim, J., Giroud, J., and Perianin, A.,** Staurosporine, a protein kinase inhibitor, upregulates the stimulation of human neutrophil respiratory burst by *N*-formyl peptides and platelet activating factor, *Biochem. Biophys. Res. Commun.,* 168, 65, 1990.
153. **Travers, J. B., Li, Q., Kniss, D. A., and Fertel, R. H.,** Identification of functional platelet activating factor receptors in Raji lymphoblasts, *J. Immunol.,* 143, 3708, 1989.

154. **Brock, T. A. and Gimborne, M. A., Jr.,** Platelet activating factor alters calcium homoeostasis in cultured vascular endothelial cells, *Am. J. Physiol.,* 250, H1086, 1986.

155. **Thurston, A. W., Jr. and Shukla, S. D.,** Novel mechanisms for PAF receptor signalling in A431 cells, manuscript in preparation.

156. **Masudda, N. and Ui, M.,** Possible involvement of GTP-binding proteins in growth regulation of human epidermoid carcinoma cell line, A431, *FEBS Lett.,* 291, 9, 1991.

157. **Kroegel, C., Pleass, R., Yukawa, T., Chung, K. F., Westwick, J., and Barnes, P. J.,** Characterization of platelet-activating factor-induced elevation of cytosolic free calcium concentration in eosinophils, *FEBS Lett.,* 243, 41, 1989.

158. **Kramp, W., Pieroni, G., Pinckard, R. N., and Hanahan, D. J.,** Observations on the critical micellar concentration of 1-O-alkyl-2-acetyl-*sn*-glycero-3-phosphocholine and a series of its homologs and analogs, *Chem. Phys. Lipids,* 35, 49, 1984.

159. **Randriamampita, C. and Trautmann, A.,** Biphasic increase in intracelular calcium induced by platelet activating factor in macrophages, *FEBS Lett.,* 249, 199, 1989.

160. **Block, L. H., Imhof, E., and Peruchoud, A. P.,** Platelets of asthmatics show increased phosphatidylinositol turnover in response to PAF, *Am. Rev. Resp. Dis.,* 137, 235, 1988.

161. **Shukla, S. D., Paul, A., and Klachko, D. M.,** Hypersensitivity of diabetic human platelets to platelet activating factor, *Thromb. Res.,* 66, 239, 1992.

162. **Ng, D. S. and Wong, K.,** Effect of platelet activating factor (PAF) on cytosolic free calcium in human peripheral blood mononuclear leukocytes, *Res. Commun. Chem. Pathol. Pharmacol.,* 64, 351, 1989.

163. **Shukla, S. D. and Hanahan, D. J.,** Acetylglyceryl ether phosphorylcholine (AGEPC; platelet activating factor)-induced stimulation of rabbit platelets: correlation between phosphatidic acid level, $^{45}Ca^{2+}$ uptake and [^{3}H] serotonin secretion, *Arch. Biochem. Biophys.,* 232, 458, 1984.

164. **MacIntyre, D. E., Bushfield, M., and Shaw, A. M.,** Regulation of platelet cytosolic free calcium by cyclic nucleotides and protein kinase C, *FEBS Lett.,* 188, 383, 1985.

165. **Lee, T., Malone, B., and Snyder, F.,** Stimulation of Ca^{2+} uptake by 1-O-alkyl-2-acetyl-*sn*-glycero-3-phosphocholine (platelet activating factor) in rabbit platelets: possible involvement of the lipoxygenase pathway, *Arch. Biochem. Biophys.,* 223, 33, 1983.

166. **Homma, H., Tokumura, A., and Hanahan, D. J.,** Binding and internalization of platelet-activating factor 1-O-alkyl-2-acetyl-*sn*-glycero-3-phosphocholine in washed rabbit platelets, *J. Biol. Chem.,* 262, 10582, 1987.

167. **Tou, J.-S., Jeter, J. R., Dola, C. P., and Venkatesh, S.,** Accumulation of phosphatidic acid mass and increased *de novo* synthesis of glycerolipids in platelet-activating factor activated neutrophils, *Biochem. J.,* 280, 625, 1991.

168. **Prescott, S. M., Zimmerman, G. A., and McIntyre, T. M.,** Platelet activating factor, *J. Biol. Chem.,* 265, 17381, 1990.

169. **Shukla, S. D.,** unpublished data.

Chapter 6

POLYMORPHONUCLEAR NEUTROPHIL RESPONSES TO AND PROCESSING OF PLATELET ACTIVATING FACTOR

Joseph T. O'Flaherty

TABLE OF CONTENTS

ISBN 0-8493-7299-2
© 1993 by CRC Press, Inc.

I. INTRODUCTION

Platelet-activating factor (PAF) was first described as a humoral mediator of acute anaphylactic, allergic, and inflammatory reactions. Its primary targets seemed to be platelets, polymorphonuclear neutrophils (PMN), and smooth muscle wherein it elicited a burst of aggregatory, secretory, and/or contractile activity.[1,2] More recent work, however, has expanded the range of PAF bioactions to include diverse tissues and more sustained responses. Thus, we now know that PAF induces lymphocytic and neurocytic tissues not only to release intercellular mediators, but also to transcribe protooncogenes and differentiate over hours into more mature forms.[3-14] This chapter examines how PAF interacts with one particularly responsive cell type, PMN. As the text emphasizes, the findings with PMN apply to many, it not all, PAF-sensitive cells. Furthermore, among the large variety of cell agonists, PAF possesses unique structural and physiochemical properties, is extraordinarily sensitive to metabolic inactivation, flows through processing pathways that do not handle any other known class of stimuli, and uses response mechanisms that are unexplained by standard transductional pathways. Exemplifying the last point, studies suggest PAF-stimulated PMN regulate their Ca^{2+} and, in turn, this cellular Ca^{2+} regulates PAF bioactions in novel ways. The PAF interaction with PMN, then, provides an exciting arena for determining how a pathophysiologically important mediator operates as well as for challenging old and examining new stimulus-response coupling schemes.

II. STRUCTURE AND PHYSIOCHEMISTRY

Antigen-challenged rabbit leukocytes release a PAF mixture composed of 1-O-octadecyl- and 1-O-hexadecyl-2-acetyl-GPCs (GPC is *sn*-glycero-3-phosphocholine).[15] Other tissues produce not only a larger array of alkyl ether acetyl GPCs but also many acetylated phospholipids[16-25] that can be and are mistaken for PAF. For example, stimulated PMN produce 1-O-hexadecyl- (~40%) and 1-O-octadecyl-2-acetyl-GPC (20%), several other C-14 to C-20 saturated and unsaturated alkyl ether acetyl GPCs (~10%), 1-O-alkyl/alkenyl-2-acetyl-*sn*-glycerol-3-phosphatidylethanolamines (~20%), and 1-O-acyl-2-acetyl-GPCs (~10%). Mast cells[26] and endothelial cells,[27,28] on the other hand, produce up to 97% 1-O-acyl-2-acetyl-GPCs with only small or trace amounts of alkyl ether acetyl GPCs. Since only long-chain alkyl ether acetyl GPCs possess appreciable PAF activity,[24,25] the role of acetylated phospholipids in, for example, endothelial cell function,[29] requires clarification. Here, the term PAF is limited to acetylated GPCs containing long-chain alkyl ethers at *sn*-1.

PAF has limited aqueous solubility. Critical micellar concentrations (CMC) for 1-O-hexadecyl-2-acetyl-GPC, 1-O-octadecyl-2-acetyl-GPC, 1-O-hexadecanoyl-2-acetyl-GPC, 1-O-hexadecyl-2-lyso-GPC, and 1,2-diacyl-GPCs are 1.1, 0.25, 1.3, 4, and <0.001 μM, respectively.[30] Above their CMC, GPCs disorganize membranes to produce cytolysis.[32-34] Below their CMC, they stick to surfaces.[35-38] The latter process reduces PAF bioavailability. Accordingly, PAF must be solubilized with a carrier protein, generally albumin, before presentation to cells. Human albumin has four high affinity (K_d ~100 nM) PAF acceptor sites plus larger numbers of less specific PAF absorbing sites.[36] Other carriers, e.g., C-reactive protein and α-acidic glycoprotein, also bind PAF firmly.[37] Clearly, the *in vivo* as well as *in vitro* actions of PAF are modified by ambient proteins. Excesses of these carriers can totally abrogate PAF bioactions.[35,37,38-44]

III. STRUCTURE-ACTIVITY RELATIONS

The relative stimulating potencies of 1-O-octadecyl-, 1-O-cis-9′-hexadecenyl-, 1-O-cis-9′-octadecenyl-, 1-O-*cis,cis*-9′,12′-octadecadienyl-, and 1-O-pentadecyl-2-acetyl-GPCs are

100, 15, 80, 60, 90, and 90, respectively.[23,45,46] Acetyl GPCs with longer or shorter sn-1-alkyl ethers are relatively impotent PAF agonists, while 1-O-acyl-2-acetyl-GPCs and 1-O-alkyl-2-acetyl-sn-glycero-3-phosphatidylethanolamines are ~3000-fold weaker than PAF.[24,25,47] PAF analogues with sn-2 propionate, butyrate, hexanoate, succinate, and phthalate esters show progressive declines in activity with increasing chain size.[24] sn-2 Lyso, sn-2 methoxy, and the inverted PAF stereoisomer do not stimulate PMN, whereas sn-2-ethoxy (ethyl ether at sn-2), sn-2 propyl (no oxygen at sn-2), and sn-2-N-methycarbamoyl PAF analogues are, respectively, 30-, 200-, and 5-fold weaker than PAF.[48-54] With respect to the sn-3 position, 1-O-alkyl-2-acetylglycerols and 1-O-alkyl-2-acetyl-sn-glycero-3-phosphatidates lack PAF activity,[25,39,55] but sn-3-phosphohonocholine or sn-3-N',N',N'-triethyl phosphocholine PAF analogues are 30- and 2-fold weaker than PAF.[56] Many of these structure-activity relations apply to other diverse tissues than PMN.[45,51,52,57-59] Thus, cells generally have very similar PAF recognition requirements and, of the biologically produced PAF molecular species, 1-O-hexadecyl-2-acetyl-GPC has optimal activity. Nevertheless, 1-O-(3-tetradecyl)phenyl-2-acetyl-GPC, 1-O-(4-azido-2-hydroxy-3-iodobenzamido)undecyl-2-acetyl-GPC, 1-O-(11-phthalimido)undecyl-2-acetyl-GPC, and several 1-O-heterocyclic-2-acetyl-GPCs exceed PAF in potency.[60-62] Moreover, 1-O-alkyl-2-methoxy-GPC, although inactive on PMN and platelets, is as potent as PAF in stimulating monocytes.[63] Naturally occurring PAF molecular species, then, are not necessarily the most potent of all possible PAF analogues and recognition systems for PAF do show some cell-specific differences. The PAF analogues with sn-1 heterocyclic residues may prove to be useful photoaffinity labels.[61,62]

IV. UPTAKE AND METABOLISM

Cells have a prodigious capacity to take up and metabolize GPCs. With respect to PAF, this processing may proceed by receptor-independent endocytosis, receptor-dependent endocytosis, or routes that bypass endocytosis.[64-71] Recent studies suggest that PAF is processed principally by the latter pathway. Thus, erythrocytes take up but do not metabolize PAF. Incorporated PAF initially extracts with albumin washes and therefore localizes to the plasma membrane outer leaflet. Gradually, however, the PAF sequesters from extracellular albumin and thus has internalized.[72,73] Internalization rates increase when erythrocytes are albumin loaded,[73] suggesting that cytosolic carrier proteins can modulate PAF movements. In PMN suspended at 4°C, PAF likewise enters plasmalemma[56] and remains albumin extractable for hours.[41,42] In contrast, at 37°C, PMN-incorporated PAF rapidly ($t_{1/2}$ ~1 min) becomes albumin insensitive, yet remains plasmalemma associated.[40,42,56] The cells soon deacetylate and acylate ($t_{1/2}$ ~2.5 min) plasma membrane PAF, and slowly ($t_{1/2}$ ~20 min) move acylated metabolite to Golgi/granule storage sites.[56] This sequence is opposite to standard endocytotic pathways wherein ligands move to Golgi/granules before becoming metabolized.[65] Indeed, cellular attack of PAF generally employs cytosolic acetylhydrolase and particulate (possibly plasmalemma) transacylase.[35,40,56,73-80] Classical endocytosis pathways would not deliver PAF to these metabolic sites. Moreover, PMN treated with proteases, PAF antagonists, or excess PAF lose >90% of their specific PAF binding capacity but metabolize PAF almost normally.[74] Note that stimulated PMN metabolize PAF quicker than resting PMN and this effect pertains to PAF, i.e., the rate of PAF metabolism rises far above that expected by a mass affect in PMN exposed to stimulatory, compared to substimulatory, PAF concentrations.[40,41,56,74] PAF thus induces its own degradation, and blockade of PAF binding sites, by canceling this induction, may slow PAF metabolism to resting cell rates.[40,74] Finally, cells contain a heat-labile, trypsin-sensitive, and soluble 60 kDa protein that transports PAF, but not diacyl GPC analogues, between artificial[81,82] and perhaps cellular[74,81-85] membranes. Taken together, the available data suggest that PAF traverses the plasma membrane and moves across cytosol by a transfer protein-dependent, endocytotosis-independent route. PAF receptors do not directly participate in this processing, but can stimulate it by activating the ability of the parent cell to, for example, translocate the ligand across the plasmalemma.[40,41]

V. FUNCTIONAL BIOACTIONS

PAF induces PMN to migrate,[48] degranulate,[45-56] make oxygen radicals,[48,86,87] aggregate,[50,52,88] adhere with endothelium,[29,89,90] and take up hexoses.[91,92] It also primes PMN for increased responsiveness to other stimuli;[25,86,90,93-100] however, PAF-treated PMN are not primed, but rather desensitized to a second PAF challenge.[45-47,51,53,54,74,104-107] This stimulus-selective desensitization develops within 30 to 60 s and endures for 5 to 90 min. PAF analogues desensitize PMN to each other, but stimuli that are structurally unrelated to PAF generally do not cross-desensitize PMN to PAF. Indeed, diacylglycerols, tumor necrosis factor-α, colony stimulating factors, and chemotactic oligopeptides prime PMN to a PAF hyperresponsive state.[55,93,106-110] While the mechanisms for many of these priming effects have not been evaluated, one example of PAF cooperativity has been extensively examined. 5-Hydroxyeicosatetraenoate (5-HETE) enhances the PMN degranulating potency of PAF and PAF analogues by 100- to 1000-fold.[111] The arachidonic acid metabolite lacks appreciable intrinsic degranulating activity and fails to alter degranulation responses elicited by chemotactic peptides, for example. Various HETEs, diHETES, and triHETES have no 5-HETE-like activity, but 5,15-diHETE and 5,20-diHETE, while 30- and 100-fold weaker than 5-HETE, nevertheless do potentiate PMN responses to PAF. The unnatural stereoisomer of 5-HETE is also relatively inactive. The most recent studies find that 5-HETE enhances a broad range of PAF effects on PMN, including the earliest occurring transductional events. It dramatically enhances, for example, the ability of PAF to activate PLA_2 and PLC.[23,106,111-117] 5-HETE thus uses a stereo- and structurally specific (i.e., 5-HETE receptor mediated?) mechanism to augment PAF potency. It may act by up-regulating PAF receptors or receptor-support systems.[117]

VI. PLATELET ACTIVATING FACTOR RECEPTORS

Early studies reported on PAF binding to PMN;[118-121] however, all such assays suffer critical pitfalls. First, cells do not bind PAF unless the ligand is solubilized with albumin, yet excess albumin inhibits PAF binding.[122] Binding assays reflect PAF partitioning between cells and albumin. Second, PAF forms micelles at 300 to 1100 nM.[30] Hence, binding must be accomplished over a range of PAF concentrations that are constricted at the higher end. Third, nonspecific PAF binding far exceeds specific binding at 37°C.[56] Lower ambient temperatures greatly reduce nonspecific binding.[56] Fourth, PMN have an enormous capacity to metabolize PAF at *sn*-2.[40,56,73-75] Other cell types similarly metabolize PAF at this site[35,76-80] or at *sn*-3.[124-127] Both pathways produce bioinactive metabolites that totally obscure specific binding. At 4°C, PMN do not measurably alter PAF,[56] perhaps partly because the ligand stays in the outer leaflet of plasma membrane under these conditions.[40,41] Nevertheless, PAF binding is an endothermic reaction: observed PAF binding affinities decline with ambient temperatures.[127] Fifth, binding (e.g., filtration) assays that wash PMN may remove PAF from its binding sites to distort results.[56,128] Assays (e.g., centrifugation through silicone oil) that omit PMN washing give higher K_a and R_t PAF binding values. Based on these many considerations, PMN/PAF binding assays are best conducted at 4°C with PAF levels below ~300 nM in the presence of ~25 to 125 µg albumin per milliliter. Nonwashing methods seem preferable for separating free from bound ligands. Ultimately, however, these assays give operational binding parameters that can at best only estimate the state of PAF receptors that may exist physiologically.

We find that PMN have specific, saturable, and reversible high and low affinity PAF binding sites. These sites cosediment almost exclusively with plasmalemma markers on Percoll gradients[56] and bind PAF analogues with affinities that correlate closely with each analogue's biological potency.[54,56] The latter correlation persists even with nonmetabolizable PAF analogues.[54] The potency of PAF in stimulating, for example, PMN degranulation, therefore, does not require, and is not limited by, its metabolism. Other groups report only a single class of PAF receptors on PMN,[129-134] platelets,[122,127,129,135-139] endothelium,[139] macrophages,[140] monocytes,[141] lymphoblasts,[142] brain,[143] retina,[144] and lung.[145,146] However, these studies are based on assays using PAF concentrations ≤ 10 nM. Hwang et al.[148] found that rabbit platelet membranes, although previously reported to possess only high affinity PAF binding sites, exhibited low affinity binding sites when ligand concentrations were extended well beyond 10 nM. Similar experiments demonstrate two binding sites for PAF on macrophages[149] and eosinophils.[150] Hence, many cell types may prove to possess low as well as high affinity PAF binding sites when evaluated at PAF levels up to ~100 to 200 nM. In any case, the relative functions of the two receptor types are debatable. Some experiments suggest that high affinity PAF receptors govern PMN excitation, whereas low affinity binding sites may be spare PAF receptors or, alternatively, nonreceptor binding elements.[87,128,150] PMN and eosinophil high and low affinity receptors, on the other hand, may serve to elicit different cell responses.[120,150]

Cell-impenetrant sulfhydryl reagents and proteases depress PMN specific binding of PAF.[74,151] PAF receptors thus have critical thiol residues and peptide bonds exposed at the PMN surface. Solubilized platelet membranes have a ~200 kDa protein that binds PAF[152,153] and a photoaffinity PAF analogue tags a 52-kDa surface membrane protein on platelets.[62] The relation of these proteins to the PAF receptor is uncertain,[154] particularly because Honda et al.[155] expressed a much lower molecular weight, high affinity, and functional PAF receptor in COS-7 cells and frog oocytes using guinea pig lung cDNA. The cDNA codes for a 39-kDa amino acid sequence with extensive homology to rhodopsin-like receptors. Such receptors span plasmalemma seven times, possess a single membranous ligand acceptor site, and interact with G-proteins. The guinea pig PAF receptor contains four serine and five threonine residues that may serve as targets for intracellular protein kinases.[155] Because PAF binding exhibits tissue-specific differences in cation sensitivities, K_d values, and antagonist susceptibilities,[130,131,135,156] future cloning studies may find PAF receptor heterogeneities.

VII. RECEPTOR REGULATION

HL-60 promyelocytes do not specifically bind PAF,[74,157] but progressively develop this capacity as they mature toward PMN.[157] Similarly, rat Kupffer cells, when depleted of PAF receptors, restore normal receptor numbers over several hours by a cycloheximide-inhibitable mechanism.[158] Hence, cellular synthesis of PAF receptors and/or receptor support systems contributes to the long-term expression of PAF receptors. Several other factors impact on PAF receptors, but act much more rapidly.

Rhodopsin-like receptors increase their ligand affinity by associating with G-proteins. Agonist binding to the high affinity G-protein receptor complex causes associated G-protein to exchange its GDP for cytosolic GTP, dissociate from its receptor, and activate key excitatory enzymes such as PLC and PLA$_2$. The original receptor, now G-protein dissociated, collapses to a low affinity state. However, activated G-protein soon hydrolyzes its GTP to GDP and thus becomes available for reassociating with low affinity receptors to again promote the high affinity state.[159,160] Relevant to this scheme, PAF stimulates PMN membranes to hydrolyze GTP. Pertussis toxin (PT) which inhibits G_i- and G_o-proteins, and cholera toxin, which uncouples G_s-protein from receptor activation, block this induced GTP hydrolysis. GTP, by dissociating PAF/G-protein complexes, reduces PAF binding to PMN membranes.[131,161] Thus, PAF receptors interact with G-proteins and agents promoting this interaction may convert low affinity PAF receptors to their high affinity counterparts. Similar PAF receptor/G-protein interactions occur with other cell types.[135,148,153]

Protein kinase C (PKC), a ubiquitous effector enzyme, moves from cytosol to plasmalemma during its activation. Activated PKC stimulates response-eliciting proteins but also can down-regulate various nearby plasma membrane receptor systems.[128,162] PKC activators induce PMN and Kupffer cells, but not platelets, to lose high affinity PAF binding sites.[163,164] The kinase may achieve this by phosphorylating PAF receptors or PAF receptor support systems (for example, G-proteins). The PKC effect occurs rapidly ($t_{1/2}$ ~0.5 min) and may be involved in the physiological control of PAF receptors during PMN stimulation (see below).

Mono- and bivalent cations alter membrane binding of PAF. Such effects define subtle, tissue-specific differences in PAF receptors and implicate G-proteins in PAF binding.[129,131,132,135,136,148,153] The actions of Ca^{2+}, however, have other implications. The cation promotes PAF binding to PMN membranes.[132] Furthermore, PMN depleted of Ca^{2+} exhibit low cytosolic Ca^{2+} ($[Ca^{2+}]_i$) levels and 30% fewer high affinity receptors available to PAF. The effect is indifferent to extracellular Ca^{2+} but rapidly reverse when PMN Ca^{2+} is restored to resting cell levels.[87] Moreover, agents that stimulate PMN to increase or decrease $[Ca^{2+}]_i$ concurrently increase and decrease, respectively, the number of high affinity receptors available to PAF.[166] Hence, stimulated changes in PMN Ca^{2+} may regulate PAF receptor expression, perhaps by inducing G-proteins to convert low affinity PAF receptors to the high affinity state.

PAF causes PMN to lose high affinity PAF binding sites.[74,120] The effect develops within 90 s, endures for 5 to 60 min, parallels the onset and duration of PAF-induced desensitization, and is reduced in PMN pretreated with PKC inhibitors. On the other hand, PAF does not down-regulate rabbit platelet PAF receptors[41] and PAF-induced PAF receptor down-regulation in Kupffer cells reverses only over several hours and requires intact protein synthesis.[158] Kupffer cells also down-regulate PAF receptors following elevation of their cAMP.[167] Because PAF receptors couple to adenylcyclase[131] and agents activating adenylcyclase inhibit PMN responses to PAF,[169,170] cAMP may act on PAF receptors in PMN. Thus, PAF-induced autologous receptor down-regulation might proceed by various pathways (e.g., PKC, cAMP), produces rapidly reversing (e.g., PMN) or less reversible receptor changes (e.g., Kupffer cells), and may (e.g., PMN) or may not (e.g., PAF rapidly desensitize rabbit platelets without altering these receptors[41]) correlate with induction of desensitization.

VIII. RECEPTOR LINKAGES

PAF stimulates PMN to cleave resident phosphatidylinositols and other phospholipids at *sn*-2 and *sn*-3 by a PT-sensitive mechanism.[117,171-179] Inferentially, then, PAF receptors operate through G_i- and/or G_o-proteins to mobilize PLA_2 and PLC. Products of these cleavages have many actions: inositol triphosphate releases stored Ca^{2+} to raise $[Ca^{2+}]$; diacylglycerols bind with and activate PKC; and arachidonic acid may activate PKC or alternatively become oxygenated to cell-stimulating metabolites, such as leukotriene (LT)B_4, 5-HETE, and prostaglandins (PGs). PAF-challenged PMN rapidly make many of these products, briefly raise $[Ca^{2+}]_i$, and move cytosolic PKC to the plasma membrane.[86,88,114,128,171-173,178-187] The cells also generate endogenous PAF by a PLA_2-dependent pathway;[23,188,189] raise cAMP[168] by activating G_s-protein or elevating cell Ca^{2+};[131,190] form phosphatidic acid by a PLD-dependent mechanism;[191] and take up ambient Ca^{2+}.[182,192] Moreover, functional responses to PAF are reduced in PMN treated with PT;[95,171,173,180,193,194] drugs that inhibit LTB_4 and 5-HETE synthesis;[168,178,179,195,196] intracellular Ca^{2+} chelators;[87] agents that inhibit the effector element for Ca^{2+}, calmodulin;[45,92] Ca^{2+} channel blockers;[192] and PKC blockade.[128,183] In a general sense, therefore, the various pathways mediate PAF bioactions. However, studies produce confusing or conflicting results and we as yet have no clear ordering of mediator actions that fully explains how PAF elicits any given function. Several examples are illustrative.

First, the $[Ca^{2+}]_i$-raising actions of PAF are surprisingly resistant to PT.[173,183] This and possibly other PAF effects, therefore, either involve PT-resistant G-proteins or bypass G-proteins altogether. Second, calmodulin antagonists may inhibit PKC;[92] Ca^{2+} channel blockers antagonize PAF binding;[130,197,198] and PKC blockade has tangential effects on PMN that may alter responsiveness in unexpected ways.[128,199] Pharmacological agents, then, often lack specificity. Third, PMN incubated with LTB_4 are densitized to a second LTB_4 challenge in assays of aggregation, degranulation, and Ca^{2+} transients. The PMN concurrently lose responsiveness to PAF in aggregation assays, suggesting that endogenous LTB_4 mediates this PAF action. Nevertheless, the same LTB_4-desensitized PMN degranulate and raise $[Ca^{2+}]_i$ normally when challenged with PAF.[106,107,168,179,199-201] Thus, presumptive mediators may have response selective rather than generalized roles in cell excitation. Fourth, elevated $[Ca^{2+}]_i$ may activate adenylcyclase or PLA_2 and PLC; LTB_4 and 5-HETE promote PLA_2 activation; activated PKC can block the excitatory actions of LTB_4 and 5-HETE; and PGs depresses PMN responses to both PAF and LTB_4.[23,107,114,169,170,190,202,203] Mediators, then, promote or inhibit each other's formation and/or actions. This effect tends to blur mediator functions. Fifth, current models of rhodopsin-like receptor coupling do not explain the PAF/PMN interaction. In these models, ligand-bound receptors trigger $[Ca^{2+}]_i$ rises and diacylglycerol production. Elevated $[Ca^{2+}]_i$ then causes cytosolic PKC to bind with membrane diacylglycerol and thereby to become active in phosphorylating response-eliciting elements. Consequently, $[Ca^{2+}]_i$-fixed cells should be, and reportedly are, completely unresponsive to agonists operating through rhodopsin-like receptors. $[Ca^{2+}]_i$-fixed PMN, however, exhibit substantial, although reduced, PKC translocation, degranulation, and oxidative metabolism responses to PAF.[87,187] Moreover, these PMN experience decreases in the number of high affinity receptors available to PAF[87] and presumably will not exhibit the normal increases in PAF receptor expression that attend $[Ca^{2+}]_i$ rises.[166] Evidently, then, elevated $[Ca^{2+}]_i$ may enhance but is not essential for PMN responses to PAF; hyporesponsiveness in $[Ca^{2+}]_i$-fixed PMN may reflect PAF receptor decreases; and Ca^{2+} may contribute to PAF-induced responses by regulating PAF receptor expression in addition to, or in place of, its more accepted role in modulating postreceptor events.

The same postreceptor pathways pertain to the actions of PAF on other cell types.[8,12,103,141,149,204-211] As in PMN, however, their precise roles in mediating function are uncertain.

IX. CONCLUSIONS

The studies cited suggest a working model for PAF-PMN interaction. PAF partitions between carrier albumin and cells. Low levels of albumin favor PAF entry into the plasmalemma outer leaflet. The cellular PAF traverses to the inner leaflet rapidly and at rates that rise as the target PMN transduces the PAF challenge into excitation. Internalized PAF almost immediately becomes deacetylated and acylated before more slowly moving to Golgi/granules. This movement is likely mediated through a specific cytosolic transfer protein that picks up acylated PAF metabolite at plasmalemma and shuttles it to interior storage sites. Meanwhile, plasmalemma outer leaflet PAF binds to its high affinity receptors. The ligand-bound receptors proceed to unlease G_i-, G_o-, and/or G_s-proteins that in turn activate PLA_2 and C or adenylcyclase. Consequently, arachidonate, LTB_4, 5-HETE, PGs, endogenous PAF, diacylglycerol, and cAMP form. Additionally, the receptor triggers release of storage Ca^{2+}, Ca^{2+} uptake, rises in $[Ca^{2+}]_i$, and PKC mobilization by unknown and potentially novel mechanisms. PT-insensitive G-proteins may be responsible for altering $[Ca^{2+}]_i$, whereas arachidonate may mediate the $[Ca^{2+}]_i$-independent movements of PKC. Next, membrane PKC binds diacylglycerol and becomes active in eliciting function. PKC may operate in concert with other mediators such as arachidonate metabolites[162] to achieve these results. Elevated $[Ca^{2+}]_i$ and (possibly) endogenously formed 5-HETE, may feedback to convert low affinity PAF receptors to the high affinity state. In effect, this recruits spare PAF receptors and increases the number of high affinity PAF receptors bound by a set PAF dosage, thereby potentially promoting further cell excitation. Soon, however, $[Ca^{2+}]_i$ falls, 5-HETE is metabolized to a much less active analogue, 5,20-diHETE, and PKC phosphorylates PAF receptors or receptor-support systems. These events, along with receptor/G-protein dissociation and (perhaps) the effects of elevated cAMP, collapse high affinity PAF receptors to a low affinity, transduction element-uncoupled state. PMN excitation ceases, functional responses terminate, and desensitization occurs. The receptors, now in a low affinity configuration, release bound PAF which internalizes and becomes metabolized. As ambient PAF is cleared, cAMP levels decline, PAF receptors and/or receptor-support systems are dephosphorylated, and G-proteins regenerate the ability to promote a high affinity PAF receptor configuration. The PMN re-expresses normal PAF receptor numbers and is ready to respond anew.

REFERENCES

1. **Henson, P. M. and Pinckard, R. N.,** Basophil-derived platelet-activating factor (PAF) as an *in vivo* mediator of acute allergic reactions: demonstration of specific desensitization of platelets to PAF during IgE-induced anaphylaxis in the rabbit, *J. Immunol.,* 119, 2179, 1977.

2. **Vargaftig, B. B., Chignard, M., Benveniste, J., Lefort, J., and Wal, F.,** Background and present status of research on platelet-activating factor (PAF-acether), *Ann. N.Y. Acad. Sci.,* 370, 119, 1981.

3. **Rola-Pleszczynski, M., Pouliot, C., Turcotte, S., Pignol, B., Braquet, P., and Bouvrette, L.,** Immune regulation by platelet-activating factor. I. Induction of suppressor cell activity in human monocytes and CD8 + T and of helper cell activity in CD4 + T cells. *J. Immunol.,* 140, 3547, 1988.

4. **Vivier, E., Salem, P., Dulioust, A., Praseuth, D., Metezeau, P., Benveniste, J., and Thomas, Y.,** Immunoregulatory functions of paf-acether. II. Decrease of CD2 and CD3 antigen expression, *Eur. J. Immunol.,* 18, 425, 1988.

5. **Dulioust, A., Duprez, V., Pitton, C., Salem, P., Hemar, A., Benveniste, J., and Thomas, Y.,** Immunoregulatory functions of paf-acether. III. Down-regulation of CD4+T cells high-affinity IL-2 receptor expression, *J. Immunol.,* 144, 3123, 1990.

6. **Pignol, B., Hénane, S., Mencia-Huerta, J.-M., Rola-Pleszczynski, M., and Braquet, P.,** Effect of platelet-activating factor (paf-acether) and its specific receptor antagonist, BN 52021, on interleukin 1 (IL1) release and synthesis by rat spleen adherent monocytes, *Prostaglandins,* 33, 931, 1987.

7. **Salem, P., Deryckx, S., Duliost, A., Vivier, E., Denizot, Y., Damais, C., Dinarello, C. A., and Thomas, Y.,** Immunoregulatory functions of paf-acether. IV. Enhancement of IL-1 production by muramyl dipeptide-stimulated monocytes, *J. Immunol.,* 144, 1338, 1990.

8. **Schulam, P. G., Kuruvilla, A., Putcha, G., Mangus, L., Franklin-Johnson, J., and Shearer, W. T.,** Platelet-activating factor induces phospholipid turnover, calcium flux, arachidonic acid liberation, eicosanoid generation, and oncogene expression in a human B cell line, *J. Immunol.,* 146, 1642, 1991.

9. **Pignol, B., Hénane, S., Sorlin, B., Rola-Pleszczynski, M., Mencia-Huerta, J.-M., and Braquet, P.,** Effect of long-term treatment with platelet-activating factor on IL-1 and IL-2 production by rat spleen cells, *J. Immunol.,* 145, 980, 1990.

10. **Kornecki, E. and Ehrlich, Y. H.,** Neuroregulatory and neuropathological actions of the ether-phospholipid platelet-activating factor, *Science,* 240, 1792, 1988.

11. **Camoratto, A. M. and Grandison, L.,** Platelet-activating factor stimulates prolactin release from dispersed rat anterior pituitary cells *in vitro, Endocrinology,* 124, 1502, 1989.

12. **Junier, M. P., Tiberghien, C., Rougeot, C., Fafeur, V., and Dray, F.,** Inhibitory effect of platelet-activating factor (PAF) on leuteinizing hormone-releasing hormone and somatostatin release from rat median eminence *in vitro* correlated with the characterization of specific PAF receptor sites in rat hypothalamus, *Endocrinology,* 123, 72, 1988.

13. **Doly, M., Bonhomme, B., Braquet, P., Chabrier, P. E., and Meyniel, G.**, Effects of platelet-activating factor on electrophysiology of isolated retinas and their inhibition by BN 52021, a specific PAF-acether receptor antagonist, *Immunopharmacology,* 13, 189, 1987.

14. **Squinto, S. P., Block, A. L., Braquet, P., and Bazan, N. G.**, Platelet-activating factor stimulates a Fos/Jun/AP-1 transcriptional signaling system in human neuroblastoma cells, *J. Neurosci. Res.,* 24, 558, 1989.

15. **Hanahan, D. J., Demopoulos, C. S., Liehr, J., and Pinckard, R. N.**, Identification of platelet activating factor isolated from rabbit basophils as acetyl glyceryl ether phosphorylcholine, *J. Biol. Chem.,* 255, 5514, 1980.

16. **Pinckard, R. N., Jackson, E. M., Hoppens, C., Weintraub, S. T., Ludwig, J. C., McManus, L. M., and Mott, G. E.**, Molecular heterogeneity of platelet-activating factor produced by stimulated human polymorphonuclear leukocytes, *Biochem. Biophys. Res. Commun.,* 122, 325, 1984.

17. **Mueller, H. W., O'Flaherty, J. T., and Wykle, R. L.**, The molecular species distribution of platelet-activating factor synthesized by rabbit and human neutrophils, *J. Biol. Chem.,* 259, 14554, 1984.

18. **Haroldsen, P. E., Clay, K. L., and Murphy, R. C.**, Quantitation of lyso-platelet activating factor molecular species from human neutrophils by mass spectrometry, *J. Lipid Res.,* 28, 42, 1987.

19. **Ramesha, C. S. and Pickett, W. C.**, Species-specific variations in the molecular heterogeneity of the platelet-activating factor, *J. Immunol.,* 138, 1559, 1987.

20. **Bossant, M. J., Farrinotti, R., De Maack, F., Mahuzier, G., Benveniste, J., and Ninio, E.**, Capillary gas chromatography and tandem mass spectrometry of paf-acether and analogs: absence of 1-O-alkyl-2-propionyl-*sn*-glycero-3-phosphocholine in human polymorphonuclear neutrophils, *Lipids,* 24, 121, 1989.

21. **Satouchi, K., Oda, M., and Saito, K.**, 1-Acyl-2-acetyl-*sn*-glycero-3-phosphocholine from stimulated human polymorphonuclear leukocytes, *Lipids,* 22, 285, 1987.

22. **Tessner, T. G. and Wykle, R. L.**, Stimulated neutrophils produce an ethanolamine plasmalogen analog of platelet-activating factor, *J. Biol. Chem.,* 262, 12660, 1987.

23. **Tessner, T. G., O'Flaherty, J. T., and Wykle, R. L.**, Stimulation of platelet-activating factor synthesis by a nonmetabolizable bioactive analog of platelet-activating factor and influence of arachidonic acid metabolites, *J. Biol. Chem.,* 264, 4794, 1989.

24. **O'Flaherty, J. T., Salzer, W. L., Cousart, S., McCall, C. E., Piantadosi, C., Surles, J. R., Hammett, M. J., and Wykle, R. L.**, Platelet-activating factor and analogues: comparative studies with human neutrophils and rabbit platelets, *Res. Commun. Chem. Pathol. Pharmacol.,* 39, 291, 1983.

25. **Pinckard, R. N., Ludwig, J. C., and McManus, L. M.**, Platelet-activating factors, in *Inflammation: Basic Principles and Clinical Correlates,* Gallin, J. I., Goldstein, I. M., and Synderman, R., Eds., Raven Press, New York, 1988, 139.

26. **Triggiani, M., Hubbard, W. C., and Chilton, F. H.**, Synthesis of 1-acyl-2-acetyl-*sn*-glycero-3-phosphocholine by an enriched preparation of the human lung mast cell, *J. Immunol.,* 144, 4773, 1990.

27. **Mueller, H. W., Nollert, M. U., and Eskin, S. G.**, Synthesis of 1-acyl-2-[³H]acetyl-*sn*-glycero-3-phosphocholine, a structural analog of platelet activating factor, by vascular endothelial cells, *Biochem. Biophys. Res. Commun.,* 176, 1557, 1991.

28. **Garcia, M. C., Mueller, H. W., and Rosenthal, M. D.**, C$_{20}$ polyunsaturated fatty acids and phorbol myristate acetate enhance agonist-stimulated synthesis of 1-radyl-2-acetyl-*sn*-glycero-3-phosphocholine in vascular endothelial cells, *Biochim. Biophys. Acta,* 1083, 37, 1991.

29. **Whatley, R. E., Zimmerman, G. A., McIntyre, T. M., Taylor, R., and Prescott, S. M.**, Production of platelet-activating factor by endothelial cells, *Sem. Thromb. Hemost.,* 13, 445, 1987.

30. **Kramp, W., Pieroni, G., Pinckard, R. N., and Hanahan, D. J.**, Observations on the critical micellar concentration of 1-O-alkyl-2-acetyl-*sn*-glycero-3-phosphocholine and a series of its homologs and analogs, *Chem. Phys. Lipids,* 35, 49, 1984.

31. **Hoffman, D. R., Hajdu, J., and Synder, F.**, Cytotoxicity of platelet activating factor and related alkyl-phospholipid analogs in human leukemia cells, polymorphonuclear neutrophils, and skin fibroblasts, *Blood,* 63, 545, 1984.

32. **Sawyer, D. B. and Andersen, O. S.**, Platelet-activating factor is a general membrane perturbant, *Biochim. Biophys. Acta,* 987, 129, 1989.

33. **Bratton, D. L., Harris, R. A., Clay, K. L., and Henson, P. M.**, Effects of platelet activating factor and related lipids on phase transition of dipalmitoylphosphatidylcholine, *Biochim. Biophys. Acta,* 941, 76, 1988.

34. **Bratton, D. L., Harris, R. A., Clay, K. L., and Henson, P. M.**, Effects of platelet activating factor on calcium-lipid interactions and lateral phase separations in phospholipid vesicles, *Biochim. Biophys. Acta,* 943, 211, 1988.

35. **Cabot, M. C., Blank, M. L., Welsh, C. J., Horan, M. J., Cress, E. A., and Snyder, F.**, Metabolism of 1-alkyl-2-acetyl-*sn*-glycero-3-phosphocholine by cell cultures, *Life Sci.,* 31, 2891, 1982.

36. **Clay, K. L., Johnson, C., and Henson, P.**, Binding of platelet activating factor to albumin, *Biochim. Biophys. Acta,* 1046, 309, 1990.

37. **Randell, E., Mookerjea, S., and Nagpurkar, A.,** Interaction between rat serum phosphorylcholine binding protein and platelet activating factor, *Biochem. Biophys. Res. Commun.,* 167, 444, 1990.

38. **Ludwig, J. C., McManus, L. M., and Pinckard, R. N.,** Synthesis-release coupling of platelet activating factors (PAF) from stimulated human neutrophils, *Adv. Inflammation Res.,* 11, 111, 1986.

39. **Tokumura, A., Yoshida, J., Maruyama, T., Fukuzawa, K., and Tsukatani, H.,** Platelet aggregation induced by ether-linked phospholipids. I. Inhibitory actions of bovine serum albumin and structural analogues of platelet activating factor, *Thromb. Res.,* 46, 51, 1987.

40. **Tokumura, A., Tsutsumi, T., Yoshida, J., and Tsukatani, H.,** Translocation of exogenous platelet-activating factor and its lyso-compound through plasma membranes is a rate-limiting step for their metabolic conversions into alkylacylglycerophosphocholines in rabbit platelets and guinea-pig leukocytes, *Biochim. Biophys. Acta,* 1044, 91, 1990.

41. **Homma, H., Tokumura, A., and Hanahan, D. J.,** Binding and internalization of platelet-activating factor 1-O-alkyl-2-acetyl-*sn*-glycero-3-phosphocholine in washed rabbit platelets, *J. Biol. Chem.,* 262, 10582, 1987.

42. **Vigo, C.,** Effect of C-reactive protein on platelet-activating factor-induced platelet aggregation and membrane stabilization, *J. Biol. Chem.,* 260, 3418, 1985.

43. **Kilpatrick, J. M. and Virella, G.,** Inhibition of platelet-activating factor by rabbit C-reactive protein, *Clin. Immunol. Immunopathol.,* 37, 276, 1985.

44. **Nagpurkar, A., Randell, E., Choudhury, S., and Mookerjea, S.,** Effect of rat phosphorylcholine-binding protein on platelet aggregation, *Biochim. Biophys. Acta,* 967, 76, 1988.

45. **Surles, J. R., Wykle, R. L., O'Flaherty, J. T., Salzer, W. L., Thomas, M. J., Snyder, F., and Piantadosi, C.,** Facile synthesis of platelet-activating factor and racemic analogues containing unsaturation in the *sn*-1-alkyl chain, *J. Med. Chem.,* 28, 73, 1985.

46. **Smith, R. J., Bowman, B. J., and Iden, S. S.,** Characteristics of 1-O-hexadecyl- and 1-O-octadecyl-2-O-acetyl-*sn*-glyceryl-3-phosphorylcholine-stimulated granule enzyme release from human neutrophils, *Clin. Immunol. Immunopathol.,* 28, 13, 1983.

47. **Triggiani, M., Goldman, D. W., and Chilton, F. H.,** Biological effects of 1-acyl-2-acetyl-*sn*-glycero-3-phosphocholine in the human neutrophil, *Biochim. Biophys. Acta,* 1084, 41, 1991.

48. **Shaw, J. O., Pinckard, R. N., Ferrigni, K. S., McManus, L. M., and Hanahan, D. J.,** Activation of human neutrophils with 1-O-hexadecyl/octadecyl-2-acetyl-*sn*-glyceryl-3-phosphorylcholine (platelet activating factor), *J. Immunol.,* 127, 1250, 1981.

49. **Dewald, B. and Baggiolini, M.,** Platelet-activating factor as a stimulus of exocytosis in human neutrophils, *Biochim. Biophys. Acta,* 888, 42, 1986.

50. **O'Flaherty, J. T., Miller, C. H., Lewis, J. C., Wykle, R. L., Bass, D. A., McCall, C. E., Waite, M., and DeChatelet, L. R.,** Neutrophil responses to platelet-activating factor, *Inflammation,* 5, 193, 1981.

51. **Wykle, R. L., Miller, C. H., Lewis, J. C., Schmitt, J. D., Smith, J. A., Surles, J. R., Piantadosi, C., and O'Flaherty, J. T.,** Stereospecific activity of 1-O-alkyl-2-O-acetyl-*sn*-glycero-3-phosphocholine and comparision of analogs in the degranulation of platelets and neutrophils, *Biochem. Biophys. Res. Commun.,* 100, 1651, 1981.

52. **O'Flaherty, J. T., Wykle, R. L., Miller, C. H., Lewis, J. C., Waite, M., Bass, D. A., McCall, C. E., and DeChatelet, L. R.,** 1-O-Alkyl-*sn*-glyceryl-3-phosphorylcholines. A novel class of neutrophil stimulants, *Am. J. Pathol.,* 103, 70, 1981.

53. **Wykle, R. L., Surles, J. R., Piantadosi, C., Salzer, W. L., and O'Flaherty, J. T.,** Platelet activating factor (1-O-alkyl-2-O-acetyl-*sn*-glycero-3-phosphocholine). Activity of analogs lacking oxygen at the 2-position, *FEBS Lett.,* 141, 29, 1982.

54. **O'Flaherty, J. T., Redman, J. F., Jr., Schmitt, J. D., Ellis, J. M., Surles, J. R., Marx, M. H., Piantadosi, C., and Wykle, R. L.,** 1-*O*-Alkyl-2-*N*-methylcarbamyl-glycerophosphocholine: a biologically potent, non-metabolizable analog of platelet-activating factor, *Biochem. Biophys. Res. Commun.,* 147, 18, 1987.

55. **O'Flaherty, J. T., Schmitt, J. D., McCall, C. E., and Wykle, R. L.,** Diacylglycerols enhance human neutrophil degranulation responses: relevancy to a multiple mediator hypothesis of cell function, *Biochem. Biophys. Res. Commun.,* 123, 64, 1984.

56. **O'Flaherty, J. T., Surles, J. R., Redman, J., Jacobson, D., Piantadosi, C., and Wykle, R. L.,** Binding and metabolism of platelet-activating factor by human neutrophils, *J. Clin. Invest.,* 78, 381, 1986.

57. **Satouchi, K., Pinckard, R. N., McManus, L. M., and Hanahan, D. J.,** Modification of the polar head group of acetyl glyceryl ether phosphorylcholine and subsequent effects upon platelet activation, *J. Biol. Chem.,* 256, 4425, 1981.

58. **Blank, M. L., Cress, E. A., Lee, T.-C., Malone, B., Surles, J. R., Piantadosi, C., Hajdu, J., and Snyder, F.,** Structural features of platelet activating factor (1-alkyl-2-acetyl-*sn*-glycero-3-phosphocholine) required for hypotensive and platelet serotonin responses, *Res. Commun. Chem. Pathol. Pharmacol.,* 38, 3, 1982.

59. **Stimler, N. P., Gerard, C., and O'Flaherty, J. T.,** Contraction of human lung tissues by platelet-activating factor (AAGPC), in *Platelet-Activating Factor,* Benveniste, J. and Arnoux, B., Eds., Elsevier, Amsterdam, 1983, 195.

60. **Shen, T. Y., Hwang, S.-B., Doebber, T. W., and Robbins, J. C.,** The chemical and biological properties of PAF agonists, antagonists, and biosynthetic inhibitors, in *Platelet-Activating Factor and Related Lipid Mediators,* Snyder, F., Ed., Plenum Press, New York, 1987, 153.

61. **Bette-Bobillo, P., Bienvenue, A., Broquet, C., and Maurin, L.,** Synthesis and characterization of a radioiodinated, photoreactive and physiologically active analogue of platelet activating factor, *Chem. Phys. Lipids,* 37, 215, 1985.

62. **Chau, L.-Y., Tsai, Y.-M., and Cheng, J.-R.,** Photoaffinity labeling of platelet-activating factor binding sites in rabbit platelet membranes, *Biochem. Biophys. Res. Commun.,* 161, 1070, 1989.

63. **Rose, J. K., Debs, R. A., Philip, R., Ruis, N. M., and Valone, F. H.,** Selective activation of human monocytes by the platelet-activating factor analog 1-O-hexadecyl-2-O-methyl-*sn*-glycero-3-phosphorylcholine, *J. Immunol.,* 144, 3513, 1990.

64. **Pagano, R. E. and Sleight, R. G.,** Defining lipid transport pathways in animal cells, *Science,* 229, 1051, 1985.

65. **Zachowski, A., Favre, E., Cribier, S., Hervé, and Devaux, P. F.,** Outside-inside translocation of aminophospholipids in the human erythrocyte membrane is mediated by a specific enzyme, *Biochemistry,* 25, 2585, 1986.

66. **Zachowski, A., Herrmann, A., Paraf, A., and Devaux, P. F.,** Phospholipid outside-inside translocation in lymphocyte plasma membranes is a protein-mediated phenomenon, *Biochim. Biophys. Acta,* 897, 197, 1987.

67. **Mohandas, N., Wyatt, J., Mel, S. F., Rossi, M. E., and Shohet, S. B.,** Lipid translocation across the human erythrocyte membrane: regulatory factors, *J. Biol. Chem.,* 257, 6537, 1982.

68. **Wirtz, D. W. A. and Zilversmit, D. B.,** Exchange of phospholipids between liver mitochondria and microsomes *in vitro, J. Biol. Chem.,* 243, 3596, 1968.

69. **Yaffe, M. P. and Kennedy, E. P.,** Intracellular phospholipid movement and the role of phospholipid transfer proteins in animal cells, *Biochemistry,* 22, 1497, 1983.

70. **Moreau, P. and Morré, D. J.,** Cell-free transfer of membrane lipids. Evidence for lipid processing, *J. Biol. Chem.,* 266, 4329, 1991.

71. **Moreau, P., Rodriguez, M., Cassagne, C., Morré, D. M., and Morré, D. J.,** Trafficking of lipids from the endoplasmic reticulum to the Golgi apparatus in a cell-free system from rat liver, *J. Biol. Chem.,* 266, 4322, 1991.

72. **Schneider, E., Haest, C. W. M., and Deuticke, B.,** Transbilayer reorientation of platelet-activating factor in the erythrocyte membrane, *FEBS Lett.,* 198, 311, 1986.

73. **Bratton, D. L., Kailey, J. M., Clay, K. L., and Henson, P. M.,** A model for the extracellular release of PAF: the influence of plasma membrane phospholipid asymmetry, *Biochim. Biophys. Acta,* 1062, 24, 1991.

74. **O'Flaherty, J. T., Chabot, M. C., Redman, J., Jr., Jacobson, D., and Wykle, R. L.,** Receptor-independent metabolism of platelet-activating factor by myelogenous cells, *FEBS Lett.,* 250, 341, 1989.

75. **Chilton, F. H., O'Flaherty, J. T., Ellis, J. M., Swendsen, C. L., and Wykle, R. L.,** Metabolic fate of platelet-activating factor in neutrophils, *J. Biol. Chem.,* 258, 6357, 1983.

76. **Kramer, R. M., Patton, G. M., Pritzker, C. R., and Deykin, D.,** Metabolism of platelet-activating factor in human platelets: transacylase-mediated synthesis of 1-O-alkyl-2-arachidonoyl-*sn*-glycero-3-phosphocholine, *J. Biol. Chem.,* 259, 13316, 1984.

77. **McKean, M. L. and Silver, M. J.,** Phospholipid biosynthesis in human platelets: the acylation of lyso-platelet-activating factor, *Biochem. J.,* 225, 723, 1985.

78. **Malone, B., Lee, T.-C., and Snyder, F.,** Inactivation of platelet activating factor by rabbit platelets: lyso-platelet activating factor as a key intermediate with phosphatidylcholine as the source of arachidonic acid in its conversion to a tetraenoic acylated product, *J. Biol. Chem.,* 260, 1531, 1985.

79. **Billah, M. M., Eckel, S., Myers, R. F., and Siegel, M. I.,** Metabolism of platelet-activating factor (1-O-alkyl-2-acetyl-sn-glycero-3-phosphocholine) by human promyelocytic leukemic HL60 cells: stimulated expression of phospholipase A_2 and acetyltransferase requires differentiation, *J. Biol. Chem.,* 261, 5824, 1986.

80. **Sugiura, T., Masuzawa, Y., Nakagawa, Y., and Waku, K.,** Transacylation of lyso platelet-activating factor and other lysophospholipids by macrophage microsomes. Distinct donor and acceptor selectivities, *J. Biol. Chem.,* 262, 1199, 1987.

81. **Banks, J. B., Wykle, R. L., O'Flaherty, J. T., and Lumb, R. H.,** Evidence from protein-catalyzed transfer of platelet activating factor by macrophage cytosol, *Biochim. Biophys. Acta,* 961, 48, 1988.

82. **Lumb, R. H., Record, M., Ribbes, G., Pool, G. L., Terce, F., and Chap, H.,** PAF-acether transfer activity in HL-60 cells is induced during differentiation, *Biochem. Biophys. Res. Commun.,* 171, 548, 1990.

83. **Ribbes, G., Ninio, E., Fontan, P., Record, M., Chap, H., Benveniste, J., and Douste-Blazy, L.,** Evidence that biosynthesis of platelet-activating factor (paf-acether) by human neutrophils occurs in an intracellular membrane, *FEBS Lett.,* 191, 195, 1985.

84. **McKean, M. L., Silver, M. J., Authi, K. S., and Crawford, N.,** Formation of diacyl- and alkylacyl-phosphatidylcholine by the membranes of human platelets, *FEBS Lett.,* 195, 38, 1986.

85. **Riches, D. W., Young, S. K., Seccombe, J. F., Henson, J. E., Clay, K. L., and Henson, P. M.,** The subcellular distribution of platelet-activating factor in stimulated human neutrophils, *J. Immunol.,* 145, 3062, 1990.

86. **Ingraham, L. M., Coates, T. D., Allen, J. M., Higgins, C. P., Baehner, R. L., and Boxer, L. A.,** Metabolic, membrane, and functional responses of human polymorphonuclear leukocytes to platelet-activating factor, *Blood,* 59, 1259, 1982.

87. **O'Flaherty, J. T., Rossi, A. G., Jacobson, D. P., and Redman, J. F.,** Roles of Ca^{2+} in human neutrophil responses to receptor agonists, *Biochem. J.,* 227, 705, 1991.

88. **Dahl, M.-L.,** Aggregating and prostanoid-releasing effects of platelet-activating factor and leukotrienes on human polymorphonuclear leukocytes and platelets, *Int. Arch. Allergy Appl. Immunol.,* 76, 145, 1985.

89. **Breviario, F., Bertocchi, F., DeJana, E., and Bussolino, F.,** IL-1-induced adhesion of polymorphonuclear leukocytes to cultured human endothelial cells. Role of platelet activating factor, *J. Immunol.,* 141, 3391, 1988.

90. **Bercellotti, G. M., Wickham, N. W. R., Gustafson, K. S., Yin, H. Q., Hebert, M., and Jacob, H. S.,** Thrombin-treated endothelium primes neutrophil functions: inhibition by platelet-activating factor receptor antagonists, *J. Leukocyte Biol.,* 45, 483, 1989.

91. **O'Flaherty, J. T., Cousart, S., Swendsen, C. L., DeChatelet, L. R., Bass, D. A., Love, S. H., and McCall, C. E.,** Role of Ca^{2+} and Mg^{2+} in neutrophil hexose transport, *Biochim. Biophys. Acta,* 640, 223, 1981.

92. **McCall, C., Schmitt, J., Cousart, S., O'Flaherty, J., Bass, D., and Wykle, R.,** Stimulation of hexose transport by human polymorphonuclear leukocytes: a possible role for protein kinase C, *Biochem. Biophys. Res. Commun.,* 126, 450, 1985.

93. **Dewald, B. and Baggiolini, M.,** Activation of NADPH oxidase in human neutrophils. Synergism between fMLP and the neutrophil products PAF and LTB_4, *Biochem. Biophys. Res. Commun.,* 128, 297, 1985.

94. **Gay, J. C., Beckman, J. K., Zaboy, K. A., and Lukens, J. N.,** Modulation of neutrophil oxidative responses to soluble stimuli by platelet-activating factor, *Blood,* 67, 931, 1986.

95. **Shalit, M., Dabiri, G. A., and Southwick, F. S.,** Platelet-activating factor both stimulates and "primes" human polymorphonuclear leukocyte actin filament assembly, *Blood,* 70, 1921, 1987.

96. **Ingraham, L. M., Lafuze, J. E., Boxer, L. A., and Baehner, R. L.,** In vitro and in vivo effects of treatment by platelet-activating factor on *N*-formyl-met-leu-phe-mediated responses of polymorphonuclear leucocytes, *Br. J. Haematol.,* 66, 219, 1987.

97. **Vercellotti, G. M., Yin, H. Q., Gustafson, K. S., Nelson, R. D., and Jacob, H. S.,** Platelet-activating factor primes neutrophil responses to agonists: role in promoting neutrophil-mediated endothelial damage, *Blood,* 71, 1100, 1988.

98. **Worthen, G. S., Seccombe, J. F., Clay, K. L., Guthrie, L. A., and Johnston, R. B., Jr.,** The priming of neutrophils by lipopolysaccharide for production of intracellular platelet-activating factor. Potential role in mediation of enhanced superoxide secretion, *J. Immunol.,* 140, 3553, 1988.

99. **Warren, J. S., Mandel, D. M., Johnson, K. J., and Ward, P. A.,** Evidence for the role of platelet-activating factor in immune complex vasculitis in the rat, *J. Clin. Invest.,* 83, 669, 1989.

100. **Paubert-Braquet, M., Koltz, P., Guilbaud, J., Hosford, D., and Braquet, P.,** Platelet-activating factor amplifies tumour necrosis factor-induced superoxide generation by human neutrophils, *Adv. Exp. Med. Biol.,* 264, 275, 1990.

101. **Dubois, C., Bissonnette, E., and Rola-Pleszczynski, M.,** Platelet-activating factor (PAF) enhances tumor necrosis factor production by alveolar macrophages. Prevention by PAF receptor antagonists and lipooxygenase inhibitors. *J. Immunol.,* 143, 964, 1989.

102. **Bonavida, B., Mencia-Huerta, J.-M., and Braquet, P.,** Effects of platelet-activating factor on peripheral blood monocytes: induction and priming for TNF secretion, *J. Lipid Med.,* 2, S65, 1990.

103. **Morrison, W. J. and Shukla, S. D.,** Desensitization of receptor-coupled activation of phosphoinositide-specific phospholipase C in platelets: evidence for distinct mechanisms for platelet-activating factor and thrombin, *Mol. Pharmacol.,* 33, 58, 1988.

104. **O'Flaherty, J. T., Lees, C. J., Miller, C. H., McCall, C. E., Lewis, J. C., Love, S. H., and Wykle, R. L.,** Selective desensitization of neutrophils: further studies with 1-O-alkyl-*sn*-glycero-3-phosphocholine analogues, *J. Immunol.,* 127, 731, 1981.

105. **Smith, R. J., Bowman, B. J., and Iden, S. S.,** Stimulation of the human neutrophil superoxide anion-generating system with 1-O-hexadecyl/octadecyl-2-acetyl-*sn*-glyceryl-3-phosphorycholine, *Biochem. Pharmacol.,* 33, 973, 1984.

106. **O'Flaherty, J. T.**, Neutrophil degranulation: evidence pertaining to its mediation by the combined effects of leukotriene B$_4$, platelet-activating factor, and 5-HETE, *J. Cell. Physiol.*, 122, 229, 1985.

107. **O'Flaherty, J. T., Schmitt, J. D., Wykle, R. L., Redman, J. F., Jr., and McCall, C. E.**, Diacylglycerols and mezerein activate neutrophils by a phorbol myristate acetate-like mechanism, *J. Cell. Physiol.*, 125, 192, 1985.

108. **Schleiffenbaum, B. and Fehr, J.**, The tumor necrosis factor receptor and human neutrophil function: deactivation and cross-deactivation of tumor necrosis factor-induced neutrophil responses by receptor down-regulation, *J. Clin. Invest.*, 86, 184, 1990.

109. **Naccache, P. H., Faucher, N., Borgeat, P., Gasson, J. C., and DiPersio, J. F.**, Granulocyte-macrophage colony-stimulating factor modulates the excitation-response coupling sequence in human neutrophils, *J. Immunol.*, 140, 3541, 1988.

110. **O'Flaherty, J. T., Wykle, R. L., Thomas, M. J., and McCall, C. E.**, Neutrophil degranulation responses to combinations of arachidonate metabolites and platelet-activating factor, *Res. Commun. Chem. Pathol. Pharmacol.*, 43, 3, 1984.

111. **O'Flaherty, J. T., Thomas, M. J., Hammett, M. J., Carroll, C., McCall, C. E., Wykle, R. L.**, 5-L-Hydroxy-6,8,11,14-eicosatetraenoate potentiates the human neutrophil degranulating action of platelet-activating factor, *Biochem. Biophys. Res. Commun.*, 111, 1, 1983.

112. **O'Flaherty, J. T. and Thomas, M. J.**, Effect of 15-lipoxygenase-derived arachidonate metabolites on human neutrophil degranulation, *Prostaglandins Leukotrienes Med.*, 17, 199, 1985.

113. **O'Flaherty, J. T., Thomas, M. J., McCall, C. E., and Wykle, R. L.**, Potentiating actions of hydroxyeicosatetraenoates on human neutrophil degranulation responses to leukotriene B$_4$ and phorbol myristate acetate, *Res. Commun. Chem. Pathol. Pharmacol.*, 40, 475, 1983.

114. **O'Flaherty, J. T., Wykle, R. L., Redman, J., Samuel, M., and Thomas, M.**, Metabolism of 5-hydroxyicosatetraenoate by human neutrophils: production of a novel ω-oxidized derivative, *J. Immunol.*, 137, 3277, 1986.

115. **Rossi, A. G., Thomas, M. J., and O'Flaherty, J. T.**, Stereospecific bioactions of 5-hydroxyeicosatetraenoate, *FEBS Lett.*, 240, 163, 1988.

116. **Rossi, A. G. and O'Flaherty, J. T.**, Bioactions of 5-hydroxyicosatetraenoate and its interaction with platelet-activating factor, *Lipids*, in press.

117. **Rossi, A. G., Redman, J. F., Jacobson, D. P., and O'Flaherty, J. T.**, Enhancement of human neutrophil responses to platelet-activating factor by 5(S)-hydroxyicosatetraenoate, *J. Lipid Mediators*, in press.

118. **Shaw, J. O. and Henson, P. M.**, The binding of rabbit basophil-derived platelet-activating factor to rabbit platelets, *Am. J. Pathol.*, 98, 791, 1980.

119. **O'Flaherty, J. T., Jacobson, D. P., and Redman, J. F.**, Regulators of platelet-activating factor receptors in polymorphonuclear neutrophils, *Biochem. J.*, in press.

120. **Valone, F. H. and Goetzl, E. J.**, Specific binding by human polymorphonuclear leucocytes of the immunological mediator 1-O-hexadecyl/octadecyl-2-acetyl-*sn*-glycero-3-phosphorylcholine, *Immunology*, 48, 141, 1983.

121. **Bussolino, F., Tetta, C., and Camussi, G.**, Specific binding of 1-[^{3}H]-O-alkyl-2-acetyl-*sn*-glyceryl-3-phosphoryl choline (platelet-activating factor, PAF) by human polymorphonuclear neutrophils, *Agents Actions*, 15, 15, 1984.

122. **Korth, R. and Benveniste, J.**, BN 52021 displaced[^{3}H]PAF-acether from, and inhibits its binding to, intact human platelets, *Eur. J. Pharmacol.*, 142, 331, 1987.

123. **Nishihira, J. and Ishibashi, T.**, A phospholipase C with a high specificity for platelet-activating factor in rabbit liver light mitochondria, *Lipids*, 21, 780, 1986.

124. **Kumar, R., King, R. J., Martin, H. M., and Hanahan, D. J.**, Metabolism of platelet-activating factor (alkylacetylphosphocholine) by type-II epithelial cells and fibroblasts from rat lungs, *Biochim. Biophys. Acta*, 917, 33, 1987.

125. **Haroldsen, P. E., Voelkel, N. F., Henson, J. E., Henson, P. M., and Murphy, R. C.**, Metabolism of platelet-activating factor in isolated perfused rat lung, *J. Clin. Invest.*, 79, 1860, 1987.

126. **Kawasaki, T. and Synder, F.**, The metabolism of lyso-platelet-activating factor (1-O-alkyl-2-lyso-*sn*-glycero-3-phosphocholine) by a calcium-dependent lysophospholipase D in rabbit kidney medulla, *Biochim. Biophys. Acta*, 920, 85, 1987.

127. **Borea, P. A., Montesi, L., Muzzolini, A., and Fantozzi, R.**, Temperature dependence of [^{3}H]PAF binding to washed human platelets, *Biochem. Pharmacol.*, 41, 629, 1991.

128. **O'Flaherty, J. T., Jacobson, D. P., and Redman, J. F.**, Birdirectional effects of protein kinase C activators. Studies with human neutrophils and platelet-activating factor, *J. Biol. Chem.*, 264, 6836, 1989.

129. **Hwang, S.-B., Lee, C.-S. C., Cheah, M. J., and Shen, T. Y.**, Specific receptor sties for 1-O-alkyl-2-O-acetyl-*sn*-glycero-3-phosphocholine (platelet activating factor) on rabbit platelet and guinea pig smooth muscle membranes, *Biochemistry*, 22, 4756, 1983.

130. **Paulson, S. K., Wolf, J. L., Novotney-Barry, A., and Cox, C. P.**, Pharmacologic characterization of the rabbit neutrophil receptor for platelet-activating factor, *Proc. Exp. Biol. Med.*, 195, 247, 1990.

131. **Hwang, S.-B.**, Identification of a second putative receptor of platelet-activating factor from human poly-morphonuclear leukocytes, *J. Biol. Chem.*, 263, 3225, 1988.
132. **Marquis, O., Robaut, C., and Cavero, I.**, Evidence for the existence and ionic modulation of platelet-activating factor receptors mediating degranulatory responses in human polymorphonuclear leukocytes, *J. Pharmacol. Exp. Ther.*, 250, 293, 1989.
133. **Dent, G., Ukena, D., Chanez, P., Sybrecht, G., and Barnes, P.**, Characterization of PAF receptors on human neutrophils using the specific antagonist, WEB 2086: correlation between receptor binding and function, *FEBS Lett.*, 244, 365, 1989.
134. **Marquis, O., Robaut, C., and Cavero, I.**, [³H]52770 RP, a platelet-activating factor receptor antagonist, and tritiated platlet-activating factor label a common specific binding site in human polymorphonuclear leukocytes, *J. Pharmacol. Exp. Ther.*, 244, 709, 1988.
135. **Hwang, S.-B., Lam, M.-H., and Pong, S.-S.**, Ionic and GTP regulation of binding of platelet-activating factor to receptors and platelet-activating factor-induced activation of GTP-ase in rabbit platelet membranes, *J. Biol. Chem.*, 261, 532, 1986.
136. **Valone, F. H. and Ruis, N. M.**, Platelet-activating factor binding to human platelet membranes, *Biotechnol. Appl. Biochem.*, 8, 465, 1986.
137. **Janero, D. R., Burghardt, B., and Burghardt, C.**, Specific binding of 1-*O*-alkyl-2-acetyl-*sn*-glycero-3-phosphocholine (platelet-activating factor) to the intact canine platelet, *Thromb. Res.*, 50, 789, 1988.
138. **Duronio, V., Reany, A., Wong, S., Bigras, C., and Salari, H.**, Characterization of platelet-activating factor receptors in procine platelets, *Can. J. Physiol. Pharmacol.*, 68, 1514, 1990.
139. **Korth, R., Hirafuji, M., Keraly, C. L., Delautier, D., Bidault, J., and Benveniste, J.**, Interaction of the Paf antagonist WEB 2086 and its hetrazepine analogues with human platelets and endothelial cells, *Br. J. Pharmacol.*, 98, 653, 1989.
140. **Valone, F. H.**, Identification of platelet-activating factor receptors in P388D1 murine macrophages, *J. Immunol.*, 140, 2389, 1988.
141. **Ng, D. S. and Wong, K.**, Specific binding of platelet-activating factor (PAF) by human peripheral blood mononuclear leukocytes, *Biochem. Biophys. Res. Commun.*, 155, 311, 1988.
142. **Travers, J. B., Li, Q., Kniss, D. A., and Fertel, R. H.**, Identification of functional platelet-activating factor receptors in Raji lymphoblasts, *J. Immunol.*, 143, 3708, 1989.
143. **Domingo, M. T., Spinnewyn, B., Chabrier, P. E., and Braquet, P.**, Presence of specific binding sites for platelet-activating factor (PAF) in brain, *Biochem. Biophys. Res. Commun.*, 151, 730, 1988.
144. **Thierry, A., Doly, M., Braquet, P., Cluzel, J., and Meyniel, G.**, Presence of specific platelet-activating factor binding sites in the rat retina, *Eur. J. Pharmacol.*, 163, 97, 1989.
145. **Dent, G., Ukena, D., Sybrecht, G. W., and Barnes, P. J.**, [³H]WEB 2086 labels platelet activating factor receptors in the guinea pig and human lung, *Eur. J. Pharmacol.*, 169, 313, 1989.
146. **Gomez, J., Bloom, J. W., Yamamura, H. I., and Halonen, M.**, Characterization of receptors for platelet-activating factor in guinea pig lung membranes, *Am. J. Resp. Cell. Mol. Biol.*, 3, 259, 1990.
147. **Hwang, S.-B. and Lam, M.-H.**, Species difference in the specific receptors of platelet activating factor, *Biochem. Pharmacol.*, 35, 4511, 1986.
148. **Hwang, S.-B., Lam, M.-H., and Hsu, A. H.-M.**, Characterization of platelet-activating factor (PAF) receptor by specific binding of [³H]L-659,989, a PAF receptor antagonist, to rabbit platelet membranes: possible multiple conformational states of a single type of PAF receptors, *Mol. Pharmacol.*, 35, 48, 1989.
149. **Prpic, V., Uhing, R. J., Weiel, J. E., Jakoi, L., Gawdi, G., Herman, B., and Adams, D. O.**, Biochemical and functional responses stimulated by platelet-activating factor in murine peritoneal macro-phages, *J. Cell. Biol.*, 107, 363, 1988.
150. **Kroegel, C., Yukawa, T., Westwick, J., and Barnes, P. J.**, Evidence for two platelet activating factor receptors on eosinophils: dissociation between PAF-induced intracellular calcium mobilization degranulation and superoxides anion generation in eosinophils, *Biochem. Biophys. Res. Commun.*, 162, 511, 1989.
151. **Ng, D. S. and Wong, K.**, Effect of sulfhydryl reagents on PAF binding to human neutrophils and platelets, *Eur. J. Pharmacol.*, 154, 47, 1988.
152. **Valone, F. H.**, Isolation of a platelet membrane protein which binds the platelet-activating factor 1-O-hexadecyl-2-acetyl-*sn*-glycero-3-phosphorylcholine, *Immunology*, 52, 169, 1984.
153. **Chau, L.-Y. and Jii, Y.-J.**, Characterization of ³H-labelled platelet activating factor receptor complex solubilized from rabbit platelet membranes, *Biochim. Biophys. Acta*, 970, 103, 1988.
154. **Matsumoto, M. and Miwa, M.**, Platelet-activating factor-binding protein in human serum, *Adv. Prosta-glandin, Thromboxane, Leukotriene Res.*, 15, 705, 1985.
155. **Honda, Z.-i., Nakamura, M., Miki, I., Minami, M., Watanabe, T., Seyama, Y., Okado, H., Toh, H., Ito, K., Miyamoto, T., and Shimizu, T.**, Cloning by functional expression of platelet-activating factor receptor from guinea-pig lung, *Nature*, 349, 342, 1991.
156. **Dive, G., Godfroid, J.-J., Lamotte-Braseur, J., Batt, J.-P., Heymans, F., Dupont, L., and Braquet, P.**, PAF-receptor. I. "Cache-coreilles" effect of selected high-potency platelet-activating factor (PAF) antagonists, *J. Lipid Mediators*, 1, 201, 1989.

157. **Vallari, D. S., Austinhirst, R., and Snyder, F.,** Development of specific functionally active receptors for platelet-activating factor in HL-60 cells following granulocytic differentiation, *J. Biol. Chem.,* 265, 4261, 1990.

158. **Chao, W., Liu, H., Hanahan, D. J., and Olson, M. S.,** Regulation of platelet-activating factor receptors in rat Kupffer cells, *J. Biol. Chem.,* 264, 20448, 1989.

159. **Taylor, C. W.,** The role of G proteins in transmembrane signalling, *Biochem. J.,* 272, 1, 1990.

160. **Bourne, H. R., Sanders, D. A., and McCormick, F.,** The GTPase superfamily: conserved structure and molecular mechanism, *Nature,* 349, 117, 1991.

161. **Ng, D. S. and Wong, K.,** GTP regulation of platelet-activating factor binding to human neutrophil membranes, *Biochem. Biophys. Res. Commun.,* 141, 353, 1986.

162. **Conquer, J. and Mahadevappa, V. G.,** Evidence for the possible involvement of protein kinase C in the activation of non-specific phospholipase A_2 in human neutrophils, *J. Lipid Med.,* 3, 113, 1991.

163. **Yamazaki, M., Gomez-Cambronero, J., Durstin, M., Molski, T. F. P., Becker, E. L., and Sha'afi, R. I.,** Phorbol 12-myristate 13-acetate inhibits binding of leukotriene B_4 and platelet-activating factor and the responses they induce in neutrophils: site of action, *Proc. Natl. Acad. Sci. U.S.A.,* 86, 5791, 1989.

164. **Chao, W., Liu, H., Hanahan, D. J., and Olson, M. S.,** Regulation of platelet-activating factor receptor and PAF receptor-mediated arachidonic acid release by protein kinase C activation in rat Kupffer cells, *Arch. Biochem. Biophys.,* 282, 188, 1990.

165. **Homma, H. and Hanahan, D. J.,** Attenuation of platelet activating factor (PAF)-induced stimulation of rabbit platlet GTPase by phorbol ester, dibutyryl cAMP, and desensitization: concomitant effects on PAF receptor binding characteristics, *Arch. Biochem. Biophys.,* 262, 32, 1988.

166. **O'Flaherty, J. T., Redman, J. F., and Jacobson, D. P.,** Interactions between cellular Ca^{2+} and the expression of receptors for platelet-activating factor and *N*-formyl-Met-leu-phe in human neutrophils, submitted.

167. **Chao, W., Liu, H., Zhou, W., Hanahan, D. J., and Olson, M. S.,** Regulation of platelet-activating factor receptor and platelet-activating factor receptor-mediated biological responses by cAMP in rat Kupffer cells, *J. Biol. Chem.,* 265, 17576, 1990.

168. **Gorman, R. R., Morton, D. R., Hopkins, N. K., and Lin, A. H.,** Acetyl glyceryl ether phosphorylcholine stimulates leukotriene B_4 synthesis and cyclic AMP accumulation in human polymorphonuclear leukocytes, *Adv. Prostaglandin, Thrmoboxane, Leukotriene Res.,* 12, 57, 1983.

169. **Rossi, A. G. and O'Flaherty, J. T.,** Prostaglandin binding sites in human polymorphonuclear neutrophils, *Prostaglandins,* 37, 641, 1989.

170. **Ney, P. and Schrör, K.,** E-type prostaglandins but not iloprost inhibit platelet activating factor-induced generation of leukotriene B_4 by human polymorphonuclear leukocytes, *Br. J. Pharmacol.,* 96, 186, 1989.

171. **Verghese, M. W., Charles, L., Jakoi, L., Dillon, S. B., and Snyderman, R.,** Role of a guanine nucleotide regulatory protein in the activation of phospholipase C by different chemoattractants, *J. Immunol.,* 138, 4374, 1987.

172. **Rossi, A. G., McMillan, R. M., and MacIntyre, D. E.,** Agonist-induced calcium flux, phosphoinositide metabolism, aggregation and enzyme secretion in human neutrophils, *Agents Actions,* 24, 272, 1988.

173. **Naccache, P. H., Molski, M. M., Volpi, M., Becker, E. L., and Sha'afi, R. I.,** Unique inhibitory profile of platelet activating factor induced calcium mobilization, polyphosphoinositide turnover and granule enzyme secretion in rabbit neutrophils towards pertussis toxin and phorbol ester, *Biochem. Biophys. Res. Commun.,* 130, 677, 1985.

174. **Nakashima, S., Suganuma, A., Sato, M., Tohmatsu, T., and Nozawa, Y.,** Mechanism of arachidonic acid liberation in platelet-activating factor-stimulated human polymorphonuclear neutrophils, *J. Immunol.,* 143, 1295, 1989.

175. **Tao, W., Molski, T. F. P., and Sha'afi, R. I.,** Arachidonic acid release in rabbit neutrophils, *Biochem. J.,* 257, 633, 1989.

176. **Tou, J.-S.,** Platelet-activating factor promotes arachidonate incorporation into phosphatidylinositol and phosphatidylcholine in neutrophils, *Biochem. Biophys. Res. Commun.,* 127, 1045, 1985.

177. **Tou, J.-S.,** Platelet-activating factor modulates phospholipid acylation in human neutrophils, *Lipids,* 22, 333, 1987.

178. **Chilton, F. H., O'Flaherty, J. T., Walsh, C. E., Thomas, M. J., Wykle, R. L., DeChatelet, L. R., and Waite, B. M.,** Platelet activating factor: stimulation of the lipoxygenase pathway in polymorphonuclear leukocytes by 1-O-alkyl-2-O-acetyl-*sn*-glycero-3-phosphocholine, *J. Biol. Chem.,* 257, 5402, 1982.

179. **Lin, A. H., Morton, D. R., and Gorman, R. R.,** Acetyl glyceryl ether phosphorylcholine stimulates leukotriene B_4 synthesis in human polymorphonuclear leukocytes, *J. Clin. Invest.,* 70, 1058, 1982.

180. **Lad, P. M., Olson, C. V., Grewal, I. S., and Scott, S. J.,** A pertussis toxin-sensitive GTP-binding protein in the human neutrophil regulates multiple receptors, calcium mobilization and lectin-induced capping, *Proc. Natl. Acad. Sci. U.S.A.,* 82, 8643, 1985.

181. **Hartiala, K. T., Scott, I. G., Viljanen, M. K., and Akerman, K. E. O.,** Lack of correlation between calcium mobilization and respiratory burst activation induced by chemotactic factors in rabbit polymorphonuclear leukocytes, *Biochem. Biophys. Res. Commun.,* 144, 794, 1987.

182. **Merritt, J. E., Jacob, R., and Hallam, T. J.,** Use of manganese to discriminate between calcium influx and mobilization from internal stores in stimulated human neutrophils, *J. Biol. Chem.,* 264, 1522, 1989.

183. **O'Flaherty, J. T. and Nishihira, J.,** Arachidonate metabolites, platelet-activating factor, and the mobilization of protein kinase C in human polymorphonuclear neutrophils, *J. Immunol.,* 138, 1889, 1987.

184. **Gay, J. C. and Stitt, E. S.,** Platelet-activating factor induces protein kinase activity in the particulate fraction of human neutrophils, *Blood,* 71, 159, 1988.

185. **Gay, J. C. and Stitt, E. S.,** Enhancement of phorbol ester-induced protein kinase activity in human neutrophils by platelet-activating factor, *J. Cell Physiol.,* 137, 439, 1988.

186. **Gay, J. C.,** Priming of neutrophil oxidative responses by platelet-activating factor, *J. Lipid Med.,* 2, S161, 1990.

187. **O'Flaherty, J. T., Redman, J. F., Jacobson, D. P., and Rossi, A. G.,** Stimulation and priming of protein kinase C translocation by a Ca^{2+} transient-independent mechanism. Studies in human neutrophils challenged with platelet-activating factor and other receptor agonists, *J. Biol. Chem.,* 265, 21619, 1990.

188. **Doebber, T. W. and Wu, M. S.,** Platelet-activating factor (PAF) stimulates the PAF-synthesizing enzyme acetyl-CoA: 1-alkyl-*sn*-glycero-3-phosphocholine O^2-acetyltransferase and PAF synthesis in neutrophils, *Proc. Natl. Acad. Sci. U.S.A.,* 84, 7557, 1987.

189. **Sugiura, T., Fukuda, T., Masuzawa, Y., and Waku, K.,** Ether lysophospholipid-induced production of platelet-activating factor in human polymorphonuclear leukocytes, *Biochim. Biophys. Acta,* 1047, 223, 1990.

190. **Verghese, M. W., Fox, K., McPhail, L. C., and Snyderman, R.,** Chemoattractant-elicited alterations of cAMP levels in human polymorphonuclear leukocytes require a Ca^{2+}-dependent mechanism which is independent of transmembrane activation of adenylate cyclase, *J. Biol. Chem.,* 260, 6769, 1985.

191. **Reinhold, S. L., Prescott, S. M., Zimmerman, G. A., and McIntyre, T. M.,** Activation of human neutrophil phospholipase D by three separable mechanisms, *FASEB J.,* 4, 208, 1990.

192. **O'Flaherty, J. T., Swendsen, C. L., Lees, C. J., and McCall, C. E.,** Role of extracellular calcium in neutrophil degranulation responses to 1-O-alkyl-2-O-acetyl-*sn*-glycero-3-phosphocholine, *Am. J. Pathol.,* 105, 107, 1981.

193. **Lad, P. M., Olson, C. V., and Grewal, I. S.,** Platelet-activating factor mediated effects on human neutrophil function are inhibited by pertussis toxin, *Biochem. Biophys. Res. Commun.,* 129, 632, 1985.

194. **O'Flaherty, J. T., Jacobson, D., and Redman, J.,** Mechanism involved in the mobilization of neutrophil calcium by 5-hydroxyeicosatetraenoate, *J. Immunol.,* 140, 4323, 1988.

195. **O'Flaherty, J. T., Wykle, R. L., Lees, C. J., Shewmake, T., McCall, C. E., and Thomas, M. J.,** Neutrophil-degranulating action of 5,12-dihydroxy-6,8,10,14-eicosatetraenoic acid and 1-O-alkyl-2-O-acetyl-*sn*-glycero-3-phosphocholine, *Am. J. Pathol.,* 105, 264, 1981.

196. **Smith, R. J. and Bowman, B. J.,** Stimulation of human neutrophil degranulation with 1-O-octadecyl2-O-acetyl-*sn*-glyceryl-3-phosphorylcholine: modulation by inhibitors of arachidonic acid metabolism, *Biochem. Biophys. Res. Commun.,* 104, 1495, 1982.

197. **Wade, P. J., Lunt, D. O., Lad, N., Tuffin, D. P., and McCullagh, K. G.,** Effect of calcium and calcium antagonists on [^{3}H]-PAF-acether binding to washed human platelets, *Thromb. Res.,* 41, 251, 1986.

198. **Valone, F. H.,** Inhibition of platelet-activating factor binding to human platelets by calcium channel blockers, *Thromb. Res.,* 45, 427, 1987.

199. **O'Flaherty, J. T., Redman, J. F., and Jacobson, D. P.,** Cyclical binding, processing, and functional interactions of neutrophils with leukotriene B$_4$, *J. Cell. Physiol.,* 142, 299, 1990.

200. **O'Flaherty, J. T., Hammett, M. J., Shewmake, T. B., Wykle, R. L., Love, S. H., McCall, C. E., and Thomas, M. J.,** Evidence for 5,12-dihydroxy-6,8,10,14-eicosatetraenoate as a mediator of human neutrophil aggregation, *Biochem. Biophys. Res. Commun.,* 103, 552, 1981.

201. **O'Flaherty, J. T., Wykle, R. L., McCall, C. E., Shewmake, T. B., Lees, C. J., and Thomas, M.,** Desensitization of the human neutrophil degranulation response: studies with 5,12-dihydroxy-6,8,10,14-eicosatetraenoic acid, *Biochem. Biophys. Res. Commun.,* 101, 1290, 1981.

202. **Billah, M. M., Bryant, R. W., and Siegel, M. I.,** Lipoxygenase products of arachidonic acid modulate biosynthesis of platelet-activating factor (1-O-alkyl-2-acetyl-*sn*-glycero-3-phosphocholine) by human neutrophils via phospholipase A$_2$, *J. Biol. Chem.,* 260, 6899, 1985.

203. **Saito, H., Hirai, A., Tamura, Y., and Yoshida, S.,** The 5-lipoxygenase products can modulate the synthesis of platelet-activating factor (alkyl-acetyl GPC) in Ca-ionophore A23187-stimulated rat peritoneal macrophages, *Prostaglandins Leukotrienes Med.,* 18, 271, 1985.

204. **Uhing, R. J., Prpic, V., Hollenbach, P. W., and Adams, D. O.,** Involvement of protein kinase C in platelet-activating factor-stimulated diacylglycerol accumulation in murine peritoneal macrophages, *J. Biol. Chem.,* 264, 9224, 1989.

205. **Kadiri, C., Cherqui, G., Masliah, J., Rybkine, T., Etienne, J., and Béréziat, G.,** Mechanism of N-formyl-methionyl-leucyl-phenylalanine- and platelet-activating factor-induced arachidonic acid release in guinea pig alveolar macrophages: involvement of a GTP-binding protein and role of protein kinase A and protein kinase C, *Mol. Pharmacol.,* 38, 418, 1990.

206. **Barzaghi, G., Sarau, H. M., and Mong, S.,** Platelet-activating factor-induced phosphoinositide metabolism in differentiated U-937 cells in culture, *J. Pharmacol. Exp. Ther.,* 248, 559, 1988.

207. **Murphy, S. and Welk, G.,** Hydrolysis of polyphosphoinositides in astrocytes by platelet-activating factor, *Eur. J. Pharmacol.,* 188, 399, 1990.

208. **Grandison, L.,** Platelet activating factor induces inositol phosphate accumulation in cultures of rat and bovine anterior pituitary cells, *Endocrinology,* 127, 1786, 1990.

209. **Yue, T.-L., Gleason, M. M., Hallenbeck, J., and Feuerstein, G.,** Characterization of platelet-activating factor-induced elevation of cytosolic free-calcium level in neurohybrid NCB-20 cells, *Neuroscience,* 41, 177, 1991.

210. **Söling, H.-D., Eibl, H., and Fest, W.,** Acetylcholine-like effects of 1-O-alkyl-2-acetyl-*sn*-glycero-3-phosphocholine ("platelet-activating factor") and its analogues in exocrine secretory glands, *Eur. J. Biochem.,* 144, 65, 1984.

211. **Shukla, S. D. and Hanahan, D. J.,** AGEPC (platelet activating factor) induced stimulation of rabbit platelets: effects on phosphatidylinositol, di- and tri-phosphoinositides and phosphatidic acid metabolism, *Biochem. Biophys. Res. Commun.,* 106, 697, 1982.

Chapter 7

CHARACTERIZATION AND REGULATION OF PLATELET ACTIVATING FACTOR RECEPTORS IN THE LIVER

Merle S. Olson

TABLE OF CONTENTS

ISBN 0-8493-7299-2
© 1993 by CRC Press, Inc.

I. INTRODUCTION

For nearly a decade my laboratory has been attempting to identify and to characterize the receptor(s) for platelet activating factor (PAF) in the hepatic vasculature. In this chapter, I would like to summarize the role of PAF as a signaling molecule in the liver and to discuss the progress that we have made in characterizing PAF receptors in liver-derived cells. In this discussion I make no attempt to review the literature in this area comprehensively; rather I concentrate on the contribution that my laboratory group has made to this specific area of research.

II. HEPATIC EFFECTS OF PLATELET ACTIVATING FACTOR

The liver plays a crucial role in the maintenance of glucose homeostasis both during physiological feeding and fasting cycles[1,2] and during pathophysiological episodes.[3,4] The hormonal signaling molecules and mechanisms employed during physiological glucoregulatory scenarios are, of course, primarily the pancreatic peptide hormones, glucagon and insulin, and adrenergic agonists of either adrenal or sympathetic neuronal derivation. It is becoming increasingly evident that during either systemic or actual hepatic pathophysiological situations various lipid and peptide autacoid mediators assume a prominent role in the regulation of hepatic glycogenolysis/gluconeogenesis and subsequent enhanced glucose output necessary to produce the requisite hyperglycemia observed in the early phases of, for instance, sepsis or anaphylaxis.

Because of our interest in hepatic regulatory mechanisms, we became intrigued by the possibility that the potent lipid autacoid PAF, or 1-O-alkyl-2-acetyl-*sn*-glycero-3-phosphocholine (AGEPC), may be a key regulatory factor during trauma responses by the liver. In 1983 we demonstrated[5] that PAF at extremely low concentrations (i.e., 2×10^{-10} M) resulted in nearly a threefold increase in glucose output from the perfused liver derived from a fed rat (Figure 1). Removing the acetyl moiety from the *sn*-2 position of PAF or employing the *sn*-1 stereoisomer of PAF at 500 times the concentration obliterated the hepatic responses in perfused liver preparation. Coincident with, even slightly preceding, the increase in hepatic glucose output occurred an increase in hepatic portal pressure (vascular resistance) in response to PAF,[7] suggesting but not proving that the glucoregulatory response elicited by PAF was derived from the potent vasoconstrictive characteristics of this substance. This observation coupled with the observation that glycogenolysis in preparations of isolated rat hepatocytes was not stimulated at any concentration of PAF, even though these cells were fully competent in their glycogenolytic responses to glucagon and α-adrenergic agonists. The same result was obtained in attempts to stimulate glucose output in rat liver slices. In other words, an intact hepatic vasculature was required in order for PAF to elicit this sequence of responses.

Other experiments were performed which indicated that the increased glucose output resulting from PAF infusion was (1) dependent upon the perfusate Ca^{2+} concentration;[8] (2) a transient response involving an initial sharp peak of glucose release followed by an elevated, more prolonged rate of glucose release;[8] (3) mediated by the conversion of relatively inactive phosphorylase b to active phosphorylase a coincident with an increase in the ADP level of the tissue; and (4) inhibited by several well-defined PAF receptor antagonists such as the PAF analogues U66985 and CV3988.[9] It was demonstrated that the PAF-mediated glycogenolytic response in the perfused liver was inhibited strongly by the infusion of β-adrenergic agonists, but not by α-adrenergic agonists or glucagon.[10,11] Moreover, evidence was generated that the "response elements" or receptors for PAF were localized on vascular cells of the small portal venules instead of on parenchymal cells,[12] which was consistent with our findings that PAF infusion into a retrograde perfused liver (i.e., vena cava to portal)

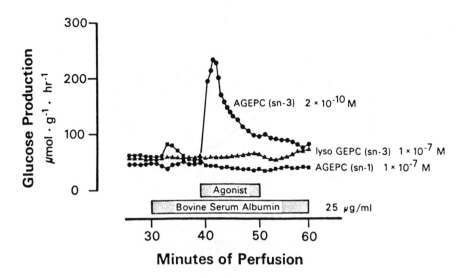

FIGURE 1. The effect of PAF [AGEPC (*sn*-3)], •; [lysoPAF (*sn*-3)], ▲; and [AGEPC (*sn*-1)], ■, on glucose production in the perfused rat liver. (Reprinted with permission of the *Journal of Biological Chemistry*.)

required nearly 1000 times more than the concentration of PAF in the anterograde perfused liver to elicit the glycogenolytic response, and that PAF was unable to stimulate hepatic glycogenolysis in isolated hepatocytes.

Several other interesting characteristics of the hepatic PAF response were defined in this series of papers from my laboratory. First, it was discovered that PAF infusion resulted in an increased production of uric acid by the perfused liver.[13] The implication of this finding is that the extensive vasoconstriction induced as a result of PAF treatment of the liver caused transient ischemia in selected sinusoids. This action resulted in an increased output of uric acid as a result of enhanced oxygen radical production. Second, it was demonstrated (Figure 2) that PAF was capable of mobilizing a small pool of hepatic calcium (probably of non-parenchymal cell origin).[14] These data were acquired in livers equilibrated with $^{45}Ca^{2+}$ prior to mediator challenge; they suggested that a small pool of calcium localized in sinusoidal cells was stimulated or mobilized upon mediator application to the liver. Third, we were able to demonstrate that the signaling mechanism(s) involved in the hepatic response to PAF probably involved vicinal dithiol moieties in that both the hemodynamic and metabolic responses to PAF in the liver were completely inhibited by very low concentrations of the trivalent arsenical, phenylarsine oxide.[15]

Finally, an extensive series of experiments was performed in order to assess whether either the hemodynamic or the glycogenolytic effects of PAF on the perfused liver were direct vs. indirect responses. In this regard other laboratories have either suggested or implied that the heptic PAF response is actually mediated by PAF-induced activation of phospholipase A_2 (PLA_2), with the resultant production of several cyclooxygenase metabolites. These eicosanoids then stimulate receptors on the hepatocyte to activate phosphorylase activity and subsequent hepatic glycogenolysis.[16-19] Our twofold position in this controversy has always been that PAF or particulate substances cause eicosanoid synthesis in sinusoidal cells of the liver, and that PAF, particulates, and certain eicosanoids, can cause independent hemodynamic effects on the hepatic vasculature (e.g., vasoconstriction) resulting in ischemia-induced glycogenolysis. The latter contention was made in a study in which we were able to inhibit eicosanoid synthesis in response to PAF infusion into the perfused liver with the cyclooxygenase inhibitor, ibuprofen, without a significant effect on the hemodynamic or glycogenolytic response of the perfused liver to PAF (Figure 3).[20]

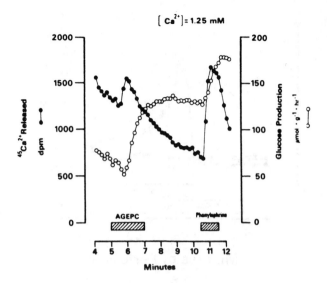

FIGURE 2. AGEPC- and phenylephrine-stimulated release of calcium and glucose from liver preloaded with $^{45}Ca^{2+}$. Livers were loaded with $^{45}Ca^{2+}$ for 50 min. After the livers were loaded, washout proceeded for 4 min prior to sample collection. At 5 min into the washout, a 2-min infusion of AGEPC (20 nM) was begun; at 10.5 min; a 1-min infusion of phenylephrine (10 µM) was started. Samples were collected at 12-s intervals. $^{45}Ca^{2+}$ and glucose concentrations were determined. (Reprinted with permission of *Biochemistry*.) Perfusate $[Ca^{2+}]$ = 1.25 mM.

Another recent finding supports our suggested sequelae of events in the hepatic PAF response. Fisher and colleagues[21] demonstrated that nitric oxide (i.e., a potent vasodilator) infusion completely inhibited both the hemodynamic and the glycogenolytic effects of PAF infusion, again suggesting direct PAF effects on the hepatic microcirculation as being key to the glycogenolytic response of the lipid autacoid.

III. SYNTHESIS OF PLATELET ACTIVATING FACTOR IN THE LIVER

We employed several experimental approaches to ascertain whether PAF was synthesized in the perfused liver or in liver-derived cultured cells following stimulation or challenge. We were able to demonstrate that challenge of the isolated perfused rat liver with heat-aggregated immunoglobulin G (IgG),[22] zymosan,[23] or bacterial lipopolysaccharide[24] (Figure 4) cause the synthesis and release of PAF as well as various eicosanoids. It is likely that either phagocytosis or endocytosis of such particulate substances activates (at least) a PLA_2 leading to the conversion of alkylacyl-PAF to lyso-PAF prior to final conversion to PAF itself. The hemodynamic and glycogenolytic effects of IgG, zymosan, and lipopolysaccharide mimic the PAF response in the perfused liver. Interestingly, or curiously, depending upon your perspective, the sensitivity of the hepatic particulate responses to either cyclooxygenase or lipooxygenase inhibitors or to PAF receptor antagonists provide somewhat mixed (read: complex) results. Whereas the IgG and zymosan glycogenolytic responses could be partially inhibited by cyclooxygenase inhibitors, neither a cyclooxygenase inhibitor nor PAF receptor antagonists could inhibit to any great extent the lipopolysaccharide-induced hepatic responses. This series of experiments has led us to believe that particulate challenge of the liver certainly causes an increase in lipid (and possibly peptide) autacoid synthesis by the sinusoidal cells of the liver (Figure 5). Further, it is now our suggestion that the particulates themselves (e.g., lipopolysaccharide) can independently evoke the hemodynamic and sub-

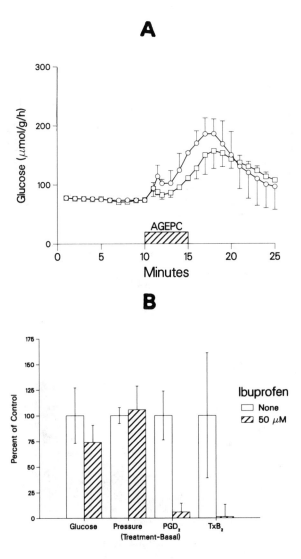

FIGURE 3. (A) Effects of varying concentrations of ibuprofen on glucose output stimulated by AGEPC. Ibuprofen (50 μM) was infused into the liver 15 min prior to beginning the AGEPC infusion. Each curve represents the mean glucose output of three livers perfused under identical conditions, whith the standard deviations of the data indicated. Livers were perfused and glucose release into perfusate was determined. ○, control; □, 50 μM ibuprofen. (B) Effect of 50 μM ibuprofen on AGEPC-stimulated changes in glucose output, vascular resistance, PGD$_2$, and thromboxane B$_2$ (TxB$_2$). Changes in glucose output, vascular resistance, and perfusate PGD$_2$ and TxB$_2$ were measured and represent the difference between values obtained during AGEPC exposure (2 to 3 min) and values prior to AGEPC exposure. The values for each condition represent the mean of three separate perfusions under identical conditions. The control values (no ibuprofen) for the differences are glucose, 135 μmol/g/h; vascular resistance, 9.9 mmHg; prostaglandin D$_2$, 61,963 pg/min/g; TxB$_2$, 174 pg/min/g. (Reprinted with permission of the *Journal of Biological Chemistry*.)

sequent glycogenolytic responses without necessarily involving mediator synthesis. To what extent the lipid mediators may be involved in signal propagation in the hepatic sinusoids is currently under careful scrutiny.

In two recent studies we have been able to demonstrate the capability of the liver to synthesize PAF under pathophysiological conditions such as during obstructive jaundice[25] and as a consequence of hepatic ischemia/reperfusion injury[26] in intact rat models of these

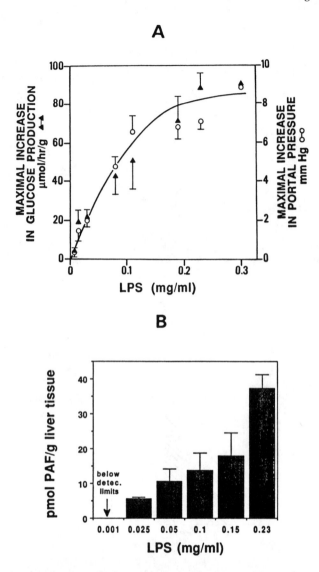

FIGURE 4. (A) The effect of lipopolysaccharide (LPS) on glucose output and portal pressure changes in the perfused rat liver. Rat livers were perfused for 30 min prior to challenge with a 2-min infusion of *S. typhosa* at the final concentration noted. Each point represents the mean ($\pm$ SEM) of from 3 to 10 livers. (B) The effect of LPS on PAF synthesis in perfused rat liver. Livers were perfused, as indicated in A, and were freeze-clamped, extracted, and assayed for PAF using a standard platelet aggregation-based bioassay. PAF values in picomoles per gram of tissue represent the mean ($\pm$ SEM) of 3 to 6 livers.

situations. Ligating the common bile duct causes obstructive jaundice in the rat and results in a 6-fold increase in hepatic PAF levels within 7 d following duct ligation. Rendering animals neutropenic did not diminish PAF accumulation in the livers of duct-obstructive animals; however, pretreatment and maintenance of animals with neomycin and polymixin B prior to duct ligation in order to minimize the release of endotoxin from the gastrointestinal tracts of jaundiced animals largely prevented the hepatic synthesis of PAF. Treatment of jaundiced animals with PAF receptor antagonists BN52021 and WEB2170 minimized the hepatic inflammation and deterioration of hepatic function, suggesting a central role for PAF in hepatic pathophysiology.

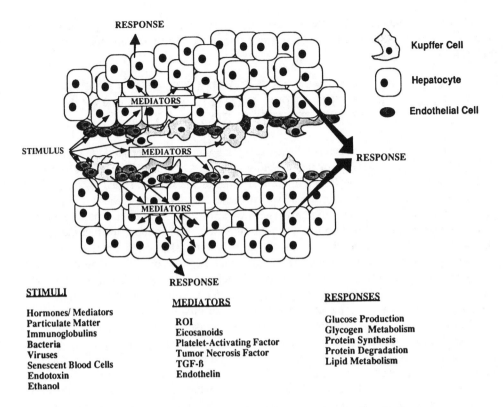

STIMULI

Hormones/ Mediators
Particulate Matter
Immunoglobulins
Bacteria
Viruses
Senescent Blood Cells
Endotoxin
Ethanol

MEDIATORS

ROI
Eicosanoids
Platelet-Activating Factor
Tumor Necrosis Factor
TGF-ß
Endothelin

RESPONSES

Glucose Production
Glycogen Metabolism
Protein Synthesis
Protein Degradation
Lipid Metabolism

FIGURE 5. Representation of hepatic sinusoidal and parenchymal cells.

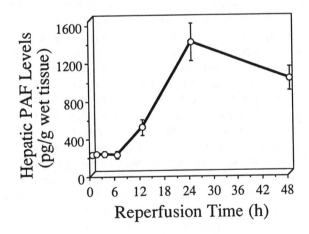

FIGURE 6. PAF levels in ischemic/reperfused rat livers. Rats were exposed to 60 min of hepatic ischemia and allowed to reperfuse for the time periods indicated.

In another study[26] an *in vivo* model of hepatic ischemia/reperfusion injury PAF levels in the liver were increased 7-fold with 24 h of reperfusion following 60 min of ischemic challenge (Figure 6). Again, neutropenic animals demonstrated the same response, eliminating the circulating neutrophil as the cellular source of the PAF. Disrupting hepatic Kupffer cell function by infusing animals with gadolinium chloride and treating animals with allopurinol to minimize the impact of active oxygen species in this response minimized the hepatic PAF accumulation. Finally, pretreatment of animals with PAF receptor antagonists prior to ischemia minimized the inflammatory responses resulting from reperfusion of the ischemic liver.

IV. IDENTIFICATION AND CHARACTERIZATION OF PLATELET ACTIVATING FACTOR RECEPTORS ON HEPATIC-DERIVED CELLS

An extensive study has been conducted in my laboratory to understand the nature of the receptors and the complexities of the signaling responses in which PAF is involved in the liver. Because we were able to determine that most of the hepatic signaling responses to PAF were localized to sinusoidal cells and we knew that Kupffer cells were able to synthesize[27] and to metabolize[28] PAF, our initial approach was to identify and then to characterize PAF receptors on sinusoidal cells in primary culture. Our studies have indicated that the Kupffer cell possesses PAF receptors that are highly specific with a K_d of approximately 0.45 nM and with a receptor density of between 10,000 and 12,000 per cell[29] (Figure 7). These receptors are coupled via specific G-proteins to both PLC and PLA$_2$ signaling mechanisms[30] which result in the production of inositol polyphosphates and diacylglycerol with intracellular calcium release and arachidonic acid metabolites, respectively.

Further, characterization of the regulatory characteristics of the PAF receptor indicated that cAMP analogues or forskolin (an activator of adenylate cyclase) also down-regulate the PAF receptor.[32] In all cases using Scatchard analysis down-regulation equates to a decrease in the number of receptors that can be detected by ligand-binding analyses with no effect observed on the affinity of the ligand for the surface receptor. Also, in all cases, the down-regulation of the PAF receptor causes a decrease in the biological response(s) of PAF on these cells (e.g., arachidonic acid release and/or eicosanoid synthesis is diminished).

In addition to being sensitive to cAMP-mediated regulation the Kupffer cell PAF receptor appears to be down-regulated following exposure to phorbol esters [e.g., protein kinase C (PKC) activation][33] (Figure 8). This down-regulation is transient (e.g., 50% reduction within 60 min of phorbol ester exposure); due to a decrease in the number of surface receptors with no appreciable change in the affinity of the receptor for its ligand; independent of new protein synthesis; and coupled to a decrease in the rate of arachidonic acid release.

Finally, in our ongoing experimental effort we have shown that the Kupffer cell PAF receptor is down-regulated by exposure to incubation conditions resulting in an increased level of phosphorylation of tyrosine residues on cellular proteins.[34-36] In these studies a very close correlation is apparent between the level of tyrosine phosphorylation and the surface expression of PAF receptors. Moreover, studies are currently being pursued to identify the various protein/enzyme substrates for the tyrosine kinases obviously active in controlling the PAF receptor and its subsequent signaling pathways. At present we have no data proving that the activation of various types of protein kinases actually phosphorylate the PAF receptor itself. In the absence of an immunological probe for the PAF receptor, such experiments are not feasible.

V. CONCLUSION

Nearly one decade ago we began an effort to establish the liver and its various constituent cell types as models for investigating various facets of the physiological/pathophysiological signaling mechanisms in which PAF is involved. Our conclusion after prosecuting this rather large body of work is that the liver is an exquisite model exhibiting a myriad of PAF-mediated effects crucial to trauma responses in which the liver plays a role. We remain

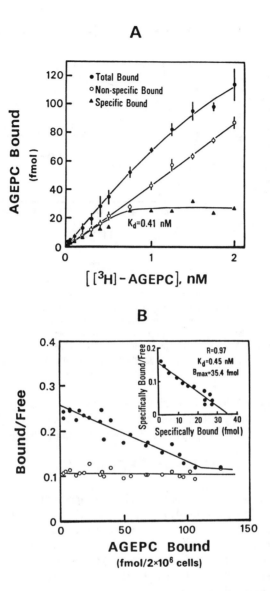

FIGURE 7. (A) Saturation curve of [³H]AGEPC binding to rat Kupffer cells. [³H]AGEPC in concentrations between 0.025 and 2.0 nM were incubated with 2×10^6 Kupffer cells in the presence or absence of 2 μM unlabeled AGEPC, at 25°C for 60 min. Specific binding (▲) was determined by subtracting nonspecific binding (○) from total binding (●). Each data point and bar represent the mean value ± standard error of measurements from three to six separate experiments which were performed in duplicate. (B) Scatchard analysis of the [³H]AGEPC binding to rat Kupffer cells. The results from the experiments performed in A were analyzed using a Scatchard plot. The total binding (●) and nonspecific binding (○) of [³H]AGEPC to the Kupffer cells were determined in the presence and absence, respectively, of 2 μM unlabeled AGEPC. The data shown here are the combination of the results from three experiments. (Inset) Scatchard plot of specific [³H]AGEPC binding to rat Kupffer cells. The specific binding is determined by subtracting nonspecific binding from total binding. The data in the inset are the mean value of measurements from three experiments which were performed in duplicate or triplicate. (Reprinted with permission of the *Journal of Biological Chemistry*.)

convinced that among the panoply of mediators produced during hepatic stress/trauma PAF and its receptor(s) are key in the molecular signaling that occurs between the cells of the hepatic sinusoid and parenchyma. The next phase of activity in our laboratory will be to employ the information made possible by the successful cloning and sequencing of the PAF receptor[37] to investigate receptor expression and regulation again in both normal physiological

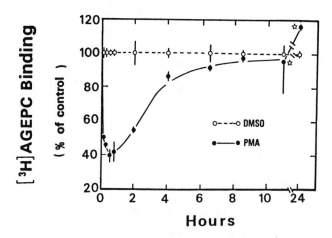

FIGURE 8. Time course of phorbol myristate acetate (PMA) inhibition of [³H]AGEPC binding to cultured Kupffer cells. Kupffer cells were incubated at 37°C in RPMI 1640 culture medium in the presence of DMSO (○) or PMA (40 nM, ●) for the indicated time period. The cells were then washed three times with Hank's buffer containing 0.1% bovine serum albumin at 25°C and incubated with 1.0 nM [³H]AGEPC at 25°C for 60 min in the absence or in the presence of an excess of unlabeled AGEPC (1.0 μM), after which the specific [³H]AGEPC binding was quantified. The data are presented as percentages of the control (51.2 ± 3.6 fmol, from 10 time points, measured in triplicate), which was preincubated in the absence of PMA. Star symbols indicate that 40 nM PMA was included in the binding medium during the [³H]AGEPC binding assay. (Reprinted with permission of *Archives of Biochemistry and Biophysics.*)

(Figure 9) and pathophysiological situations. Also of crucial importance is elucidating the relationships of both synergy and apposition that exist between the various lipid and peptide mediators elaborated by cells responsive to tissue injury and inflammation.

ACKNOWLEDGMENTS

The author would like to acknowledge funding in support of this research from the NIH (DK-19473 and DK-33538) and the Robert A. Welch Foundation. The author would also like to acknowledge the close collaboration between my laboratory and that of Donald J. Hanahan. Finally, this research activity would not have been possible without the outstanding contributions of R. Behal, D. Buxton, W. Chao, M. DeBuysere, R. Duffy-Krywicki, R. Fisher, C. R. Gandhi, K. Hill, M. Kester, R. Kumar, D. Lapointe, B. Levine, H. Liu, M. McCollum, T. Nouchi, S. Robertson, M. Steinhelper, S. Shukla, and W. Zhou.

Extracellular Space

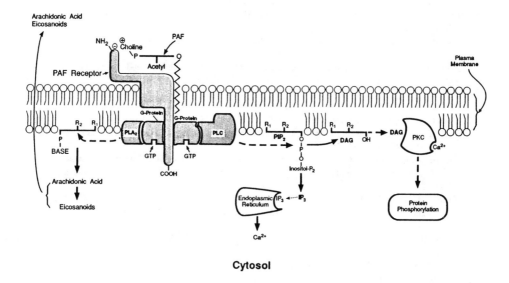

FIGURE 9.   Representation of the PAF receptor and its various signal transduction mechanisms.

REFERENCES

1. **Huijing, F.,** Glycogen metabolism and glycogen-storage diseases, *Physiol. Rev.,* 55, 609, 1975.
2. **Hers, H. G.,** The control of glycogen metabolism in the liver, *Annu. Rev. Biochem.,* 45, 167, 1976.
3. **Decker, K.,** Biologically active products of stimulated liver macrophages (Kupffer cells), *Eur. J. Biochem.,* 192, 245, 1990.
4. **Steinhelper, M. E., Duffy-Krywicki, R. H., and Olson, M. S.,** Regulation of hepatic glycogenolysis by vasoactive autacoid mediators, in *Perfused Liver,* Ballet, F. and Thurman, R. G., Eds., INSERM/John Libby, Paris, 1991, 121.
5. **Shukla, S. D., Buxton, D. B., Olson, M. S., and Hanahan, D. J.,** Acetylglyceryl ether phosphorylcholine. A potent activator of hepatic phosphoinositide metabolism and glycogenolysis, *J. Biol. Chem.,* 258, 10212, 1983.
6. **Fisher, R. A., Shukla, S. D., DeBuysere, M. S., Hanahan, D. J., and Olson, M. S.,** The effect of acetylglyceryl ether phosphorylcholine on glycolysis and phosphatidylinositol 4,5-bisphosphate metabolism in rat hepatocytes, *J. Biol. Chem.,* 259, 8685, 1984.
7. **Buxton, D. B., Fisher, R. A., Hanahan, D. J., and Olson, M. S.,** Platelet activating factor-mediated vasoconstriction and glycogenolysis in the perfused rat liver, *J. Biol. Chem.,* 261, 644, 1986.
8. **Buxton, D. B., Shukla, S. D., Hanahan, D. J., and Olson, M. S.,** Stimulation of hepatic glycogenolysis by acetylglyceryl ether phosphorylcholine, *J. Biol. Chem.,* 259, 1468, 1984.
9. **Buxton, D. B., Hanahan, D. J., and Olson, M. S.,** Specific antagonists of platelet activating factor-mediated vasoconstriction and glycogenolysis in the perfused rat liver, *Biochem. Pharmacol.,* 35, 893, 1986.
10. **Fisher, R. A., Kumar, R., Hanahan, D. J., and Olson, M. S.,** Effects of β-adrenergic stimulation on 1-O-hexadecyl-2-acetyl-*sn*-glycero-3-phosphocholine-mediated vasoconstriction and glycogenolysis in the perfused rat liver, *J. Biol. Chem.,* 261, 8817, 1986.
11. **Steinhelper, M. E., Fisher, R. A., Revtyak, G. E., Hanahan, D. J., and Olson, M. S.,** β_2-Adrenergic agonist regulation of immune aggregate- and PAF-stimulated hepatic metabolism, *J. Biol. Chem.,* 264, 10976, 1989.
12. **Hill, C. E., Sheridan, P. J., Hanahan, D. J., and Olson, M. S.,** Localization of platelet activating factor binding in the perfused rat liver, *Biochem. J.,* 253, 651, 1988.

13. **Hill, C. E. and Olson, M. S.,** Stimulation of uric acid release from the perfused rat liver following stimulation by platelet activating factor or potassium, *Biochem. J.,* 247, 207, 1987.

14. **Lapointe, D. S., Hanahan, D. J., and Olson, M. S.,** Mobilization of hepatic calcium pools by platelet activating factor, *Biochemistry,* 26, 1568, 1987.

15. **Steinhelper, M. E. and Olson, M. S.,** Regulation of immune-aggregate-stimulated hepatic glycogenolysis and vasoconstriction by vicinal dithiols, *Biochem. J.,* 249, 631, 1988.

16. **Altin, J. G., Dieter, P., and Bygrave, F. L.,** Evidence that Ga^{2+} fluxes and respiratory, glycogenolytic and vasoconstrictive effects induced by the action of platelet-activating factor and L-α-lysophosphatidyl-choline in the perfused rat liver are mediated by products of the cyclo-oxygenase pathway, *Biochem. J.,* 245, 145, 1987.

17. **Casteleijn, K., Kuiper, J., van Rooij, H. C. J., Kamps, J. A. A. M., Koster, J. F., and van Berkel, T. J. C.,** Hormonal control of glycogenolysis in parenchymal liver cells by Kupffer and endothelial liver cells, *J. Biol. Chem.,* 263, 2699, 1988.

18. **Casteleijn, E., Kuiper, J., van Rooij, H. C. J., Kamps, J. A. A. M., Koster, J. F., and van Berkel, T. J. C.,** Endotoxin stimulates glycogenolysis in liver by means of intercellular communication, *J. Biol. Chem.,* 263, 6953, 1988.

19. **Kuiper, J., DeRijke, Y. B., Zijlstra, F. J., Van Wass, M. P., and van Berkel, T. J. C.,** The induction of glycogenolysis in the perfused liver by PAF is mediated by PGD_2 from Kupffer cells, *Biochem. Biophys. Res. Commun.,* 157, 1288, 1988.

20. **Lapointe, D. S. and Olson, M. S.,** PAF-stimulated hepatic glycogenolysis is not mediated through cyclooxygenase-derived metabolites of arachidonic acid, *J. Biol. Chem.,* 264, 12130, 1989.

21. **Moy, J. A., Bates, J. N., and Fisher, R. A.,** Effects of nitric oxide on platelet-activating factor and α-adrenergic-stimulated vasoconstriction and glycogenolysis in the perfused rat liver, *J. Biol. Chem.,* 266, 8092, 1991.

22. **Buxton, D. B., Hanahan, D. J., and Olson, M. S.,** Stimulation of glycogenolysis and platelet activating factor production by heat-aggregated immunoglobulin G in the perfused rat liver, *J. Biol. Chem.,* 259, 13758, 1984.

23. **Fisher, R. A., Robertson, S. M., Steinhelper, M. E., Revtyak, G., Kumar, R., Hanahan, D. J., and Olson, M. S.,** Autocoid production and metabolic/hemodynamic responses to zymosan in the perfused rat liver, *Arch. Biochem. Biophys.,* submitted for publication.

24. **Duffy-Krywicki, R. H., Tasumi, Y., Kumar, R., Lapointe, D. S., and Olson, M. S.,** The effect of lipopolysaccharide on the synthesis of platelet activating factor and eicosanoids in the perfused rat liver, *Am. J. Physiol.,* submitted for publication.

25. **Zhou, W., Chao, W., Levine, B. A., and Olson, M. S.,** Platelet activating factor mediates hepatic injury during obstructive jaundice in the rat, *Am. J. Physiol.,* in press.

26. **Zhou, W., McCollum, M. O., Levine, B. A., and Olson, M. S.,** Inflammation and platelet activating factor production during hepatic ishemic/reperfusion, *Hepatology,* in press.

27. **Chao, W., Siafaka-Kapadai, A., Olson, M. S., and Hanahan, D. J.,** Biosynthesis of platelet activating factor by cultured rat Kupffer cells stimulated with calcium ionophore A23187, *Biochem. J.,* 257, 823, 1989.

28. **Chao, W., Siafaka-Kapadai, A., Hanahan, D. J., and Olson, M. S.,** Metabolism of platelet activating factor (PAF) and lyso-PAF by rat Kupffer cells, *Biochem. J.,* 261, 77, 1989.

29. **Chao, W., Liu, H., DeBuysere, M. S., Hanahan, D. J., and Olson, M. S.,** Identification of receptors for platelet activating factor in rat Kupffer cells, *J. Biol. Chem.,* 264, 13591, 1989.

30. **Gandhi, C. R. and Olson, M. S.,** Two distinct pathways of platelet activating factor-induced hydrolysis of phosphoinositides in cultures of rat Kupffer cells, *J. Biol. Chem.,* 265, 18234, 1990.

31. **Chao, W., Liu, H., Hanahan, D. J., and Olson, M. S.,** Regulation of platelet activating factor receptors in rat Kupffer cells, *J. Biol. Chem.,* 264, 20448, 1989.

32. **Chao, W., Liu, H., Zhou, W., Hanahan, D. J., and Olson, M. S.,** Regulation of platelet activating factor (PAF) receptors and PAF-receptor-mediated biological responses by cAMP in rat Kupffer cells, *J. Biol. Chem.,* 265, 17576, 1990.

33. **Chao, W., Liu, H., Hanahan, D. J., and Olson, M. S.,** Regulation of platelet activating factor (PAF) receptor and PAF receptor-mediated arachidonic acid release by protein kinase C activation in rat Kupffer cells, *Arch. Biochem. Biophys.,* 282, 188, 1990.

34. **Chao, W., Liu, H., Hanahan, D. J., and Olson, M. S.,** Platelet activating factor-stimulated protein tyrosine phosphorylation and eicosanoid synthesis in rat Kupffer cells: evidence for calcium-dependent and protein kinase C-dependent and -independent pathways, *J. Biol. Chem.,* 267, 6725, 1992.

35. **Chao, W., Liu, H., Hanahan, D. J., and Olson, M. S.,** Protein tyrosine phosphorylation and regulation of the receptor for platelet activating factor in rat Kupffer cells: effect of sodium vanadate, *Biochem. J.,* in press.

36. **Chao, W., Liu, H., Hanahan, D. J., and Olson, M. S.,** Tyrosine phosphorylation of GTPase-activating protein in cultured rat Kupffer cells stimulated with platelet activating factor and sodium vanadate, *J. Biol. Chem.,* submitted for publication.

37. **Nakamura, M., Honda, Z., Izumi, T., Sakanaka, C., Mutoh, H., Minami, M., Bito, H., Seyama, Y., Matsumoto, T., Noma, M., and Shimizu, T.,** Molecular cloning and expression of platelet-activating factor receptor from human leukocytes, *J. Biol. Chem.,* 266, 20400, 1991.

Chapter 8

PLATELET ACTIVATING FACTOR RECEPTOR-MEDIATED SIGNAL TRANSDUCTION MECHANISM IN NEUROHYBRID CELLS

Tian-Li Yue, Paul G. Lysko, Eitan Friedman, and Giora Feuerstein

TABLE OF CONTENTS

ISBN 0-8493-7299-2
© 1993 by CRC Press, Inc.

I. INTRODUCTION

Platelet activating factor (PAF) has been found in the central nervous system (CNS),[1-3] and its production by neuronal cells was confirmed recently in our laboratory[4] and others.[5] Specific binding sites for PAF have been found in synaptosomes and microsomal fractions of rat cerebral cortex[6] as well as gerbil brain tissue.[7] The effects of PAF on cerebral circulation and brain function have been observed *in vivo* and *in vitro*.[8,9] More recently, a role for PAF as a putative mediator in CNS injury, particularly in brain ischemia and traumatic injury-induced neuronal damage, has been suggested because the levels of PAF have significantly increased and the PAF antagonists have protective effects in these CNS pathological states (for a review, see Reference 10). However, little information is available regarding functional studies of PAF at the cellular level of neuronal tissues, in particular, signal transduction mechanisms. To this end, we have studied the effect of PAF on second messenger systems in two different neuronal derived cell lines: NG108-15 cells, a hybrid of mouse neuroblastoma/rat glioma cells, and NCB20, a hybrid of mouse neuroblastoma/Chinese hamster embryo brain cells. Both cell lines have been successfully used to study the neuronal regulation of intracellular Ca^{2+}.[11-13]

II. PLATELET ACTIVATING FACTOR-INDUCED INTRACELLULAR FREE Ca^{2+} ($[Ca^{2+}]_i$) ELEVATION[14,15]

PAF induced an immediate and concentration-dependent increase in $[Ca^{2+}]_i$ in both NG108-15 and NCB20 cells with EC_{50} values of 6.8 and 2.6 nM, respectively (Figure 1). The PAF metabolite/precusor, lyso-PAF, was ineffective at concentrations up to 20 μM. PAF-induced $[Ca^{2+}]_i$ elevation was inhibited by several structurally unrelated PAF antagonists such as BN50739, WEB2086, SRI63-441, and BN52021, in a concentration-dependent manner. The basal levels of $[Ca^{2+}]_i$ were not affected by the PAF antagonists and the PAF antagonists did not affect the bradykinin-, ATP-, or endothelin-1-induced increase in $[Ca^{2+}]_i$. The voltage-sensitive calcium channel blockers, nifedipine and diltiazem, up to 10 μM had no effect on the PAF-induced increase in $[Ca^{2+}]_i$; however, extracellular Ca^{2+} depletion caused an 82 and a 64% reduction of PAF-induced $[Ca^{2+}]_i$ elevation in NG108-15 and NCB20 cells, respectively. The remainder, contributed from intracellular sources, was inhibited by TMB8 (2.5 to 50 μM), an intracellular free-Ca^{2+} scavenger. Both cell lines exhibited homologous desensitization to the sequential addition of PAF, but no heterologous desensitization between PAF and other agonists such as bradykinin, endothelin, angiotensin II, and ATP was observed. The response of the two fusion parents of the NG108-15 cell line to PAF was different. PAF only induced $[Ca^{2+}]_i$ elevation in the fusion parent N18TG2 cells, a neuroblastoma cell line, but not in the fusion parent C6 glioma cells.

III. PLATELET ACTIVATING FACTOR-INDUCED PHOSPHATIDYLINOSITOL TURNOVER[15,16]

In both NG108-15 and NCB20 cells, PAF induced a concentration-dependent increase in phosphatidylinositol (PI) metabolism and the EC_{50} values for IP_3 formation was 5.1 and 1.96 nM, respectively (Figure 2). The maximal production of IP_3 was 159% over basal at 100 nM PAF in NG108-15 cells and 254% over basal at 50 nM PAF in NCB20 cells. The PAF-induced formation of IP_3 mainly was 1,4,5-IP_3, which was confirmed by HPLC, and the peak of 1,4,5-IP_3 was clearly apparent at 10 s after the addition of PAF. The PAF-induced PI metabolism in both NG108-15 and NCB20 cells was inhibited by the PAF antagonist BN50739 in a concentration-dependent manner with IC_{50} values of 3.6 and 6.5

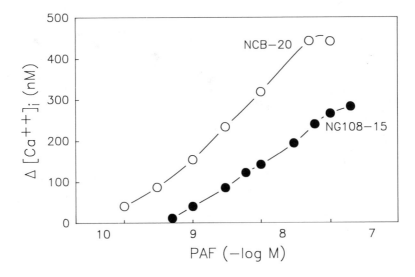

FIGURE 1. Concentration dependence of PAF-stimulated increase in $[Ca^{2+}]_i$ in NG108-15 and NCB20 cells.

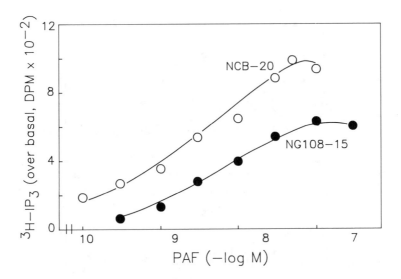

FIGURE 2. Concentration dependence of PAF-stimulated production of IP_3 in NG108-15 and NCB20 cells.

nM, respectively. The production of other PI metabolites such as IP_1 and IP_2 was also stimulated by PAF and inhibited by BN50739. In addition, PAF antagonists had no effect on the basal levels of PI metabolites in both cell lines.

IV. PROTEIN KINASE C IN THE REGULATION OF PLATELET ACTIVATING FACTOR-INDUCED Ca²⁺ SIGNAL AND PHOSPHOINOSITIDE TURNOVER

PAF at concentrations of 1 pM to 10 nM, dose-dependently stimulated protein kinase C (PKC) translocation in NCB20 cells. This redistribution in cellular PKC from cytosol to membrane-bound enzyme was inhibited by BN50739 (Figure 3). Furthermore, the PKC activator, phorbol 12,13-dibutyrate (PDBu) inhibited PAF-induced PI metabolism and $[Ca^{2+}]_i$

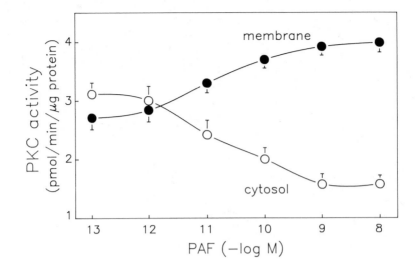

FIGURE 3. PAF-induced PKC translocation in NCB20 cells.

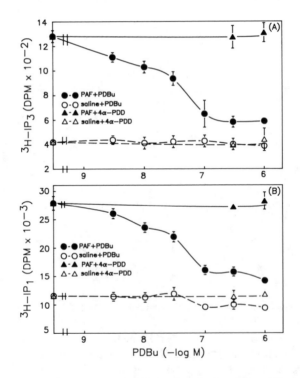

FIGURE 4. Effects of phorbol ester on PAF-induced production of IP_3 and IP_1 in NCB20 cells.

mobilization in both NCB20 and NG108-15 cells in a concentration-dependent manner. The maximal inhibition for IP_3 and IP_1 formation in NCB20 cells was 87 and 74%, respectively, in the presence of 1 μM PDBu (Figure 4). The basal accumulation of IP_3 and IP_1 was not affected by PDBu. The dose-response curve of PAF for inducing $[Ca^{2+}]_i$ elevation in NCB20 cells was shifted to the right and the maximal response of PAF was reduced by 81%. This suggested that PDBu inhibited PAF-induced $[Ca^{2+}]_i$ elevation not only via inhibition of PAF-induced IP_3 formation, but also by affecting PAF receptor-operated Ca^{2+} channels. However, the basal levels of $[Ca^{2+}]_i$ were not affected by PDBu. Neither PAF-induced PI metabolism nor PAF-induced $[Ca^{2+}]_i$ mobilization was affected by the biologically inactive 4α-phorbol (4α-PDD). The inhibitory effects of PDBu on both the PAF-induced increase in $[Ca^{2+}]_i$ and PI turnover were partially reversed by the PKC inhibitor H-7. These results seem to suggest that PAF-induced PKC activation may serve as a negative feedback to protect against cellular overstimulation.

V. G-PROTEINS COUPLED TO PLATELET ACTIVATING FACTOR RECEPTORS IN NEURONS

Receptor-mediated activation of phospholipase C (PLC) involves a GTP binding protein (G-protein) which serves as a coupling unit between the receptor and the effector PLC.[17] Studies with human neutrophils point to the existence of pertussis toxin (PT)-sensitive G-protein coupled to the PAF receptor.[18] Conversely, treatment of human platelet membranes with PT had no effect on GTPase activity stimulated by PAF.[19] Similar results were also recently reported in U937 cells, a human monocytic leukemic cell line, in which neither $[Ca^{2+}]_i$ mobilization nor PI turnover induced by PAF was sensitive to PT.[20] These data suggest that not only are the G-proteins coupled to various receptors different, but that the G-proteins coupled to the same receptor in diverse cell types may also be different. Pretreatment of NCB20 cells with PT significantly reduced PAF-induced production of IP_3 and IP_1 in a concentration-dependent manner. The maximal inhibition of PAF-induced IP_3 and IP_1 formation was 66.9 ± 3.5 and $45.8 \pm 4.3\%$, respectively, with a PT concentration of 300 ng/ml (n = 4). Increasing the PT concentration further did not increase the inhibitory effect on PAF-induced PI turnover. The PAF-induced increase in $[Ca^{2+}]_i$ in NCB20 cells was only moderately reduced ($16.6 \pm 6.5\%$) by PK (300 ng/ml) when the cells were suspended in KRH buffer containing 1 mM Ca^{2+}; however, the inhibitory effect of PT on the PAF-induced intracellular Ca^{2+} release increased substantially when the cells were suspended in Ca^{2+}-free KRH buffer, suggesting that the PAF receptor-operated Ca^{2+} channel appears to be insensitive to PT. Exposure of membranes prepared from NCB20 cells to [^{32}P]NAD and preactivated PT resulted mainly in a single band of radioactivity with an apparent mass of approximately 38 kDa, indicating the incorporation of [^{32}P]NAD into the protein due to PT-induced ADP-ribosylation of the substrate.[21] Pretreatment of the cells with various concentrations of PT inhibited, in a dose-dependent manner, the incorporation of [^{32}P]ADP-ribose into the substrate protein during the subsequent membrane labeling experiment. The maximal inhibition was observed when the concentration of PT reached 300 ng/ml; nearly all the ADP-ribosylation was inhibited, correlating well with the concentration of PT for producing maximal inhibition of PAF-induced PI metabolism and intracellular Ca^{2+} release. Figure 5 compares the effects of pretreatment of NCB20 cells to those of PT on PAF-induced IP_3 formation and [^{32}P]ADP-ribosylation, indicating that an additional PT-insensitive G-protein or mechanism exists for a portion of PAF-induced PI turnover. Using immunoprecipitation procedures, we confirmed that at least three α-subunits of the G-proteins ($G_{\alpha i(1,2)}$, $G_{\alpha s}$, and $G_{\alpha o}$) exist in NCB20 cells. Incubation of NCB20 cell membranes with increasing concentrations of PAF (0.01 to 10 nM) elicited a concentration-related stimulation in [^{35}S]GTPγS-binding to $G_{\alpha i(1,2)}$-protein; increased binding to $G_{\alpha s}$ and $_{\alpha o}$ was observed only at the highest concentration of PAF tested (Figure 6). PAF-induced [^{35}S]GTPγS-binding to $G_{\alpha i(1,2)}$-protein was markedly inhibited by the PAF antagonist, BN50739 (Figure 7). In addition PAF-evoked activation of $G_{\alpha i(1,2)}$ was significantly reduced by preincubation with PT (Table 1), but not by CTX. These results suggest that the PAF receptor couples selectively to $G_{\alpha i(1,2)}$ as compared to $G_{\alpha s}$ or $G_{\alpha o}$, especially at low concentrations of PAF; the PT-sensitive response to PAF in NCB20 cells is likely to be mediated mainly through the

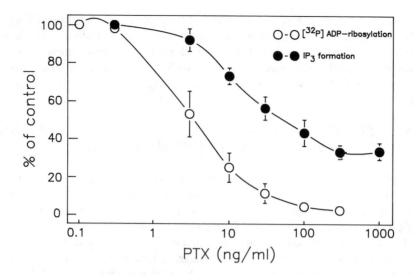

FIGURE 5. Inhibition of PAF-stimulated IP$_3$ formation and [^{32}P]ADP-ribosylation of 38-kDa membrane protein by PT.

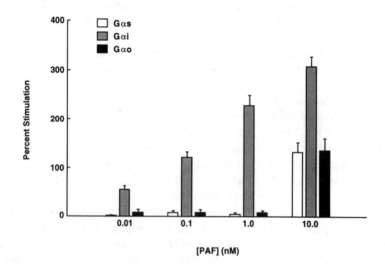

FIGURE 6. The effect of PAF on activation of G$_\alpha$-proteins in NCB20 cells.

activation of membrane G$_{\alpha i(1,2)}$-protein. This is in agreement with the results that pretreatment of NCB20 cells with PT resulted in a significant reduction of PAF-induced increase in IP$_3$ and IP$_1$ formation, and intracellular Ca^{2+} release.

VI. SUMMARY

Both in NG108-15 and NCB20 cells, PAF stimulates [Ca^{2+}]$_i$ elevation and PI metabolism through receptor activation, and the PAF-induced production of IP$_3$ is correlated with PAF-induced [Ca^{2+}]$_i$ mobilization. Phorbol ester inhibits the PAF-induced increase in PI turnover and rise in [Ca^{2+}]$_i$, which can be partially prevented by the PKC inhibitor H-7, indicating the involvement of PKC in the regulation of the PAF-induced signal transduction. PAF receptors appear to be selectively coupled to G$_{\alpha i}$-proteins and PAF signal transduction is mediated by both PT-sensitive and -insensitive pathways.

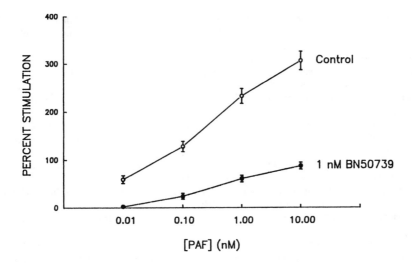

FIGURE 7. The effect of PAF antagonist, BN50739, on PAF-induced [^{35}S]GTPγS binding to membrane $G_{\alpha i(1,2)}$-protein of NCB20 cells.

TABLE 1
Effects of Pertussis Toxin (PT) on PAF-Induced [^{35}S]GTPγS Binding to Membrane G-Proteins

Percent Stimulation

	PAF (1 nM) n = 10	**PAF (10 nM) n = 10**
$G_{\alpha s}$	3.5 ± 2.8	110.3 ± 25.8
$G_{\alpha i(1,2)}$	230.8 ± 21.2	296.7 ± 20.7
$G_{\alpha o}$	7.0 ± 5.9	112.2 ± 29.3
	PTX + PAF (1 nM) **n = 4**	**PTX + PAF (10 nM)** **n = 4**
$G_{\alpha s}$	0.0 ± 0.0	88.8 ± 3.2
$G_{\alpha i(1,2)}$	38.0 ± 10.2	70.3 ± 16.4
$G_{\alpha o}$	0.0 ± 0.0	30.5 ± 4.6

REFERENCES

1. **Tokumura, A., Kamiyasu, K., Takauchi, K., and Tsukatani, H.,** Evidence for existence of various homologues and analogues of platelet-activating factor in a lipid extract of bovine brain, *Biochem. Biophys. Res. Commun.*, 145, 415, 1987.
2. **Kumar, R., Harvey, S. A. K., Kester, M., Hanahan, D. J., and Olson, M. S.,** Production and effects of platelet-activating factor in the rat brain, *Biochim. Biophys. Acta*, 963, 375, 1988.
3. **Lindsberg, P. J., Yue, T. L., Frerichs, K. U., Hallenbeck, J. M., and Feuerstein, G.,** Evidence of platelet-activating factor (PAF) as a noval mediator in experimental stroke in rabbits, *Stroke*, 21, 1452, 1990.
4. **Yue, T. L., Lysko, P. G., and Feuerstein, G.,** Production of platelet-activating factor from rat cerebellar granule cells in culture, *J. Neurochem.*, 54, 1809, 1990.
5. **Sogos, V., Bussolino, F., Pilia, E., Torelli, S., and Gremo, F.,** Acetylcholine-induced production of platelet-activating factor by human fetal brain cells in culture, *J. Neurosci. Res.*, 27, 706, 1990.

6. **Marcheselli, V. L., Rossowska, M. J., Domingo, M. T., Braquet, P., and Bazan, N. G.,** Distinct platelet-activating factor binding sites in synaptic endings and in intracellular membranes of rat cerebral cortex, *J. Biol. Chem.,* 265, 9140, 1990.

7. **Domingo, M. T., Spinnewyn, B., Chabrier, P. E., and Braquet, P.,** Presence of specific binding sites for platelet-activating factor (PAF) in brain, *Biochem. Biophys. Res. Commun.,* 151, 730, 1988.

8. **Kochanek, P. M., Nemoto, E. M., Melick, J. A., Evans, R. W., and Burke, D. F.,** Cerebrovascular and cerebrometabolic effects of intracarotid infused platelet-activating factor in rats, *J. Cereb. Blood Flow Metab.,* 8, 546, 1988.

9. **Lindsberg, P. J., Jacobs, T. P., Paakkari, I. A., Hallenbeck, J. M., and Feuerstein, G.,** Effect of systemic platelet-activating factor (PAF) on the rabbit spinal cord microcirculation, *J. Lipid Mediators,* 2, 41, 1990.

10. **Feuerstein, G., Yue, T. L., and Lysko, P. G.,** Platelet-activating factor. A putative mediator in central nervous system injury?, *Stroke,* 21(Suppl. 3), 90, 1990.

11. **Kornecki, E. and Ehrlich, Y. H.,** Neuroregulatory and neuropathological actions of the ether-phospholipid platelet-activating factor, *Science,* 240, 1792, 1988.

12. **Chuang, D. M. and Dillon-Carter, O.,** Characterization of bradykinin-induced phosphoinositide turnover in neurohybrid NCB-20 cell, *J. Neurochem.,* 51, 505, 1988.

13. **Noronha-Blob, L., Richard, C., and U'Prichard, D. C.,** Voltage-sensitive calcium channels in differentiated neuroblastoma × glioma hybrid (NG 108-15) cells: characterization by Quin 2 fluorescence, *J. Neurochem.,* 50, 1381, 1988.

14. **Yue, T. L., Gleason, M. M., Hallenbeck, J., and Feuerstein, G.,** Characterization of platelet-activating factor-induced elevation of cytosolic free-calcium level in neurohydbrid NCB-20 cells, *Neurscience,* 41, 177, 1991.

15. **Yue, T. L., Gleason, M. M., Gu, J. L., Lysko, P. G., Hallenbeck, J., and Feuerstein, G.,** Platelet-activating factor (PAF) receptor-mediated calcium mobilization and phosphoinositide turnover in neurohybrid NG 108-15 cells: studies with BN50739, a new PAF antagonist, *J. Pharmacol. Exp. Ther.,* 257, 374, 1991.

16. **Yue, T. L., Stadel, J. M., Sarau, H. M., Friedman, E., Gu, J. L., Powers, D. A., Gleason, M. M., Feuerstein, G., and Wang, H. Y.,** Platelet-activating factor (PAF) stimulates phosphoinositide turnover in neurohybrid NCB-20 cells. Involvement of pertussis toxin-sensitive G proteins and inhibition by protein kinase C, *Mol. Pharmacol.,* 41, 281, 1992.

17. **Birnbaumer, L., Abramowitz, J., and Brown, A. M.,** Receptor-effector coupling by G proteins, *Biochem. Biophys. Acta,* 1031, 163, 1990.

18. **Hwang, S. B.,** Identification of a second putative receptor of platelet-activating factor from human polymorphonuclear leukocytes, *J. Biol. Chem.,* 263, 3225, 1988.

19. **Houslay, M. D., Bojanic, D., Gawler, D., O'Hagan, S., and Wilson, A.,** Thrombin, unlike vasopressin, appears to stimulate two distinct guanine nucleotide regulatory proteins in human platelets, *Biochem. J.,* 238, 109, 1986.

20. **Barzaghi, G., Sarau, H. M., and Mong, S.,** Platelet-activating factor-induced phosphoinositide metabolism in differentiated U-937 cells in culture, *J. Pharmacol. Exp. Ther.,* 248, 559, 1989.

21. **Clark, M. A., Conway, T. M., Bennett, C. F., Crooke, S. T., and Stadel, J. M.,** Islet-activating protein inhibits leukotriene D$_4$- and leukotriene C$_4$- but not bradykinin- or calcium ionophore-induced prostacyclin systhesis in bovine endothelial cells, *Proc. Natl. Acad. Sci. U.S.A.,* 83, 7320, 1986.

Chapter 9

ACTIONS OF PLATELET ACTIVATING FACTOR ON SMOOTH AND CARDIAC MUSCLE: INTER- AND INTRACELLULAR SIGNALING MECHANISMS

A. G. Stewart and L. M. Delbridge

TABLE OF CONTENTS

ISBN 0-8493-7299-2
© 1993 by CRC Press, Inc.

I. INTRODUCTION

The discovery of platelet activating factor (PAF) as an additional mediator of immediate hypersensitivity reactions[1] has spawned an extensive effort to determine its contribution to the dysfunction of both cardiac and smooth muscle which figure prominently in anaphylaxis. The data that have emerged over the last 2 decades have provided unequivocal evidence of a role for PAF in animal models of cardiovascular shock of various etiologies, gastric ulceration, and the bronchopulmonary manifestations of immediate hypersensitivity reactions (see References 1 to 5 for reviews). PAF is also considered to have physiological roles in parturition[6-8] and possibly in the regulation of blood pressure.[9]

The involvement of PAF in models of disease has been established by examining the effects of exogenous PAF *in vivo* and in isolated tissue preparations, and by the modulatory effects of a wide range of PAF receptor antagonists.[10,11] This chapter focuses on evidence derived from functional studies for the existence of PAF receptors on smooth and cardiac muscle and, where possible, the direct effects of PAF are distinguished from those that are secondary to the release of other mediators, most notably the eicosanoids.

II. VASCULAR SMOOTH MUSCLE

A. SYSTEMIC HYPOTENSIVE ACTIONS

Intravenous administration of PAF elicits a dose-related and protracted decrease in systemic arterial blood pressure in a range of species including rat, guinea pig, rabbit, dog, pig, sheep, and nonhuman and human primates.[3,12,13] The mechanism(s) underlying the hypotensive effects include decreased cardiac output due to reduced cardiac contractility[14-16] and dilatation of resistance vessels,[17-19] resulting in a decrease in total peripheral vascular resistance.[20,21] However, in certain vascular beds PAF has well-documented vasoconstrictor actions, particularly in the coronary,[20,22-27] pulmonary,[28-30] cerebral,[13,31] and renal[20,32-34] circulations and in the microcirculation of the hamster cheek pouch.[35-37]

Pharmacological studies indicate that neither the central nor the autonomic nervous systems are required for the hypotensive actions of PAF,[38] although the activity of the latter modifies the duration of these responses.[39,40] In addition, the vasodilator responses of the gastric and mesenteric circulations are prolonged by indomethacin treatment, whereas those of the femoral circulation are curtailed, suggesting the involvement of thromboxane A_2 (TXA_2) and prostacyclin (PGI_2), respectively.[18]

B. VASODILATATION

Administration of PAF into the femoral arterial circulation of anesthetized dogs induced an increase in femoral blood flow which was enhanced by denervation. The peak responses were unaffected by pretreatment with indomethacin, theophylline or BW755c, excluding the involvement of PGI_2, adenosine, or lipoxygenase products, respectively.[19] In the rat autoperfused hindlimb preparation, PAF (1 to 10 pmol, intraarterial bolus) elicits a dose-related decrease in perfusion pressure without affecting systemic blood pressure, indicating a local vasodilator effect (Figure 1). These vasodilator responses were competitively antagonized by BN52021 (1 to 10 μM) or WEB2086 (1 to 10 μM), whereas the vasodilator responses to acetylcholine (30 pmol) were unaffected. Thus, the PAF receptor antagonists do not appear to interfere directly with the release or actions of endothelium-derived relaxing factor (EDRF; closely related or identical to nitric oxide). Similarly, WEB2086 had no effect on the release of EDRF from cultured bovine aortic endothelial cells stimulated with bradykinin.[41] The recent availability of inhibitors of nitric oxide biosynthesis should enable a clear definition of the role of this ephemeral vasodilator in the responses to PAF. It is of

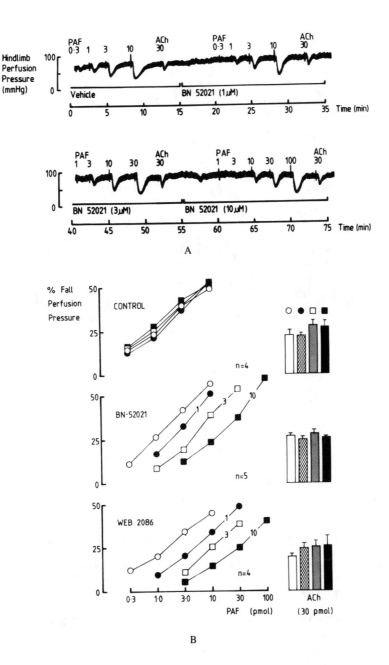

FIGURE 1. Vasomotor actions of PAF and PAF antagonists in the rat autoperfused hindlimb. (A) Bolus injections of PAF (0.3 to 10 pmol) induced dose-related decreases in hindlimb perfusion pressure, the duration of which was related to dose. (B) Infusion of BN52021 (1 to 10 μM) or WEB2086 (1 to 10μM) produced a apparently competitive antagonism, without influencing the vasodilator response to acetylcholine (30 pmol, open histograms) (Meinig, Dusting and Stewart, unpublished observations).

interest that both PAF receptor antagonists[42-45] and nitric oxide biosynthesis inhibitors[46] attenuate the profound fall in systemic arterial blood pressure in endotoxin shock, suggesting a link between these substances. Furthermore, PAF-induced vasoconstrictor responses in the hepatic circulation are attenuated by concomitant infusion of nitric oxide.[47] Thus, the ultimate response to PAF may represent a balance between the vasoconstrictor and vasodilator mechanisms that it initiates (see Figure 2).

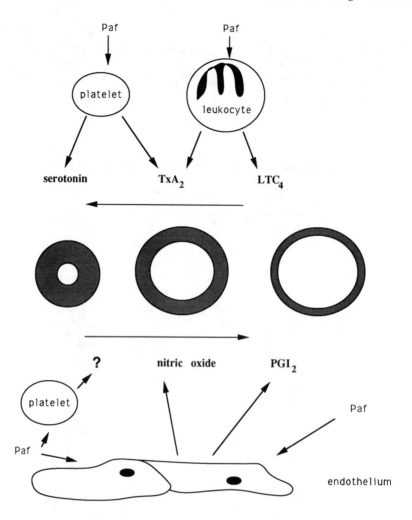

FIGURE 2. Vasomotor actions of PAF are highly dependent on interaction with endothelium, platelets, and leukocytes. Direct actions of PAF on vascular smooth muscle are unlikely at levels that may be encountered pathophysiologically. However, marked vasoconstrictor actions of PAF in blood-free perfused organs indicate that microvascular smooth muscle may be particularly sensitive to PAF. On the other hand, inhibition of these responses with eicosanoid antagonists and inhibitors suggests that resident inflammatory cells are the target.

C. SITES OF ACTION OF PLATELET ACTIVATING FACTOR IN THE VASCULATURE

1. Platelet Dependence of Vasoactivity

The observation of a hypotensive action of PAF in rats suggested a direct effect on the vasculature, because the platelets of this species are insensitive to PAF.[20] Nevertheless, it is evident from a number of studies that platelet activation products have a profound influence on the vasoactivity of PAF: the rabbit coronary and pulmonary circulations failed to respond to PAF unless platelets were included in the perfusion medium;[16,48] intracoronary administration of PAF in pigs and dogs resulted in a biphasic response, a brief dilator response followed by a vasoconstriction.[49,50] The initial response has been attributed to the release of a substance from platelets[51] which has yet to be characterized, and the later coronary vasoconstrictor response appears to be mediated exclusively by TXA_2 in pigs,[3,52] and by both TXA_2 and cysteinyl leukotrienes in dogs.[19,50] Extensive evidence can be found in buffer-perfused isolated hearts of rats and guinea pigs that indicates that PAF evokes vasoconstriction independently of platelets.[22-25,53] Similarly, PAF elicits an increase in perfusion pressure in isolated guinea pig or rat lungs perfused with physiological salt solutions[28,29] that is independent of platelets, but in the guinea pig it does depend on the generation of TXA_2.[29]

2. Endothelium-Dependent Vasodilation

More recent studies using buffer-perfused preparations have established that the pulmonary and renal circulations show a vasodilator response to relatively low doses of PAF.[54-56] It is not yet established whether this is a general phenomenon, because in other circulations, such as the hepatic, only vasoconstrictor responses have been reported.[47]

The finding that PAF was able to induce relaxation of the pulmonary artery only when the endothelium was intact suggested the involvement of an endothelium-derived relaxing substance.[54] Furthermore, Gillespie and Bowdy[57] showed that PAF infusion in rat isolated buffer-perfused lungs reduced vascular responsiveness to angiotensin II, but not to potassium chloride. In addition in lungs with elevated perfusion pressure due to angiotensin II infusion, PAF induced a decrease in perfusion pressure. Collectively, these data provided evidence consistent with the possibility that PAF released EDRF, which is increasingly being recognized as a major influence on the control of systemic blood pressure.[58]

Several lines of evidence suggest the existence of PAF receptors on endothelial cells. Radioligand binding studies,[59] evidence of receptor-mediated ultrastructural changes in human cultured umbilical vein endothelial cells,[60-62] and PAF-induced increases in intracellular Ca^{2+} [59,61,63] indicate a potential for PAF to induce nitric oxide release. However, EDRF/nitric oxide secretagogues (acetylcholine, bradykinin) almost invariably relax precontracted, endothelium-intact isolated arterial smooth muscle preparations,[64,65] whereas PAF appears to be inactive in most large arteries,[66-68] and in endothelial cells cultured from aorta.[69] In two of the four studies that show endothelium-dependent relaxation induced by PAF, extremely high doses were used in one study (10 μM),[70] and in the second no correlation existed between the potency of PAF analogues in inducing hypotension and their ability to relax isolated arterial preparations.[71]

In pulmonary and mesenteric arteries, PAF induced endothelium-dependent relaxations at a concentration range consistent with a specific effect.[54,72] In preparations of human pulmonary artery without endothelium, PAF at a concentration of 1 μM evoked small contractile responses in two of seven tissues. Preparations with an intact endothelial layer showed a diminished contractile response to histamine or $PGF_{2\alpha}$ in the presence of PAF (100 nM) which was not reduced by indomethacin, consistent with the involvement of EDRF.[73] PAF is reported to contract human isolated pial and feline isolated basilar arteries and to have relaxant actions when the arteries are preconstricted with $PGF_{2\alpha}$, the latter action being unaffected by indomethacin.[74]

Microvascular endothelial cells may express PAF receptors that are linked to EDRF/nitric oxide generation, explaining the ability of low concentrations of PAF to decrease the perfusion pressure in isolated lungs[54,58] and kidney.[55,75] In support of this possibility, it has been shown that PAF elicits a vasodilator response in the mesenteric circulation of the rat and relaxes isolated mesenteric arteries at a threshold concentration of 3 pM by a mechanism, which is sensitive to inhibitors of EDRF/nitric oxide biosynthesis.[72] Further evidence for a role for EDRF/nitric oxide in these relaxations was provided by Kamata et al.,[76] who demonstrated that the relaxations were insensitive to indomethacin and therefore were not due to PGI_2, but could be prevented by removal of the endothelium with short periods of exposure to detergents. On the other hand, PAF is known to release leukotrienes, and may release other vasoactive factors such as neuropeptides, that could in turn elicit the release of EDRF. Hence, the absence of an EDRF response in large arteries may reflect an absence of the cellular targets for PAF found in whole organs that release secondary mediators which, in turn, elicit the release of EDRF.

3. Direct Effects of Platelet Activating Factor on Vascular Smooth Muscle

As a consequence of the (usually) weak actions of PAF in isolated blood vessels, very few studies have been conducted of the direct effect of PAF on vascular smooth muscle. Cervoni et al.[70] reported direct relaxant actions of PAF in rat isolated aorta, but only at concentrations in excess of 10 μM and these responses may therefore represent nonspecific effects. Braquet and colleagues[67] examined both direct and indirect effects of PAF and the PAF receptor antagonist, BN52021, on rabbit aortic preparations with and without endothelium. Both PAF and BN52021 were inactive, irrespective of the presence of the endothelium, but PAF was reported to contract a longitudinal preparation of the rat portal vein[67] in which the integrity of the endothelium was not tested.

D. PLATELET ACTIVATING FACTOR RECEPTORS AND SIGNAL TRANSDUCTION IN VASCULAR SMOOTH MUSCLE

Despite the evidence that PAF has little, if any, direct effect on vascular smooth muscle, clear evidence is found of PAF receptors on rat vascular smooth muscle cells maintained in culture, in which PAF elicits the release of preloaded $^{45}Ca^{2+}$.[77] Direct evidence of Ca^{2+} mobilization was provided by studies of FURA-2-loaded rat aortic vascular smooth muscle cells showing that PAF (1 to 100 nM) increased intracellular calcium via receptors that were blocked by the PAF antagonists, CV6209 and WEB2086.[78] In contrast, PAF receptors linked to transmembrane Ca^{2+} movement were not detected in bovine cultured aortic vascular smooth muscle.[61] Human cultured vascular smooth muscle cells from aortic or coronary arteries express receptors for PAF that have also been shown to be linked to phosphoinositide (PI) hydrolysis.[79] Evidence for PAF receptors in vascular smooth muscle has come from studies of functional effects of PAF, rather than from PAF binding studies. Indirect evidence for an overlap in the signal transduction mechanisms for angiotensin II and PAF receptors was provided by Schwertschlag and Whorton,[80] who showed that PAF (1 to 100 nM) itself, induced a rise in intracellular Ca^{2+} in cultured vascular smooth muscle cells and that subsequent responses to angiotensin II (but not Arg-vasopressin) were desensitized, probably via activation of protein kinase C (PKC). In the latter study, PAF was found to elicit a transient rise in Ca^{2+} which preceded the rise in IP$_3$ and diacylglycerol, indicating that although PAF stimulates phospholipase C (PLC) in this cell type, the IP$_3$ is unlikely to contribute to the rise in Ca^{2+}. A mechanism for the rise in Ca^{2+} was not suggested, and in those cell types that have been investigated variability exists in the dependence of the increase in intracellular Ca^{2+} on extracellular Ca^{2+}, with activation of receptor-operated Ca^{2+} channels in macrophages,[81] neutrophils,[82,83] eosinophils,[84] and platelets,[85] and mobilization from intracellular stores in cultured endothelial cells.[61]

E. IS PLATELET ACTIVATING FACTOR A MEDIATOR OF ENDOTHELIN-INDUCED HEMODYNAMIC EFFECTS?

Endothelin-induced lethality in rats,[86] in which the initial hypertension is followed by hypotension, shows some similarity to the sudden death induced by PAF in rabbits which comprises a cessation of respiration, a precipitous fall in blood pressure, and a marked rise in plasma TXA$_2$.[87] Endothelin-induced lethality in rats is reported to be inhibited by pretreatment with PAF antagonists.[86] The reduction by PAF antagonists of the endothelin-stimulated increases in intracellular Ca^{2+} in rat cultured vascular smooth muscle provided a potential explanation for the protective effects of PAF receptor antagonists *in vivo*.[86] Furthermore, these findings suggested a role for PAF in the endothelin-induced increases in intracellular Ca^{2+}, possibly as a second messenger.[78] In a further study, PAF and endothelin were found to stimulate increases in both PGI_2 and TXA_2 biosynthesis in cultured vascular smooth muscle, and CV6209 inhibited the increase in PGI_2 levels.[88] PAF itself was previously demonstrated to stimulate PGI_2 synthesis by vascular ring preparations from several species, including humans.[89] The inhibition of PGI_2 generation in endothelin-stimulated vascular smooth muscle by CV6209 was proposed to occur by an intracellular action of PAF receptor antagonists on endogenous PAF,[88] similar to earlier suggestions regarding a relationship between PAF and eicosanoid generation in macrophages,[90,91] endothelial cells,[92] and neutrophils.[41] It is important, however, that the latter three cell types are known producers of PAF. Our recent studies have identified PAF production in porcine vascular smooth muscle in response to stimulation with bradykinin or endothelin as detected by bioassay, thin-layer chromatography (TLC), immunoassay, and gas chromatography/mass spectroscopy (GC/MS).[93,94] In addition rat cultured vascular smooth muscle produces PAF in response to endothelin and other vasoconstrictor peptides.[202] The time course of the endothelin-induced increase in intracellular Ca^{2+} is rapid (within 2 to 3 s); hence, it will be important to determine whether PAF synthesis occurs within such a short period.

Endothelin was originally identified as a vasoconstrictor peptide,[95] but several studies now indicate a stimulatory effect on the proliferation of cultured vascular smooth muscle.[96] Similarly, PAF is reported to stimulate the proliferation of porcine pulmonary vascular smooth muscle and to synergize with platelet-derived growth factor (PDGF).[97] These activities may underlie the apparent contribution of PAF to the intimal thickening in rabbits made atherosclerotic by cholesterol feeding.[98]

F. CORONARY CIRCULATION

Interest has grown considerably in the coronary vasomotor actions of PAF, as this mediator may contribute to the vascular and myocardial manifestations of cardiac anaphylaxis,[23,99-101] graft rejection, and myocardial ischemia.[102-106]

Initially, Levi et al.[23] reported that infusion of PAF into guinea pig isolated hearts elicited vasoconstrictor responses that were insensitive to inhibition by indomethacin or the leukotriene antagonist, FPL55712. In rat hearts, PAF induced the release of leukotriene C_4 (LTC_4) and TXA_2, which made a substantial contribution to the coronary vasoconstriction.[24,25] A number of subsequent studies have sought to resolve the relative roles of eicosanoids and a possible direct coronary vasoconstriction induced by PAF.[26,107] The eicosanoid release by PAF-stimulated rat hearts was confirmed as was the contribution of these products to the vasoconstriction and other cardiac effects.[27,108] In addition, *in vivo* studies in pigs[52] and dogs[16,19,49,50,109] provided clear evidence of a contribution of TXA_2 and to a lesser extent, LTC_4, in the reduction in coronary blood flow and other cardiac effects induced by PAF. The apparent decrease in importance of LTC_4 in *in vivo* as compared to *in vitro* studies may reflect an increase in TXA_2 generation and contribution due to the presence of platelets *in vitro*.

In guinea pig hearts, the contribution of eicosanoids has been observed when PAF is given as a bolus challenge,[53,110,111] but not when given by infusions.[23,112] The release of eicosanoids by guinea pig buffer-perfused hearts is controversial; Piper and Stewart[110,111] observed both TXB_2 and LTC_4 release, Stahl et al.[112] reported that infusion of 50 nM PAF failed to release detectable levels of either LTC_4 or TXB_2, Viosatt et al.[113] reported that a 100-nmol bolus dose of PAF induced TXB_2, but not LTC_4 release, and Felix et al.[53] reported that a 0.23-nmol bolus dose of PAF markedly stimulated TXB_2 release, but did not assay for leukotriene release.[53] In relation to the contribution of eicosanoids to the coronary vasoconstriction induced by PAF in guinea pig hearts, it is important to note that the vasoconstriction is protracted, whereas the release of leukotrienes is transient.[26,111] It is likely that the protracted vasoconstriction induced by PAF results from an eicosanoid-independent action which remains dependent on PAF receptor activation. The increase in perfusion pressure induced by a single bolus dose of PAF was reversible by infusion of a PAF receptor antagonist up to 30 min later, suggesting either prolonged activation of PAF receptors or autogeneration of PAF in response to the original bolus dose.[26] A contribution of both cyclooxygenase and lipoxygenase products to the dysrhythmogenic effects of PAF has been reported.[107,114,115] In addition, some agreement is seen that TXA_2 is partially responsible for the coronary vasoconstriction induced by PAF.[53,110,111] Thus, studies examining PAF infusions may fail to detect a contribution of leukotrienes and thromboxane to the early peak vasoconstriction. The reasons for variable findings with respect to eicosanoid release and participation in the coronary constrictor effects of PAF may relate to differences in dosage, in the detection limits of the assays, and to the different methods of coronary perfusion.

III. CARDIAC MUSCLE

The proposal that PAF acts directly on the myocardium to exert its negative inotropic action has been difficult to evaluate. The profound hypotension elicited by systemic administration of PAF is associated with a depression of cardiac performance, usually measured as reductions in cardiac output and left ventricular pressure development[116-118] and the coincident occurrence of conduction abnormalities. These alterations in cardiac function may reflect the major hemodynamic disturbances, the specific actions of PAF on coronary blood flow, and/or a direct negative inotropic influence on the myocardium exerted either by PAF or by secondary mediators released in response to PAF. The inotropic effects of PAF in various preparations are presented in Table 1.

A. CORONARY VASCULAR RESPONSES AND MYOCARDIAL CONTRACTILITY

In vivo and *in vitro* investigations have indicated that PAF may elicit coronary vasoconstriction and/or vasodilation depending on the species, dose, and experimental conditions. When intracardiac infusion or injection of PAF elicits sustained vasoconstriction, it is invariably linked with a reduction in myocardial contractile performance. In the guinea pig isolated heart, a number of studies have demonstrated that PAF induces a reduction in coronary flow coupled with diminished contractility.[22,119,120] In contrast, a sustained increase in circumflex coronary artery blood flow has been recorded in the dog in response to intracoronary injection of PAF. In this instance, elevated flow was not associated with a negative inotropic effect.[51] Studies using isolated heart preparations from the rabbit have indicated that in the absence of blood perfusate, this species is unresponsive to intracoronary PAF injection as evidenced by the lack of effect on electrical and mechanical parameters.[16,105] In the pig, *in vivo* recordings during intracoronary PAF infusion have documented a triphasic change in coronary blood flow (initial increase followed by a precipitous decrease preceding partial recovery) accompanied by a decline in regional contractile shortening fraction throughout.[52]

In experiments using guinea pig and rat isolated Langendorff hearts perfused at constant flow, PAF induced a decrease in left ventricular contractile parameters, suggesting that the negative inotropic action was not a consequence of reduced flow.[23-27,112,121] In the guinea pig the response to PAF was not modified by the cysteinyl leukotriene receptor antagonists FPL55712[23] or LY-171,883,[112] by inhibition of the cyclooxygenase pathway with indomethacin,[23,26] or by thromboxane synthase inhibition with OKY-1581.[112] Pretreatment with various PAF antagonists was able to prevent the impairment of contractility by PAF.[26,112,121] In these studies in which the perfusion of the coronary vasculature was controlled, the

TABLE 1
Species, Tissue, and Concentration-Related Variability in Inotropic
Responses to PAF

Species	Tissue/Preparation	Conc/dose	Inotropic action[a]	Ref.
Guinea pig	Langendorff heart	Bolus, intraaortic	NIE	22, 23, 120
Dog	*In vivo*	Bolus, intracoronary	No effect	51
Rabbit	Langendorff heart	Infusion, intracoronary	No effect	105
Pig	*In vivo*	Infusion, intracoronary	NIE	52
Guinea pig	Lang. heart, const. flow	Bolus, intracoronary	NIE	23, 26, 112, 121
Rat	Lang. heart, const. flow	Bolus, intracoronary	NIE	24, 25, 27
Rabbit	Lang. heart, const. flow	Bolus, intracoronary	No effect	16
Guinea pig	Papillary muscle	0.1 nM	Biphasic PIE/NIE	122
		0.01–0.1 nM	PIE	125
		1–100 nM	NIE	125
		1–1000 nM	NIE	126
		10 μM	NIE	23
		10 μM	PIE	127
		<1 μM	No effect	127
	Isolated atria	<1 nM	PIE	129
		≥1 nM	NIE	203
		0.1 nM–10 μM	NIE	23
		0.1–100 μM	No effect	130
Rat	Isolated atria	0.1–100 μM	PIE	130
		100 μM	PIE	70
		≤10 μM	No effect	70
Dog	Purkinje fibres	1–10 μM	Biphasic PIE/NIE	127
		>10 μM	NIE	127
Human	Papillary muscle	0.1–1000 nM	Biphasic PIE/NIE	131
	Atrial muscle	0.1–1000 nM	NIE	132

[a] NIE (negative inotropic effect), PIE (positive inotropic effect).

negative inotropic effect of PAF could not be attributed to the secondary actions of released eicosanoids. Of additional interest was the observation in one study[121] that PAF impaired myocardial relaxation more markedly than contraction — a finding that implies a role for PAF in the modulation of diastolic compliance. In the rat Langendorff perfused heart results have conflicted regarding the involvement of eicosanoids as secondary mediators of the negative inotropic effect. In one study[24] the PAF-induced decrease in cardiac contractility was prevented by indomethacin, but not by FPL55712. This contrasts with other findings indicating that neither cyclooxygenase inhibitors nor thromboxane receptor antagonists abolished the reduction in contractility elicited by PAF.[27]

Although these results in isolated hearts are suggestive of a direct effect of PAF on the myocardium, the maintenance of global coronary flow cannot preclude the possibility of local ischemia. Variation in microvascular tone and regional shunting may underlie the impaired mechanical function observed in response to PAF, even under "constant flow" conditions.

B. EFFECTS OF PLATELET ACTIVATING FACTOR ON ISOLATED CARDIAC TISSUES

To eliminate the potentially confounding effects of variation in perfusion associated with measurement of intact heart function, a number of studies have investigated the effect of PAF on isolated cardiac tissue preparations. Notwithstanding species differences, a confusing spectrum of mechanical and electrophysiological responses have been reported.

Guinea pig papillary muscles are reported to exhibit a biphasic response to relatively low concentrations of PAF (about 0.1 n*M*) characterized by an initial positive and subsequent negative inotropism.[122] At the same concentration, an increase followed by a decrease in action potential duration has been observed.[118] Because the duration of the action potential plateau is controlled largely by the magnitude of the inward calcium current, these data suggest an involvement of the L-type Ca^{2+} channel in mediating the effects of PAF. This suggestion, however, is difficult to reconcile with the additional observation in the former study that the negative, but not the positive, inotropic phase was suppressed by the Ca^{2+} channel blocker verapamil. Verapamil may not be an appropriate tool to use in attempting to characterize the L-type Ca^{2+} channel involvement in the response to PAF as it is established that compounds of this class bind to PAF binding sites and may therefore act as receptor antagonists.[123,124] In the same preparation, concentrations of 10 and 100 p*M* monophasically increased isometric force development, while reduced force development was observed within the concentration range of 1 to 100 n*M*.[125] At a slightly higher concentration range (1 to 1000 n*M*), Robertson et al.[126] reported a negative inotropic effect and a shortened action potential duration which they correlated with reduced intracellular Na^+ levels. This observation prompted the suggestion that the Na^+/Ca^{2+} exchanger may be involved by producing a calcium efflux coupled to a sodium influx in response to a depleted intracellular Na^+ concentration.[126] At an even higher concentration (10 μ*M*), in two conflicting studies, PAF produced a negative[23] and a positive[127] inotropic effect. In the latter report, in which PAF applied at lower concentrations failed to elicit any response, the increased contractility was linked with a shorter action potential duration. Because the effects of PAF in this study were similar to those of lysophosphatidylcholine and acyl carnitine, it was concluded that the influence of all three agents could be attributed to the nonspecific interaction of amphiphiles with the sarcolemmal membrane. Indeed, PAF is known to perturb membranes and induce ion channel formation at these pharmacological concentrations.[128]

In guinea pig atrial preparations a diverse range of effects have also been recorded. One group of investigators has reported a positive inotropic response to PAF levels lower than 1 n*M* and a negative inotropic effect at higher concentrations.[129] In this instance, however, verapamil blocked the positive inotropism. No effect on the action potential configuration was observed over the entire concentration range and Ca^{2+} flux measurements indicated an increased Ca^{2+} uptake at the lower concentration range only. The failure to observe a reduction in Ca^{2+} uptake at the higher concentration range suggests that neither the Na^+/Ca^{2+} exchanger nor the Ca^{2+}-L channel is involved in the negative inotropic action. All inotropic responses were selectively inhibited by the specific PAF antagonist BN52021, but were unaffected by pretreatment with adrenoceptor and muscarinic receptor blockers or by cyclooxygenase inhibition.[129] In other experiments using the same tissue, contradictory results have been obtained. A consistent reduction in the contractility of isolated left atria over the range 10 p*M* to 10 μ*M* PAF has been described,[23] as has a lack of effect of PAF on contractile performance at concentrations between 0.1 and 100 μ*M*.[130]

Fewer studies have been undertaken in other species. PAF was observed to substantially enhance the contractility of rat atria[70,130] with no evidence of a depressor effect. This action was blocked by propranolol,[70] suggesting that locally released catecholamines may be responsible.[127] In dog purkinje fibers a dose-dependent biphasic inotropic response to PAF has been reported. At concentrations of 1 to 10 μ*M* PAF elicited a transient positive inotropic effect followed by a maintained decrease in twitch amplitude, but at higher concentrations only the negative inotropic effect was observed. Action potential amplitude, upstroke velocity, and resting membrane potential were decreased by PAF. All these elctrophysiological and mechanical effects were ascribed to nonspecific amphiphilic effects.[127] Finally, the study of human tissues has also produced disparate results. Papillary muscle fragments exhibited biphasic responses to PAF applied at concentrations of 100 p*M* to 1 μ*M*. The initial increase in contractility was blocked by propranolol, and the succeeding negative inotropism was only partially suppressed by indomethacin.[131] Over an identical concentration range, PAF elicited a monophasic negative inotropic response in human atrial pectinate muscle, which was unaffected by application of indomethacin or FPL55712, but blocked by PAF antagonists.[132]

Considerable uncertainties thus remain in the interpretation of data derived from isolated tissues exposed to PAF. In particular, the contribution to the inotropic responses of PAF-induced release of mediators from nonmyocardial cell types (i.e., epithelial, neural, and inflammatory) present in these preparations is unclear. Indeed, the evidence above suggests that the occurrence of biphasic inotropism may be a consequence of transient catecholamine release. The use of cumulative concentration-response protocols[129] under these circumstances may obscure some components of the response. It is interesting that biphasic responses were observed in both atrial and ventricular preparations, possibly reflecting the dense noradrenergic innervation of both these tissues.

Electrophysiological studies have also generated confusing data. Apparently both prolongation and shortening of the action potential duration can be associated with a positive inotropic influence. Attention has focused on seeking a role for the L-type Ca^{2+} channel, but it is feasible that alterations in K^+ channel activity underlie PAF-induced changes in action potential plateau configuration. Other phospholipid-derived mediators have been identified as modulators of K^+ channel conductance in cardiac cells.[133] Altered K^+ channel currents may in fact constitute what have been designated as 'nonspecific amphiphilic effects'.

C. PLATELET ACTIVATING FACTOR EXERTS A DIRECT NEGATIVE INOTROPIC EFFECT ON ISOLATED CARDIOMYOCYTES

In view of the inconclusive nature of data derived from experiments *in vivo* and from isolated tissues *in vitro*, we have investigated the effect of PAF on the isotonic contraction of ventricular cells acutely isolated from the adult guinea pig. PAF induced a marked and significant negative inotropic effect, reducing maximum shortening by 23% (Figure 3A). The onset of this effect was relatively slow. The changes in the cell contraction profile (Figure 3B) included a significant reduction in the maximum rate of shortening and in the overall duration of the contraction cycle. In these experiments we were unable to find evidence of a selective effect of PAF on relaxation parameters as reported to occur in guinea pig papillary muscle.[121] In addition, no detectable positive inotropic (i.e., biphasic) component of the response was found at this concentration. A complete characterization of cell contractile responses over an extended concentration range would be necessary to confirm that biphasic responses observed in multicellular preparations arise indirectly from actions on other cell types.

With the use of the isolated cardiac cell model, we have been able to demonstrate that PAF has the capacity to exert a direct negative inotropic effect on the myocardium, independent of its capacity to modulate coronary vascular tone or to release secondary mediators from noncardiomyocyte cell types. The role of PAF as a physiologic/pathologic regulator of myocardial cell contractility is unclear. Other phospholipase A_2 (PLA_2) metabolic products have been recently identified as modulators of membrane permeability in cardiac cells. It is possible that PAF has a homeostatic function as an intra- or extracellular mediator in controlling cell contractile status.

IV. GASTROINTESTINAL SMOOTH MUSCLE

In common with many low molecular weight mediators of anaphylaxis, PAF causes contraction of smooth muscle preparations obtained from a number of different sites in the gatrointestinal tract (GIT) including the stomach,[134,135] the ileum,[56,135] duodenum, jejunum,

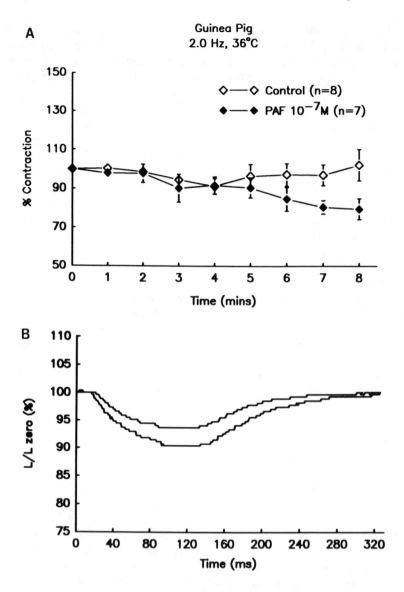

FIGURE 3.   Isolated myocytes were prepared by an enzymatic dissociation procedure[199] from the left ventricles of adult guinea pigs killed by cervical dislocation. Cells were transferred to a temperature (36°C) and flow (2.0 ml/min) controlled superfusion chamber[200] on the stage of an inverted microscope and stimulated to contract at 2.0 Hz using platinum field electrodes. A rapid computer-based imaging technique with high temporal (1 ms) and spatial (0.4 μm) resolution was used to locate cell boundaries during the contraction/relaxation cycle and to generate a profile of cell shortening from which contraction parameters were derived for each contractile event recorded.[201] (A) Time course of the action of PAF (100 nM in 0.25% BSA) on maximum cell contraction. An experimental protocol was designed to enable each cell to be used as its own control. After the initial stabilization of cell performance, contractions immediately prior to and during an 8-min test period were compared for a group of untreated cells and a group exposed to 100 nM PAF. Contractile performance of each cell (measured as maximum cell shortening and expressed as a proportion of resting length) was normalized to 100% at time "0", immediately prior to test period. (B) Contraction profile of an individual PAF (100 nM) -treated cell recorded immediately prior to (lower trace) and after an 8-min test period (upper trace). Cell shortening during the contraction cycle is shown as a proportion of resting cell length (L_{zero}).

and colon.[135] The use of the ascending colon as an alternative and highly sensitive bioassay tissue for PAF has been proposed,[136] but a degree of tachyphylaxis may limit its usefulness for some purposes. The receptor dependence of the contractile action of PAF has been established by the susceptibility of these responses to inhibition with specific PAF receptor antagonists and by the presence of specific binding sites.[137,138] In contrast, one study found that PAF (10 nM) -induced contractile responses in the guinea pig ileum were only partially and nonspecifically antagonized by high (10 to 100 μM) concentrations of PAF antagonists such as alprazolam and L-652,731, suggesting the existence of PAF receptor subtypes in this tissue.[56] Contrary to the frequent observation of contractile actions of PAF, it was reported that PAF induced relaxation of guinea pig *taenia coli* strips, but this action required concentrations in excess of 1 μM and was not shown to be dependent on receptor activation.[139]

Induction of increased gastric motility by local intraarterial PAF infusion could be attenuated by a histamine H_2 receptor antagonist and methysergide, indicating the involvement of histamine and serotonin and a possible direct contractile effect.[140] A second phase of gastric contractility was attenuated by tetrodotoxin, but not by antagonists of α- or β-adrenoceptors, or muscarinic, or nicotinic receptors, consistent with the involvement of nonadrenergic noncholinergic nerves.[140] It has been proposed that local release of PAF and the ensuing contractile response may play a role in the regulation of gastric emptying and elicit an increase in duodenal reflux.[140]

In relation to the possible role of PAF in the GIT, it may be significant that PAF is a normal constituent of the stomach[141,142] and while it is present in the highest concentration in the mucosa, it is also detectable in muscular regions.[142] The physiological role of this constitutive PAF production is not known, but interestingly, water-immersion stress of rats causes a profound fall in antral levels of PAF.[142]

The contractile effects of PAF on the GIT, in concert with its other effects on the mucosal blood flow and leukocyte chemotaxis, indicate that PAF is a strong candidate for contributing to a number of GIT inflammatory disorders.[5,143]

V. AIRWAYS SMOOTH MUSCLE

PAF is a potent bronchoconstrictor with the additional capacity to induce a relatively long-lasting increase in nonspecific bronchial reactivity. The mechanism of the bronchoconstriction seems to depend on the route of administration and the species being investigated. Many of the bronchomotor actions of PAF appear to be secondary to the activation of local and circulating inflammatory cells.

A. PARENCHYMAL LUNG STRIPS

Preparations of the parenchyma mounted in organ baths provide a means of investigating the pulmonary actions of PAF. However, it must be remembered that these preparations are heterogeneous in cellular composition with blood vessels and resident inflammatory cells as potential targets for the actions of PAF other than airways smooth muscle.

PAF has been reported to contract the guinea pig lung parenchymal strip independently of arachidonic acid metabolites or histamine and the responses were unaffected by neutrophil depletion.[144] Furthermore, contractile responses of rat lung strips (platelets insensitive to PAF) and lack of contractile material in supernatants of PAF-stimulated guinea pig platelets suggested that platelets were not involved in these responses and led the authors to propose a direct contractile action.[144] In contrast, partial inhibition of PAF-induced guinea pig lung strip contractions by tetrodotoxin or atropine and enhancement by physostigmine together with a lack of effect of hexamethonium suggested that PAF activation of postganglionic parasympathetic nerves contributes to its airways constrictor action.[145] Although indirect evidence has been found that PAF may enhance cholinergic transmission *in vivo* as a component of its ability to induce bronchial hyperreactivity,[146] no evidence has been found to suggest a quantitatively important role for parasympathetic nerves in the acute bronchoconstrictor effects of PAF.

Some of the more recent studies of PAF-induced contractions of lung strips do suggest a role for eicosanoids, because the contractions are inhibited by the flavonoid, gossypol,[147] and by high concentrations of the dual cyclooxygenase/lipoxygenase inhibitor, BW755c, but not by TXA_2 antagonists, despite the generation of significant levels of TXB_2 in response to PAF.[148] Similarly, PAF-induced contraction of rabbit lung strip has been ascribed to lipoxygenase rather than cyclooxygenase products.[149] In contrast, the leukotriene synthesis inhibitor/receptor antagonist REV5901 did not inhibit PAF-induced contractions of guinea pig lung strips.[150] McManus and co-workers[151] reported that rabbit lung strips fail to respond to PAF, and suggested that this was due to the lack of a single layer of pleural smooth muscle present in and essential for the PAF-induced contraction of guinea pig lung strips.

B. CONDUCTING AIRWAYS SMOOTH MUSCLE

Relatively high concentrations of PAF (0.07 to 0.7 μM) were found to elicit contractile responses of variable magnitude in human isolated airways which were inhibited by 1 μM WEB2086.[152] Interestingly, PAF induced an increased responsiveness to histamine which was also blocked by WEB2086.[152] The ratio of antagonist to PAF (~1:1) in the latter study contrasts with the usual WEB2086:PAF ratio required for antagonism of between 100 to 1000:1 (e.g., platelet responses), suggesting that receptors in these human airways might differ in affinity or accessibility compared with those on platelets. Recent studies of the mechanism of PAF-induced contraction failed to reveal any correlation between the magnitude of the response to PAF and the presence of inflammatory cells in the human isolated airway preparation.[153]

Studies of canine tracheal segments *in situ* suggested that PAF-induced constriction was at least partly mediated by the activation of cholinergic nerves.[146,154,155] However, canine isolated tracheal smooth muscle failed to respond to PAF, and the contractions observed in the presence of platelets were not inhibited by atropine, but were sensitive to methysergide or CV3988, implying that PAF mediated release of platelet serotonin.[156] Further studies in the dog demonstrated that a component of the tracheal contraction elicited by local intraarterial injection could be explained by the activation of postganglionic parasympathetic nerves, but bronchoconstrictor responses (changes in airways resistance, compliance) were not measured.[154] Local injection of PAF into the tracheal circulation results in a contractile response which correlated strongly with the arteriovenous difference in serotonin, but serotonin does not mediate the parasympathetic component of the PAF response, since muscarinic receptor antagonism had no effect on the constrictor effect of serotonin.[157]

The difficulty in reconciling *in vitro* and *in vivo* observations on the contractile responses to PAF may be related to the absence of a tonic vagal parasympathetic outflow in the isolated preparation. Synergism between exogenous bronchoconstrictors and neural mechanisms is an important consideration in analyzing the effects of drugs *in vivo*.

In contrast to the lack of effect of PAF on canine isolated trachea, PAF reduced the resting tone in guinea pig trachea[158,159] by an epithelium-dependent mechanism,[160] which is at least partially explained by the generation of a relaxant cyclooxygenase product.[161,162] In the absence of the epithelium, PAF was reported to induce a contraction of guinea pig trachea.[160] Not all workers have observed relaxant responses: Jancar et al.[162] reported a contractile response of tracheas and bronchi which were followed by relaxant responses to subsequent PAF exposure; Malo et al.[163] also reported a contractile effect which was enhanced by treatment with indomethacin, whereas those observed by Medeiros et al.[164] were prevented by indomethacin. Similarly, Chand et al.[165] reported that PAF induced contractile responses in both guinea pig and rat tracheas. The variation in these observations may well relate to the integrity of the epithelial layer which appears to be essential for relaxation responses.[160]

C. BRONCHIAL HYPERREACTIVITY

It is now well established that *in vivo* administration of PAF to experimental animals results in a heightened bronchial responsiveness that resembles the bronchial hyperreactivity in asthmatics, but is of a considerably lesser magnitude (see Reference 166 for a review). However, some debate continues as to whether PAF has a similar effect in either healthy or asthmatic humans.[167]

1. *In Vivo* Mechanisms of Bronchial Hyperreactivity

The mechanism of PAF-induced bronchial hyperreactivity at the cellular level is not fully understood. It appears that isolated airways smooth muscle preparations obtained from animals made hyperreactive to histamine and acetylcholine by PAF infusion *in vivo* do not show any hyperreactivity *in vitro*, nor are there detectable changes in affinity or numbers of binding sites for histamine or muscarinic receptor ligands.[168] Similarly, PAF-induced bronchial hyperreactivity is associated with a diminished bronchodilator efficacy of iso-prenaline *in vivo*, but no differences in the relaxant potency for isoprenaline on *in vitro* airways preparations were observed and β-adrenoceptor numbers and affinity on membranes from these preparations appeared to be unaffected.[169]

In contrast to the lack of *in vitro* hyperresponsiveness seen following single PAF infusions *in vivo*,[168] daily exposure of guinea pigs to PAF aerosols resulted in a sensitization of isolated trachea to histamine.[170] A number of explanations such as decreased histamine-H_2 receptor sensitivity, altered resting membrane potential, or altered eicosanoid generation were excluded, but observation of eosinophil infiltration of the submucosa suggested a role for this cell type;[170] the effect of epithelium removal on the hyperresponsiveness was not investigated.

2. Induction of Hyperreactivity *In Vitro*

PAF at concentrations that had no effect on resting tone, enhanced contractile responses of guinea pig isolated tracheas to LTD_4, and the thromboxane mimetic, U46619, but not to histamine, acetylcholine, PGD_2, or LTC_4.[163] In the rat trachea, PAF induced contraction, and unlike the guinea pig trachea, induced a diminished responsiveness to isoprenaline.[165]

A role for PAF in the development of hyperresponsiveness to cold provocation of rat isolated trachea following recovery from antigen challenge was suggested by the ability of L-652,731 to inhibit contractions induced by temperature lowering.[171] Further evidence of a link between PAF and cholinergic mechanisms was provided by the observation that atropine was also an effective inhibitor of cold-induced contractions. This model was extended by using PLA_2 exposure to induce responsiveness of rat trachea to cold provocation. Once again, atropine was an effective inhibitor, as were verapamil and diltiazem, but the effects of a specific PAF receptor antagonist were not evaluated.[172]

D. ENDOTHELIN-INDUCED AIRWAYS SMOOTH MUSCLE CONSTRICTION

The vasoconstrictor peptide, endothelin, has been shown to be a potent airways smooth muscle spasmogen in the guinea pig[173] by a mechanism partly involving TXA_2 generation.[174] Recent studies of the constrictor effect of endothelin on guinea pig isolated trachea suggest that PAF contributes to the constriction, since BN52021 inhibited the response and a degree of cross-desensitization of constrictor responses between PAF and endothelin was evident.[175] It has yet to be determined whether tracheal smooth muscle produces PAF in response to endothelin, and what cell type(s) might be involved, but there seems to be a close analogy to observations made in vascular smooth muscle (see Section II.E).

VI. OTHER SMOOTH MUSCLE TYPES

In an extensive study of responses of isolated smooth muscle preparations from rat and guinea pig, PAF was reported to contract all preparations from the GIT, including esophagus, stomach, jejunum, ileum, and the ascending colon.[135] Contractile responses were also observed in guinea pig aorta and vena cava, but it was not clear whether these preparations contained an intact endothelium. In trachea and bronchus, the first application of PAF induced contraction, and subsequent doses induced relaxation, whereas parenchyma contracted and then displayed a complete tachyphylaxis. PAF also contracted a longitudinal smooth muscle preparation from guinea pig bladder, rat uterus, and guinea pig vas deferens.[135]

PAF stimulated the release of arachidonic acid and PGE_2 from rabbit iris smooth muscle by activation of PLA_2.[176] This stimulation was blocked by Ca^{2+} channel antagonists such as nifedipine and verapamil, but the latter may act by preventing the binding of PAF to its receptor.[123] Later studies suggest that the PAF-induced release of arachidonic acid occurred via PLA_2 rather than PLC activation,[177] and established the presence of specific and saturable binding sites for PAF.[178,179]

A. LYMPHATIC SMOOTH MUSCLE

An important component of the action of PAF and other mediators of inflammation is their capacity to induce edema which is in part regulated by the flow in regional lymphatics.[180] Using *in vivo* video microscopy of the mesenteric lymphatic vessels of anesthetised rats it was established that topical superfusion of PAF relaxed the lymphatic smooth muscle and decreased calculated lymph flow, whereas histamine and leukotrienes had opposite actions.[180] In the anesthetized sheep, however, PAF induced an increase in lymph flow,[181-184] presumably because of a dominant action of PAF on increasing microvascular permeability, as suggested by an increase in lymph to plasma protein ratios.[183]

B. UTERINE SMOOTH MUSCLE

PAF has been ascribed a role in the initiation of parturition following its release by maturing lung.[185,186] PAF-induced contractile responses of guinea pig isolated myometrium were highly dependent on the formation of cyclooxygenase, and to a lesser extent lipoxygenase products, and were blocked by CV3988, suggesting a specific action.[187] The characteristics of the contraction depended on whether the tissue was quiescent or displayed phasic contractile activity; in the former state, PAF induced a rapid (0.5 to 2.0 min) contraction which was sustained for a short period (0.5 to 2.0 min), followed by a rapid relaxation. In spontaneously active strips, PAF increased the amplitude of the phasic activity.[188] In addition this group demonstrated that PAF induced contractile activity on myometrial strips obtained from pregnant women at term (39th week) by mechanism(s) involving eicosanoid formation.[188] Although PAF was found to contract myometrium from nonpregnant rats, it was less potent in pregnant rats, and in ~75% of the latter preparations it had no effect.[189]

PAF appears to be constitutively present in the normal rat uterus[190,191] as are two inhibitors (mixtures of alkyl-lyso and acyl-lyso GPCs) of PAF-induced platelet aggregation in relative quantities that would provide a balance of activity.[192] Furthermore, rabbit uterine PAF levels increase 15- to 20-fold in pregnancy, but the majority of this PAF is associated with the endometrium.[191] Rat uterus contains predominantly an acyl PAF as detected by GC/MS.[193]

The role of PAF in parturition, its tissue source (uterine or fetal?), and the mechanism of uterine smooth muscle contraction all require further elucidation.

VII. CONCLUSION

In view of the lack of direct effects of PAF in many smooth muscle preparations, it is not surprising to find that little is known of PAF receptor signal transduction mechanisms in this cell type. However, it is clear that smooth muscle cells do express PAF receptors, the activation of which may serve to regulate cellular responsiveness to other agonists, and as such, it could be expected that the signaling mechanisms will differ from those induced by substances that evoke pronounced direct effects.

As yet no studies exist of PAF or PAF antagonists binding to vascular smooth muscle and there are few studies on other nonairway smooth muscle tissues. The mechanism(s) by which the PAF receptor is linked to increases in intracellular calcium has not yet been elucidated. Furthermore little is known about the biochemical effects of PAF in smooth muscle including phospholipased (PLD) activation, Na^+/Ca^{2+} exchange, Na^+/H^+ exchange, activation of K^+ channels, protein kinase activation, and pH regulation.

In most instances of PAF stimulation of inflammatory cells the secondary mediators are either cyclooxygenase or lipoxygenase products, with clearly established roles for TXA_2 and LTC_4 in vascular smooth muscle contractile responses. Serotonin, TXA_2, and possibly other platelet products together with acetylcholine contribute to the PAF-induced constriction of bronchial smooth muscle. Nevertheless, at least in vascular smooth muscle, PAF directly stimulates a number of cellular responses, including a relatively small increase in intracellular Ca^{2+} at low concentrations (nanomolar) that may be achieved in pathological events such as shock or locally upon stimulation of inflammatory cells. Consideration should now be given to the possibility that PAF exerts more subtle influences on functions of smooth muscle other than contractile status.

In cardiac muscle, greater progress toward identifying the mechanism of PAF-induced inotropic and chronotropic effects has been achieved. Further studies are required to resolve the many contradictory observations that have been made in tissues of varying complexity from the isolated myocyte studies reported in this chapter to studies using intact animals.

A wide range of cell types, not normally regarded as primary participants in inflammatory responses, produce and in many cases retain PAF intracellularly.[93,94,142,190,191,194] The role of PAF production within smooth muscle (vascular, gastrointestinal, and uterine) and cardiac muscle remains to be established, but a contribution to signal transduction seems likely.[41,90,195,196]

The recent cloning of the PAF receptor from guinea pig lung[197] will provide a means for detecting expression of PAF receptors in various smooth muscle preparations and will assist in the identification of receptor subtypes. The development of an anti-idiotypic antibody to PAF will enable an assessment of receptor specific actions of PAF and provide a more suitable ligand for the autoradiographic mapping of PAF receptors.[198]

Finally, and most importantly, the capacity of PAF to activate platelets and leukocytes at concentrations orders of magnitudes less than those that evoke responses on smooth or cardiac muscle should remain foremost in analyzing the mechanism of action of PAF upon release *in vivo*.

ACKNOWLEDGMENTS

We thank the NH & MRC (Australia) and the National Heart Foundation (Australia) for financial support of the authors' work cited in this review. We also thank Lauren Williams for secretarial assistance in the preparation of this manuscript and Trudi Harris for preparation of the figures.

REFERENCES

1. **Braquet, P., Touqui, L., Shen, T. Y., and Vargaftig, B. B.,** Perspectives in platelet-activating factor research, *Pharmac. Rev.,* 39, 97, 1987.
2. **Braquet, P. and Rola-Plesczynski, M.,** The role of PAF in immunological responses: a review, *Prostaglandins,* 34, 143, 1987.
3. **Feuerstein, G. and Hallenbeck, J. M.,** Prostaglandins, leukotrienes, and platelet-activating factor in shock, *Annu. Rev. Pharmacol. Toxicol.,* 27, 301, 1987.
4. **Page, C. P. and Coyle, A. J.,** The interaction between PAF, platelets and eosinophils in bronchial asthma, *Eur. Respir. J. Suppl.,* 6, 483s, 1989.
5. **Esplugues, J. V. and Whittle, B. J.,** Gastric effects of PAF, *Methods Fund. Exp. Clin. Pharmacol.,* 11(Suppl. 1), 61, 1989.
6. **O'Neill, C., Gidley-Baird, A. A., Pike, I. L., and Saunders, D. M.,** Use of a bioassay for embryo-derived platelet-activating factor as a means of assessing quality and pregnancy potential of human embryos, *Fertil. Steril.,* 47, 969, 1987.
7. **Hoffman, D. R., Truong, C. T., and Johnston, J. M.,** The role of platelet-activating factor in human fetal lung maturation, *Am. J. Obstet. Gynecol.,* 155, 70, 1986.
8. **Harper, M. J.,** Platelet-activating factor: a paracrine factor in preimplantation stages of reproduction?, *Biol. Reprod.,* 40, 907, 1989.
9. **Masugi, F., Ogihara, T., Saeki, S., Otsuka, A., and Kumahara, Y.,** Role of acetyl glyceryl ether phosphorylcholine in blood pressure regulation in rats, *Hypertension,* 7, 742, 1985.
10. **Page, C. P. and Spina, D.,** The therapeutic relevance of PAF atagonists, *Agents Actions. Suppl.,* 28, 313, 1989.
11. **Casals-Stenzel, J. and Heuer, H.,** Pharmacology of PAF antagonists, *Prog. Biochem. Pharmacol.,* 22, 58, 1988.
12. **Feuerstein, G. and Siren, A. L.,** Platelet-activating factor and shock, *Prog. Biochem. Pharmacol.,* 22, 181, 1988.
13. **Piper, P. J., Stanton, A. W., and Stewart, A. G.,** Mechanisms of vascular actions of PAF, *Int. J. Tissue React.,* 9, 15, 1987.
14. **Stanton, A. W., Izumi, T., Antoniw, J. W., and Piper, P. J.,** Platelet-activating factor (Paf) antagonist, WEB 2086, protects against Paf-induced hypotension in *Macaca fascicularis, Br. J. Pharmacol.,* 97, 643, 1989.
15. **Laurindo, F. R., Goldstein, R. E., Davenport, N. J., Ezra, D., and Feuerstein, G. Z.,** Mechanisms of hypotension produced by platelet-activating factor, *J. Appl. Physiol.,* 66, 2681, 1989.
16. **Kenzora, J. L., Perez, J. E., Bergman, S. R., and Lange, L. G.,** Effects of acetyl glyceryl ether phosphorylcholine (platelet-activating factor) on ventricular preload, afterload and contractility in dogs, *J. Clin. Invest.,* 74, 1193, 1984.
17. **Goldstein, B. M., Gabel, R. A., Huggins, F. J., Cervoni, P., and Crandall, D. L.,** Effect of platelet activating factor (PAF) on blood flow distribution in the spontaneously hypertensive rat, *Life Sci.,* 35, 1373, 1984.
18. **Chu, K. M., Gerber, J. G., and Nies, A. S.,** Local vasodilator effect of platelet activating factor in the gastric, mesenteric and femoral arteries of the dog, *J. Pharmacol. Exp. Ther.,* 246, 996, 1988.
19. **Sybertz, E. J., Watkins, R. W., Baum, T., Pula, K., and Rivelli, M.,** Cardiac, coronary and peripheral vascular effects of acetyl glyceryl ether phosphoryl choline in the anaesthetized dog, *J. Exp. Pharmacol. Ther.,* 232, 156, 1985.
20. **Sanchez Crespo, M., Alonso, F., Inarrea, P., and Egido, J.,** Non-platelet-mediated vascular actions of 1-O-alkyl-2-acetyl-sn-3-glyceryl phosphorycholine (a synthetic PAF), *Agents Actions,* 11, 565, 1981.
21. **Sanchez Crespo, M., Alonso, F., Inarrea, P., Alvarez, V., and Egido, J.,** Vascular actions of synthetic PAF-acether (a synthetic platelet-activating factor) in the rat: evidence for a platelet independent mechanism, *Immunopharmacology,* 4, 173, 1982.
22. **Benveniste, J., Boullet, C., Brink, C., and Labat, C.,** The actions of Paf-acether (platelet-activating factor) on guinea-pig isolated heart preparations, *Br. J. Pharmacol.,* 80, 81, 1983.
23. **Levi, R., Burke, J. A., Guo, Z-G., Hattori, Y., Hoppens, C. M., McManus, L. M., Hanahan, D. J., and Pinckard, R. N.,** Acetyl glyceryl ether phosphorylcholine (AGEPC): a putative mediator of cardiac anaphylaxis in the guinea-pig, *Circ. Res.,* 54, 117, 1984.
24. **Piper, P. J. and Stewart, A. G.,** Coronary vasoconstriction in the rat, isolated perfused heart induced by platelet-activating factor is mediated by leukotriene C4, *Br. J. Pharmacol.,* 88, 595, 1986.
25. **Stewart, A. G. and Piper, P. J.,** Platelet-activating factor-induced vasoconstriction in rat isolated, perfused hearts: contribution of cyclo-oxygenase and lipoxygenase arachidonic acid metabolites, *Pharmacol. Res. Commun.,* 18(Suppl.), 163, 1986.

26. **Piper, P. J. and Stewart, A. G.,** Antagonism of vasoconstriction induced by platelet-activating factor in guinea-pig perfused hearts by selective platelet-activating factor receptor antagonists, *Br. J. Pharmacol.,* 90, 771, 1987.

27. **Stahl, G. L. and Lefer, A. M.,** mechanisms of platelet-activating factor-induced cardiac depression in the isolated perfused rat heart, *Circ. Shock,* 23, 165, 1987.

28. **Voelkel, N. F., Worthen, S., Reeves, J. T., Henson, P. M., and Murphy, R. C.,** Nonimmunological production of leukotrienes induced by platelet-activating factor, *Science,* 218, 286, 1982.

29. **Hamasaki, Y., Mojarad, M., Saga, T., Tai, H. H., and Said, S. I.,** Platelet-activating factor raises airway and vascular pressures and induces edema in lungs perfused with platlet-free solution, *Am. Rev. Respir. Dis.,* 129, 742, 1984.

30. **Neuwirth, R., Satriano, J. A., DeCandido, S., Clay, K., and Schlondorff, D.,** Angiotensin II causes formation of platelet activating factor in cultured rat mesangial cells, *Circ. Res.,* 64, 1224, 1989.

31. **Kochanek, P., Nemoto, E. M., Melick, J. A., Evans, R. W., and Burke, D. F.,** Cerebrovascular and cerebrometabolic effects of intracarotid infused platelet-activating factor in rats, *J. Cereb. Blood Flow Metab.,* 8, 546, 1988.

32. **Plante, G. E., Hebert, R. L., Lamoureux, C., Braquet, P., and Sirois, P.,** Hemodynamic effects of PAF-acether, *Pharmacol. Res. Commun.,* 18(Suppl.), 173, 1986.

33. **Daurius, H., Smith, J. B., and Lefer, A. M.,** Inhibition of the platelet activating factor mediated component of guinea pig anaphylaxis by receptor antagonists, *Int. Arch. Allergy Appl. Immunol.,* 80, 369, 1986.

34. **Baer, P. G. and Cagen, L. M.,** Platelet activating factor vasoconstriction of dog kidney. Inhibition by alprazolam, *Hypertension,* 9, 253, 1987.

35. **Bjork, J. and Smedegard, G.,** Acute microvascular effects of PAF-acether, as studied by intravital microscopy, *Eur. J. Pharmacol.,* 96, 87, 1983.

36. **Dillon, P. K. and Duran, W. N.,** Effect of platelet-activating factor on microvascular permselectivity: dose-response relations and pathways of action in the hamster cheek pouch microcirculation, *Circ. Res.,* 62, 732, 1988.

37. **Dillon, P. K., Ritter, A. B., and Duran, W. N.,** Vasoconstrictor effects of platelet-activating factor in the hamster cheek pouch microcirculation: dose-related relations and pathways of action, *Circ. Res.,* 62, 722, 1988.

38. **Tanaka, S., Kasuya, Y., Masuda, Y., and Shigenobu, K.,** Studies on the hypotensive effects of platelet activating factor (PAF, 1-O-alkyl-2-acetyl-*sn*-glyceryl-3-phosphorylcholine) in rats, guinea pigs, rabbits, and dogs, *J. Pharmacobiodyn.,* 6, 866, 1983.

39. **Zukowska Grojec, Z., Blank, M. L., Snyder, F., and Feuerstein, G.,** The adrenergic system and the cardiovascular effects of platelet activating factor (1-O-hexadecyl-2-acetyl-*sn*-glycero-3-phosphocholine) in SHR and WKY rats, *Clin. Exp. Hypertens. A.,* 7, 1015, 1985.

40. **Myers, A. K. and Bader, T. J.,** Role of adrenal steroids in the recovery from platelet activating factor challenge, *Circ. Shock,* 23, 143, 1987.

41. **Stewart, A. G., Dubbin, P. N., Harris, T., and Dusting, G. J.,** Platelet-activating factor may act as a second messenger in the release of icosanoids and superoxide anions from leukocytes and endothelial cells, *Proc. Natl. Acad. Sci. U.S.A.,* 87, 3215, 1990.

42. **Terashita, Z., Imura, Y., Nishikawa, K., and Sumida, S.,** Is platelet activating factor (PAF) a mediator of endotoxin shock?, *Eur. J. Pharmacol.,* 109, 257, 1985.

43. **Toyofuku, T., Kubo, K., Kobayashi, T., and Kusama, S.,** Effects of ONO-6240, a platelet-activating factor antagonist, on endotoxin shock in unanesthetized sheep, *Prostaglandins,* 31, 271, 1986.

44. **Lagente, V., Fortes, Z. B., Garcia-Leme, J., and Vargaftig, B. B.,** PAF-acether and endotoxin display similar effects on rat mesenteric microvessels: inhibition by specific antagonists, *J. Pharmacol. Exp. Ther.,* 247, 254, 1988.

45. **Yue, T. L., Farhat, M., Rabinovici, R., Perera, P. Y., Vogel, S. N., and Feuerstein, G.,** Protective effect of BN 50739, a new platelet-activating factor antagonist, in endotoxin-treated rabbits, *J. Pharmacol. Exp. Ther.,* 254, 976, 1990.

46. **Thiemermann, C. and Vane, J.,** Inhibition of nitric oxide synthesis reduces the hypotension induced by bacterial lipopolysaccharides in the rat *in vivo, Eur. J. Pharmacol.,* 182, 591, 1990.

47. **Moy, J. A., Bates, J. N., and Fisher, R. A.,** Effects of nitric oxide on platelet-activating factor- and alpha-adrenergic-stimulated vasoconstriction and glycogenolysis in the perfused rat liver, *J. Biol. Chem.,* 266, 8092, 1991.

48. **Heffner, J. E., Shoemaker, S. A., Canham, E. M., Patel, M., McMurtry, I. F., Morris, H. G., and Repine, J. E.,** Acetyl glyceryl ether phosphorylcholine-stimulated human platelets cause pulmonary hypertension and edema in isolated rabbit lungs: role of thromboxane A2, *J. Clin. Invest.,* 71, 351, 1983.

49. **Mehta, J., Wargovich, T., and Nichols, W. W.,** Biphasic effects of platelet-activating factor on coronary blood flow in anesthetized dog, *Prostaglandins, Leukotrienes, Med.,* 21, 87, 1986.

50. **Fiedler, V. B., Mardin, M., and Abram, T. S.,** Comparison of cardiac and hemodynamic effects of platelet-activating factor-acether and leukotriene D4 in anesthetized dogs, *Basic Res. Cardiol.,* 82, 197, 1987.

51. **Jackson, C. V., Schumaker, W. A., Kunkel, S. L., Driscoll, E. M., and Lucchesi, B. R.,** Platelet-activating factor and the release of a platelet-derived coronary artery vasodilator substance in the canine, *Circ. Res.,* 58, 218, 1986.

52. **Ezra, D., Laurindo, F. R., Czaja, J. F., Snyder, F., Goldstein, R. E., and Feuerstein, G.,** Cardiac and coronary consequences of intracoronary platelet activating factor infusion in the domestic pig, *Prostaglandins,* 34, 41, 1987.

53. **Felix, S. B., Steger, A., Baumann, G., Busch, R., Ochsenfeld, G., and Berdel, W. E.,** Platelet-activating factor-induced coronary constriction in the isolated perfused guinea-pig heart and antagonistic effects of the PAF antagonist WEB 2086, *J. Lipid Med.,* 2, 9, 1990.

54. **McMurtry, I. F. and Morris, K. G.,** Platelet-activating factor causes pulmonary vasodilation in the rat, *Am. Rev. Respir. Dis.,* 134, 757, 1986.

55. **Schwertschlag, U., Scherf, H., Gerber, J. G., Mathias, M., and Nies, A. S.,** L-platelet activating factor induces changes on renal vascular resistance, vascular reactivity, and renin release in the isolated perfused rat kidney, *Circ. Res.,* 60, 534, 1987.

56. **Voelkel, N. F., Chang, S. W., Pfeffer, K. D., Worthen, S. G., McMurtry, I. F., and Henson, P. M.,** PAF antagonists: different effects on platelets, neutrophils, guinea pig ileum and PAF-induced vasodilation in isolated rat lung, *Prostaglandins,* 32, 359, 1986.

57. **Gillespie, M. N. and Bowdy, B. D.,** Impact of platelet activating factor on vascular responsiveness in isolated rat lungs, *J. Pharmacol. Exp. Ther.,* 236, 396, 1986.

58. **Umans, J. G., Lindheimer, M. D., and Barron, W. M.,** Pressor effects of endothelium-derived relaxing factor inhibition in conscious virgin and gravid rats, *Am. J. Physiol.,* 259, F293, 1990.

59. **Korth, R., Hirafuji, M., Keraly, C. L., Delautier, D., Bidault, J., and Benveniste, J.,** Interaction of the Paf antagonist WEB 2086 and its hetrazepine analogues with human platelets and endothelial cells, *Br. J. Pharmacol.,* 98, 653, 1989.

60. **Bussolino, F., Camussi, G., Aglietta, M., Braquet, P., Bosia, A., Pescarmona, G., Sanavio, F., D'Urso, N., and Marchisio, P. C.,** Human endothelial cells are target for platelet-activating factor. I. Platelet-activating factor induces changes in cytoskeleton structures, *J. Immunol.,* 139, 2439, 1987.

61. **Brock, T. A. and Gimbrone, M. A.,** Platelet activating factor alters calcium homeostasis in cultured vascular endothelial cells, *Am. J. Physiol.,* 250, H1086, 1986.

62. **Northover, A. M.,** Effects of PAF and PAF antagonists on the shape of venous endothelial cells *in vitro, Agents Actions,* 28, 142, 1989.

63. **Hirafuji, M., Maeyama, K., Watanabe, T., and Ogura, Y.,** Transient increase of cytosolic free calcium in cultured human vascular endothelial cells by platelet-activating factor, *Biochem. Biophys. Res. Commun.,* 154, 910, 1988.

64. **Luscher, T. F. and Vanhoutte, P. M.,** Endothelium-dependent responses in human blood vessels, *TIPS,* 9, 181, 1988.

65. **Moncada, S., Radomski, M. W., and Palmer, R. M. J.,** Endothelium-derived relaxing factor. Identification as nitric oxide and role in the control of vascular tone and platelet function, *Biochem. Pharmacol.,* 37, 2495, 1988.

66. **Daffonchio, L., Fano, M., and Omini, C.,** Rat pulmonary artery responses to some mediators of anaphylaxis: modification by indomethacin, *Pharmacol. Res. Commun.,* 16, 679, 1984.

67. **Baranes, J., Hellegouarch, A., Le Hegarat, M., Viossat, I., Auguet, M., Chabrier, P. E., and Braquet, P.,** The effects of PAF-acether on the cardiovascular system and their inhibition by a new highly specific PAF-acether receptor antagonist BN 52021, *Pharmacol. Res. Commun.,* 18, 717, 1986.

68. **Stahl, G. L. and Lefer, A. M.,** Heterogeneity of vascular smooth muscle responsiveness to lipid vasoactive mediators, *Blood Vessels,* 24, 24, 1987.

69. **Gryglewski, R. J., Moncada, S., and Palmer, R. M. J.,** Bioassay of prostacyclin and endotheium-derived relaxing factor (EDRF) from porcine aortic endothelial cells, *Br. J. Pharmacol.,* 87, 685, 1986.

70. **Cervoni, P., Herzlinger, H. E., Lai, F. M., and Tanikella, T. K.,** Aortic vascular and atrial responses to $(+/-)$-1-O-octadecyl-2-acetyl-glyceryl-3-phosphorylcholine, *Br. J. Pharmacol.,* 79, 667, 1983.

71. **Shiegenobu, K., Masuda, Y., Tanaka, Y., and Kasuya, Y.,** Platelet activating factor analogues: lack of correlation between their activities to produce hypotension and endothelium-mediated vasodilation, *J. Pharmacobiodyn.,* 8, 128, 1985.

72. **Chiba, Y., Mikoda, N., Kawasaki, H., and Ito, K.,** Endothelium-dependent relaxant action of platelet activating factor in the rat mesenteric artery, *Nauyn Schmiedebergs Arch. Pharmacol.,* 341, 68, 1990.

73. **Ono, S., Koike, K., Tanita, T., Kubo, H., Ashino, Y., Chida, M., Suzuki, S., Isogami, K., Nasu, G., Saitoh, H. et al.**, Possible involvement of vascular endothelium-derived relaxing factor induced by platelet-activating factor (PAF) on human pulmonary artery after contraction *in vitro, Nippon Kyobu Shikkan Gakkai Zasshi*, 27, 910, 1989.

74. **Uski, T. K. and Reinstrup, P.**, Actions of platelet-activating factor on isolated feline and human cerebral arteries, *J. Cereb. Blood Flow Metab.*, 10, 428, 1990.

75. **Schwertschlag, U. S., Dennis, V. W., Tucker, J. A., and Camussi, G.**, Nonimmunological alterations of glomerular filtration by s-PAF in the rat kidney, *Kidney Int.*, 34, 779, 1988.

76. **Kamata, K., Mori, T., Shigenobu, K., and Kasuya, Y.**, Endothelium-dependent vasodilator effects of platelet activating factor on rat resistance vessels, *Br. J. Pharmacol.*, 98, 1360, 1989.

77. **Doyle, V. M., Creba, J. A., and Ruegg, U. T.**, Platelet-activating factor mobilizes intracellular calcium in vascular smooth muscle cells, *FEBS Lett.*, 197, 13, 1986.

78. **Takayasu, M., Kondo, K., and Terao, S.**, Endothelin-induced mobilization of Ca^{2+} and the possible involvement of platelet activating factor and thromboxane A_2, *Biochem. Biophys. Res. Commun.*, 160, 751, 1989.

79. **Shirinsky, V. P., Sobolevsky, A. V., Grigorian, G. Y., Danilov, S. M., Tararak, E. M., and Tkashuk, V. A.**, Agonist-induced polyphosphoinositide breakdown in cultured human endothelial and vascular smooth muscles cells, *Health Psychol.*, 7(Suppl.), 61, 1986.

80. **Schwertschlag, U. S. and Whorton, A. R.**, Platelet-activating factor-induced homologous and heterologous desensitization in cultured vascular smooth muscle cells, *J. Biol. Chem.*, 263, 13791, 1988.

81. **Conrad, G. W. and Rink, T. J.**, Platelet activating factor raises intracellular calcium ion concentration in macrophages, *J. Cell. Biol.*, 103, 439, 1986.

82. **Naccache, P. H., Molski, M. M., Volpi, M., Shefcyk, J., Molski, T. F., Loew, L., Becker, E. L., and Sha'afi, R. I.**, Biochemical events associated with the stimulation of rabbit neutrophils by platelet-activating factor, *J. Leukocyte Biol.*, 40, 533, 1986.

83. **von Tscharner, V., Prod'hom, B., Baggiolini, M., and Reuter, H.**, Ion channels in human neutrophils activated by a rise in free cytosolic calcium concentration, *Nature*, 324, 369, 1986.

84. **Kroegel, C., Pleass, R., Yukawa, T., Chung, K. F., Westwick, J., and Barnes, P. J.**, Characterization of platelet-activating factor-induced elevation of cytosolic free calcium concentration in eosinophils, *FEBS Lett.*, 243, 41, 1989.

85. **Avdonin, P. V., Men'shikov, M. Y., Svitina-Ulitina, I. V., and Tkachuk, V. A.**, Blocking of the receptor-stimulated calcium entry into human platelets by verapamil and nicardipine, *Thromb. Res.*, 52, 587, 1988.

86. **Terashita, Z., Shibouta, Y., Imura, Y., Iwasaki, K., and Nishikawa, K.**, Endothelin-induced sudden death and the possible involvement of platelet activating factor (PAF), *Life Sci.*, 45, 1911, 1989.

87. **Lefer, A. M., Muller, H. F., and Smith, J. B.**, Pathophysiological mechanisms of sudden death induced by platelet-activating factor, *Br. J. Pharmacol.*, 83, 125, 1984.

88. **Takayasu-Okishio, M., Terashita, Z., and Kondo, K.**, Endothelin-1 and platelet activating factor stimulate thromboxane A2 biosynthesis in rat vascular smooth muscle cells, *Biochem. Pharmacol.*, 40, 2713, 1990.

89. **Acharya, S. B. and MacIntyre, D. E.**, Platelet products and vascular PGI2 production, *Prostaglandins, Leukotrienes Med.*, 10, 73, 1983.

90. **Stewart, A. G. and Phillips, W. A.**, Intracellular platelet-activating factor regulates eicosanoid generation in guinea-pig resident peritoneal macrophages, *Br. J. Pharmacol.*, 98, 141, 1989.

91. **Stewart, A. G.**, CV 6209 is a non-competitive antagonist of platelet-activating factor receptors on guinea-pig resident peritoneal macrophages, *Clin. Exp. Pharmacol. Physiol.*, 16, 813, 1989.

92. **Stewart, A. G., Dubbin, P. N., Harris, T., and Dusting, G. J.**, Evidence for an intracellular action of platelet-activating factor in bovine cultured aortic endothelial cells, *Br. J. Pharmacol.*, 96, 503, 1989.

93. **Stewart, A. G., Dubbin, P. N., Harris, T., Uman, R., and Dusting, G. J.**, Porcine and bovine cultured aortic vascular smooth muscle generate platelet activating factor following receptor stimulation, *J. Lipid Med.*, 2, 176, 1990.

94. **Stewart, A. G., Croft, K., Dubbin, P. N., Harris, T., Hughes, K., and Vivian, R.**, Identification of platelet-activating factor in porcine vascular smooth muscle using bioassay, immunoassay, [3H]-acetate labeling and GC/MS, *Clin. Exp. Pharmacol. Physiol.*, Suppl. 17, 74P, 1990.

95. **Masaki, T.**, The discovery, the present state, and the future prospects of endothelin, *J. Cardiovasc. Pharmacol.*, 13(Suppl. 5), S1, 1989.

96. **Nakaki, T., Nakayama, M., Yamamoto, S., and Kato, R.**, Endothelin-mediated stimulation of DNA synthesis in vascular smooth muscle cells, *Biochem. Biophys. Res. Commun.*, 158, 880, 1989.

97. **Stoll, L. L. and Spector, A. A.**, Interaction of platelet-activating factor with endothelial and vascular smooth muscle cells in coculture, *J. Cell. Physiol.*, 139, 253, 1989.

98. **Feliste, R., Perret, B., Braquet, P., and Chap, H.,** Protective effect of BN 52021, a specific antagonist of platelet-activating factor (PAF-acether) against diet-induced cholesteryl ester deposition in rabbit aorta, *Atherosclerosis,* 78, 151, 1989.

99. **Stewart, A. G. and Piper, P. J.,** Platelet-activating factor and the cardiovascular system: involvement in cardiac anaphylaxis, in *Biologically Active Ether Lipids,* Braquet, P., Mangold, H. K., and Vargaftig, B. B., Eds., S. Karger, Basel, 1988, 132.

100. **Tosaki, A., Koltai, M., Braquet, P., and Szekeres, L.,** Possible involvement of platelet activating factor in anaphylaxis of passively sensitised, isolated guinea pig hearts, *Cardiovasc. Res.,* 23, 715, 1989.

101. **Koltai, M., Lepran, I., Szekeres, L., Viossat, I., Chabrier, E., and Braquet, P.,** Effect of BN 52021, a specific PAF-acether antagonist, on cardiac anaphylaxis in Langendorff hearts isolated from passively sensitized guinea-pigs, *Eur. J. Pharmacol.,* 130, 133, 1986.

102. **Braquet, P., Paubert-Braquet, M., Koltai, M., Bourgain, R., Bussolino, F., and Hosford, D.,** Is there a case for PAF antagonists in the treatment of ischemic states?, *Trends Pharmacol. Sci.,* 10, 23, 1989.

103. **Stahl, G. L., Terashita, Z., and Lefer, A. M.,** Role of platelet activating factor in propagation of cardiac damage during myocardial ischemia, *J. Pharmacol. Exp. Ther.,* 244, 898, 1988.

104. **Koltai, M., Tosaki, A., Hosford, D., and Braquet, P.,** Ginkgolide B protects isolated hearts against arrhythmias induced by ischemia but not reperfusion, *Eur. J. Pharmacol.,* 164, 293, 1989.

105. **Montrucchio, G., Alloatti, G., Tetta, C., De Luca, R., Saunders, R. N., Emanuelli, G., and Camussi, G.,** Release of platelet-activating factor from ischemic-reperfused rabbit heart, *Am. J. Physiol.,* 256, H1236, 1989.

106. **Wainright, C. L., Parratt, J. R., and Bigaud, M.,** The effects of PAF antagonists on arrythmias and platelets during acute myocardial ischaemia and reperfusion, *Eur. Heart J.,* 10, 235, 1989.

107. **Riedel, A. and Mest, H. J.,** The effect of PAF (platelet-activating factor) on experimental cardiac arrhythmias and its inhibition by substances influencing arachidonic acid metabolites, *Prostaglandins, Leukotrienes Med.,* 28, 103, 1987.

108. **Mest, H. J., Schneider, S., and Riedel, A.,** Relevance of eicosanoids for biochemical regulation of cardiac rhythm disturbances, *Biomed. Biochim. Acta,* 46, S534, 1987.

109. **Apprill, P., Schmitz, J. M., Campbell, W. B., Tilton, G., Ashton, J., Raheja, S., Buja, L. M., and Willerson, J. T.,** Cyclic blood flow variations induced by platelet-activating factor in stenosed canine coronary arteries despite inhibition of thromboxane synthetase, serotonin receptors, and alpha-adrenergic receptors, *Circulation,* 72, 397, 1985.

110. **Piper, P. J. and Stewart, A. G.,** Antagonism of vasoconstriction induced by platelet-activating factor in guinea-pig perfused hearts by selective platelet-activating factor receptor antagonists, *Br. J. Pharmacol.,* 90, 771, 1987.

111. **Stewart, A. G. and Piper, P. J.,** Actions of platelet-activating factor in the coronary circulation of the guinea-pig *in vitro,* in *Prostaglandins in Clinical Research,* Sinzinger, H., Ed., Alan R. Liss, New York, 1987, 229.

112. **Stahl, G. L., Lefer, D. J., and Lefer, A. M.,** PAF-acether induced cardiac dysfunction in the isolated perfused guinea pig heart, *Naunyn Schmiedeberg's Arch. Pharmacol.,* 336, 459, 1987.

113. **Viossat, I., Chapelat, M., Chabrier, P. E., and Braquet, P.,** Effects of platelet activating factor (PAF) and its receptor antagonist BN 52021 on isolated perfused guinea-pig heart, *Prostaglandins, Leukotrienes, Essential Fatty Acids,* 38, 189, 1989.

114. **Riedel, A., Schneider, S., and Mest, H. J.,** The effect of substances influencing the arachidonic acid cascade on experimental cardiac arrhythmias, *Biomed. Biochim. Acta,* 47, S27, 1988.

115. **Mest, H. J., Riedel, A., Braquet, P., and Meyer, E.,** The arrhythmogenic effect of platelet activating factor (PAF) is inhibited by PAF antagonist and by substances influencing eicosanoids, *Biomed. Biochim. Acta,* 47, S219, 1988.

116. **Montrucchio, G., Alloatti, G., Mariano, F., Meda, E., Tetta, C., Emanuelli, G., and Camussi, G.,** The pattern of cardiovascular alterations induced by infusion of platelet-activating factor in rabbit is modified by pretreatment with H1-H2 receptor antagonists but not by cyclooxygenase inhibition, *Agents Actions,* 21, 72, 1987.

117. **Feuerstein, G.,** PAF and the cardiovascular system, in *Platelet Activating Factor and Human Disease,* Page, C. P., Barnes, P. J., and Henson, P. M., Eds., Blackwell Scientific, Oxford, 1989, 138.

118. **Alloatti, G., Montrucchio, G., Mariano, F., Tetta, C., Emanuelli, G., and Camussi, G.,** Protective effect of verapamil on the cardiac and circulatory alterations induced by platelet-activating factor, *J. Cardiovasc. Pharmacol.,* 9, 181, 1987.

119. **Levi, R., Genovese, A., and Pinckard, R. N.,** Alkyl chain homologs of platelet-activating factor and their effects on the mammalian heart, *Biochem. Biophys. Res. Commun.,* 161, 1341, 1989.

120. **Burke, J. A., Levi, R., Hanahan, D. J., and Pinckard, R. N.,** Cardiac effects of acetyl glyceryl ether phosphorylcholine, *Fed. Proc.,* 41, 823, 1982.

121. **Felix, S. B., Baumann, G., Ahmad, Z., Hashemi, T., Niemczyk, M., and Berdel, W. E.,** Effects of platelet-activating factor on myocardial contraction and myocardial relaxation of isolated, perfused guinea-pig hearts, *J. Cardiovasc. Pharmacol.,* 16, 750, 1990.

122. **Camussi, G., Alloatti, G., Montrucchio, G., Meda, M., and Emanuelli, G.,** Effect of platelet activating factor on guinea-pig papillary muscle, *Experientia,* 40, 697, 1984.

123. **Wade, P. J., Lunt, D. O., Lad, N., Tuffin, D. P., and McCullagh, K. G.,** Effect of calcium and calcium antagonists on-Paf-acether binding to washed human platelets, *Thromb. Res.,* 41, 251, 1986.

124. **Filep, J. G. and Foldes-Filep, E.,** Inhibition by calcium channel blockers of the binding of platelet-activating factor to human neutrophil granulocytes, *Eur. J. Pharmacol.,* 190, 67, 1990.

125. **Tamargo, J., Tejerina, T., Delgado, C., and Barrigon, S.,** Electrophysiological effects of platelet-activating factor (PAF-acether) in guinea-pig papillary muscles, *Eur. J. Pharmacol.,* 109, 219, 1985.

126. **Robertson, D. A., Wang, D. Y., Lee, C. O., and Levi, R.,** Negative inotropic effect of platelet-activating factor: association with a decrease in intracellular sodium activity, *J. Pharmacol. Exp. Ther.,* 245, 124, 1988.

127. **Nakaya, H. and Tohse, N.,** Electrophysiological effects of acetyl glyceryl ether phosphorylcholine on cardiac tissues: comparison with lysophosphatidyl choline and long chain acyl-carnitine, *Br. J. Pharmacol.,* 89, 749, 1986.

128. **Sawyer, D. B. and Andersen, O. S.,** Platelet-activating factor is a general membrane perturbant, *Biochim. Biophys. Acta,* 987, 129, 1989.

129. **Diez, J., Delpon, E., and Tamargo, J.,** Effects of platelet-activating factor on contractile force and ^{45}Ca fluxes in guinea-pig isolated atria, *Br. J. Pharmacol.,* 100, 305, 1990.

130. **Kamitani, T., Katamoto, M., Tatsumi, M., Katsuta, K., Ono, T., Kikuchi, H., and Kumada, S.,** Mechanisms of the hypotensive effect synthetic 1-O-octadecyl-2-O-acetyl-glycero-3-phosphorylcholine, *Eur. J. Pharmacol.,* 98, 357, 1984.

131. **Alloatti, G., Montrucchio, G., Mariano, F., Tetta, C., De Paulis, R., Morea, M., Emanuelli, G., and Camussi, G.,** Effect of platelet-activating factor (PAF) on human cardiac muscle, *Int. Arch. Allergy Appl. Immunol.,* 79, 108, 1986.

132. **Robertson, D. A., Genovese, A., and Levi, R.,** Negative inotropic effect of platelet-activating factor on human myocardium: a pharmacological study, *J. Pharmacol. Exp. Ther.,* 243, 834, 1987.

133. **Kim, D. and Clapham, D. E.,** Potassium channels in cardiac cells activated by arachidonic acid and phospholipids, *Science,* 244, 1174, 1989.

134. **Levy, J. V.,** Spasmogenic effect of platelet activating factor (PAF) on isolated rat stomach fundus strip, *Biochem. Biophys. Res. Commun.,* 146, 855, 1987.

135. **Jancar, S., Theriault, P., and Sirois, P.,** Effect of PAF on selected smooth muscle preparations, *Res. Commun. Chem. Pathol. Pharmacol.,* 63, 157, 1989.

136. **Cirino, G. and Wallace, J. L.,** A superfusion bioassay for platelet-activating factor, *Can. J. Physiol. Pharmacol.,* 67, 72, 1989.

137. **Hwang, S. B., Lee, C. S., Cheah, M. J., and Shen, T. Y.,** Specific receptor sites for 1-O-alkyl-2-O-acetyl-*sn*-glycero-3-phosphocholine (platelet activating factor) on rabbit platelet and guinea pig smooth muscle membranes, *Biochemistry,* 22, 4756, 1983.

138. **Tokumura, A., Terao, M., Okamoto, M., Yoshida, K., and Tsukatani, H.,** Study of platelet-activating factor and its antagonists on rat colon strip with a new method avoiding tachyphylaxis, *Eur. J. Pharmacol.,* 148, 353, 1988.

139. **Marx, M. H., Wiley, R. A., Satchell, D. G., and Maguire, M. H.,** Darmstoff analogues. III. Actions of choline esters of acetal phosphatidic acids on visceral smooth muscle, *J. Med. Chem.,* 32, 1319, 1989.

140. **Esplugues, J. V. and Whittle, B. J.,** Mechanisms contributing to gastric motility changes induced by PAF-acether and endotoxin in rats, *Am. J. Physiol.,* 256, G275, 1989.

141. **Fernandez-Gallardo, S., Gijon, M. A., Garcia, M. C., Cano, E., and Sanchez-Crespo-M.,** Biosynthesis of platelet-activating factor in glandular gastric mucosa. Evidence for the involvement of the "de novo" pathway and modulation by fatty acids, *Biochem. J.,* 254, 707, 1988.

142. **Sugatani, J., Fujimura, K., Miwa, M., Mizuno, T., Sameshima, Y., and Saito, K.,** Occurrence of platelet-activating factor (PAF) in normal rat stomach and alteration of PAF level by water immersion stress, *FASEB J.,* 3, 65, 1989.

143. **Wallace, J. L.,** Lipid mediators of inflammation in gastric ulcer, *Am. J. Physiol.,* 258, G1, 1990.

144. **Stimler, N. P. and O'Flaherty, J. T.,** Spasmogenic properties of platelet-activating factor: evidence for a direct mechanism in the contractile response of pulmonary tissues, *Am. J. Pathol.,* 113, 75, 1983.

145. **Stimler Gerard, N. P.,** Parasympathetic stimulation as a mechanism for platelet-activating factor-induced contractile responses in the lung, *J. Pharmacol. Exp. Ther.,* 237, 209, 1986.

146. **Bethel, R. A., Curtis, S. P., Lien, D. C., Irvin, C. G., Worthen, G. S., Leff, A. R., and Henson, P. M.,** Effect of PAF on parasympathetic contraction of canine airways, *J. Appl. Physiol.,* 66, 2629, 1989.

147. **Touvay, C., Vilain, B., Sirois, P., Soufir, M., and Braquet, P.,** Gossypol: a potent inhibitor of PAF-acether- and leukotriene-induced contractions of guinea-pig lung parenchyma strips, *J. Pharm. Pharmacol.,* 39, 454, 1987.

148. **Jancar, S., Theriault, P., Provencal, B., Cloutier, S., and Sirois, P.,** Mechanism of action of platelet-activating factor on guinea-pig lung parenchyma strips, *Can. J. Physiol. Pharmacol.,* 66, 1187, 1988.

149. **Camussi, G., Montrucchio, G., Antro, C., Bussolino, F., Tetta, C., and Emanuelli, G.,** Platelet-activating factor-mediated contraction of rabbit lung strips: pharmacologic modulation, *Immunopharmacology,* 6, 87, 1983.

150. **Anderson, G. and Fennessy, M.,** Effects of REV 5901, a 5-lipoxygenase inhibitor and leukotriene antagonist, on pulmonary responses to platelet activating factor in the guinea-pig, *Br. J. Pharmacol.,* 94, 1115, 1988.

151. **Halonen, M., Dunn, A. M., Palmer, J. D., and McManus, L. M.,** Anatomic basis for species differences in peripheral lung strip contraction to PAF, *Am. J. Physiol.,* 259, L81, 1990.

152. **Johnson, P. R., Armour, C. L., and Black, J. L.,** The action of platelet activating factor and its antagonism by WEB 2086 on human isolated airways, *Eur. Respir. J.,* 3, 55, 1990.

153. **Johnson, P. R. A., Black, J. L., and Armour, C. L.,** Is the platelet activating factor (PAF) induced contraction of human isolated airway tissue related to the presence of inflammatory cells within the tissue?, *Clin. Exp. Pharmacol. Physiol.,* Suppl. 17, 37P, 1990.

154. **Leff, A. R., White, S. R., Munoz, N. M., Popovich, K. J., Shioya, T., and Stimler-Gerard, N. P.,** Parasympathetic involvement in PAF-induced contraction in canine trachealis *in vivo, J. Appl. Physiol.,* 62, 599, 1987.

155. **Serio, R. and Daniel, E. E.,** Thromboxane effects on canine trachealis neuromuscular function, *J. Appl. Physiol.,* 64, 1979, 1988.

156. **Popovich, K. J., Sheldon, G., Mack, M., Munoz, N. M., Denberg, P., Blake, J., White, S. R., and Leff, A. R.,** Role of platelets in contraction of canine tracheal muscle elicited by PAF *in vitro, J. Appl. Physiol.,* 65, 914, 1988.

157. **Murphy, T. M., Munoz, N. M., Moss, J., Blake, J. S., Mack, M. M., and Leff, A. R.,** PAF-induced contraction of canine trachea mediated by 5-hydroxytryptamine *in vivo, J. Appl. Physiol.,* 66, 638, 1989.

158. **Prancan, A., Lefort, J., Barton, M., and Vargaftig, B. B.,** Relaxation of the guinea-pig trachea induced by platelet-activating factor and by serotonin, *Eur. J. Pharmacol.,* 80, 29, 1982.

159. **Brunelleschi, S., Haye-Legrand, I., Labat, C., Norel, X., Benveniste, J., and Brink, C.,** Platelet-activating factor-acether-induced relaxation of guinea pig airway muscle: role of prostaglandin E2 and the epithelium, *J. Pharmacol. Exp. Ther.,* 243, 356, 1987.

160. **Conroy, D. M., Samhoun, M. N., and Piper, P. J.,** Relaxations of guinea-pig isolated trachea induced by platelet-activating factor are epithelial-dependent and are antagonized by WEB 2086, *Eur. J. Pharmacol.,* 186, 315, 1990.

161. **Brunelleschi, S., Renzi, D., Ledda, F., Giotti, A., Fantozzi, R., Brink, C., and Benveniste, J.,** Interference of WEB 2086 and BN 52021 with Paf-induced effects on guinea-pig trachea, *Br. J. Pharmacol.,* 97, 469, 1989.

162. **Jancar, S., Theriault, P., Braquet, P., and Sirois, P.,** Comparative effects of platelet activating factor, leukotriene D4 and histamine on guinea pig trachea, bronchus and lung parenchyma, *Prostaglandins,* 33, 199, 1987.

163. **Malo, P. E., Wasserman, M. A., and Pfeiffer, D. F.,** Enhancement of leukotriene D4-induced contraction of guinea-pig isolated trachea by platelet activating factor, *Prostaglandins,* 33, 209, 1987.

164. **Medeiros, Y. S., Torres, R. C., and Calixto, J. B.,** Tracheal responsiveness to histamine, PAF-acether and acetylcholine in normal and actively ovalbumin-sensitized guinea pigs, *Braz. J. Med. Biol. Res.,* 22, 97, 1989.

165. **Chand, N., Diamantis, W., and Sofia, R. D.,** Effect of paf-acether on isoprenaline-induced relaxation in isolated tracheal segments of rats and guinea pigs, *Eur. J. Pharmacol.,* 158, 135, 1988.

166. **Page, C. P. and Robertson, D. N.,** The role of PAF in altered airway responsiveness, *Prog. Clin. Biol. Res.,* 263, 71, 1988.

167. **Lai, C. K. and Holgate, S. T.,** Does inhaled PAF cause airway hyperresponsiveness in humans?, *Clin. Exp. Allergy,* 20, 449, 1990.

168. **Robertson, D. N., Coyle, A. J., Rhoden, K. J., Grandordy, B., Page, C. P., and Barnes, P. J.,** The effect of platelet-activating factor on histamine and muscarinic receptor function in guinea pig airways, *Am. Rev. Respir. Dis.,* 137, 1317, 1988.

169. **Barnes, P. J., Grandordy, B. M., Page, C. P., Rhoden, K. J., and Robertson, D. N.,** The effect of platelet activating factor on pulmonary beta-adrenoreceptors, *Br. J. Pharmacol.,* 90, 709, 1987.

170. **Inoue, T. and Kannan, M. S.,** Platelet-activating factor-induced functional changes in the guinea pig trachea *in vitro, Respir. Physiol.,* 77, 157, 1989.

171. **Chand, N., Diamantis, W., Mahoney, T. P., and Sofia, R. D.,** Allergic responses and subsequent development of airway hyperreactivity to cold provocation in the rat trachea: pharmacological modulation, *Eur. J. Pharmacol.,* 150, 95, 1988.

172. **Chand, N., Diamantis, W., Mahoney, T. P., and Sofia, R. D.,** Phospholipase A2 induced airway hyperreactivity to cooling and acetylcholine in rat trachea: pharmacological modulation, *Br. J. Pharmacol.,* 94, 1057, 1988.

173. **Uchida, Y., Ninomiya, H., Saotome, M., Nomura, A., Ohtsuka, M., Yanagisawa, M., Goto, K., Masaki, T., and Hasegawa, S.,** Endothelin, a novel vasoconstrictor peptide, as potent bronchoconstrictor, *Eur. J. Pharmacol.,* 154, 227, 1988.

174. **Filep, J. G., Battistini, B., and Sirois, P.,** Endothelin induces thromboxane release and contraction of isolated guinea-pig airways, *Life Sci.,* 47, 1845, 1990.

175. **Battistini, B., Sirois, P., Braquet, P., and Filep, J. G.,** Endothelin-induced constriction of guinea-pig airways: role of platelet-activating factor, *Eur. J. Pharmacol.,* 186, 307, 1990.

176. **Yousufzai, S. Y. and Abdel, Latif, A. A.,** Effects of platelet-activating factor on the release of arachidonic acid and prostaglandins by rabbit iris smooth muscle. Inhibition by calcium channel antagonists, *Biochem. J.,* 228, 697, 1985.

177. **Abdel Latif, A. A.,** Regulation of arachidonate release, prostaglandin synthesis, and sphincter constriction in the mammalian iris-ciliary body, *Prog. Clin. Biol. Res.,* 312, 53, 1989.

178. **Van Delft, J. L., Van Haeringen, N. J., Verbeij, N. L., Domingo, M. T., Chabrier, P. E., and Braquet, P.,** Specific receptor sites for PAF in iris and ciliary body of the rabbit eye, *Curr. Eye Res.,* 7, 1063, 1988.

179. **Domingo, M. T., Chabrier, P. E., Van Delft, J. L., Verbeij, N. L., Van Haeringen, N. J., and Braquet, P.,** Characterization of specific binding sites for PAF in the iris and ciliary body of rabbit, *Biochem. Biophys. Res. Commun.,* 160, 250, 1989.

180. **Ferguson, M. K., Shahinian, H. K., and Michelassi, F.,** Lymphatic smooth muscle responses to leukotrienes, histamine and platelet activating factor, *J. Surg. Res.,* 44, 172, 1988.

181. **Sessler, C. N., Glauser, F. L., Davis, D., and Fowler, A. A.,** Effects of platelet-activating factor antagonist SRI 63-441 on endotoxemia in sheep, *J. Appl. Physiol.,* 65, 2624, 1988.

182. **Christman, B. W., Lefferts, P. L., Blair, I. A., and Snapper, J. R.,** Effect of platelet-activating factor receptor antagonism on endotoxin-induced lung dysfunction in awake sheep, *Am. Rev. Respir. Dis.,* 142, 1272, 1990.

183. **Christman, B. W., Lefferts, P. L., King, G. A., and Snapper, J. R.,** Role of circulating platelets and granulocytes in PAF-induced pulmonary dysfunction in awake sheep, *J. Appl. Physiol.,* 64, 2033, 1988.

184. **Burhop, K. E., Garcia, J. G., Selig, W. M., Lo, S. K., Van Der Zee, H., Kaplan, J. E., and Malik, A. B.,** Platelet-activating factor increases lung vascular permeability to protein, *J. Appl. Physiol.,* 61, 2210, 1986.

185. **Maki, N., Hoffman, D. R., and Johnston, J. M.,** Platelet-activating factor acetylhydrolase activity in maternal, fetal, and newborn rabbit plasma during pregnancy and lactation, *Proc. Natl. Acad. Sci. U.S.A.,* 85, 728, 1988.

186. **Hoffman, D. R., Bateman, M. K., and Johnston, J. M.,** Synthesis of platelet activating factor by cholinephosphotransferase in developing fetal rabbit lung, *Lipids,* 23, 96, 1988.

187. **Montrucchio, G., Alloatti, G., Tetta, C., Roffinello, C., Emanuelli, G., and Camussi, G.,** *In vitro* contractile effect of platelet-activating factor on guinea-pig myometrium, *Prostaglandins,* 32, 539, 1986.

188. **Tetta, C., Montrucchio, G., Alloatti, G., Roffinello, C., Emanuelli, G., Benedetto, C., Camussi, G., and Massobrio, M.,** Platelet-activating factor contracts human myometrium *in vitro, Proc. Soc. Exp. Biol. Med.,* 183, 376, 1986.

189. **Medeiros, Y. S. and Calixto, J. B.,** Effect of PAF-acether on the reactivity of the isolated rat myometrium, *Braz. J. Med. Biol. Res.,* 22, 1131, 1989.

190. **Yasuda, K., Satouchi, K., and Saito, K.,** Platelet-activating factor in normal rat uterus, *Biochem. Biophys. Res. Commun.,* 138, 1231, 1986.

191. **Angle, M. J., Jones, M. A., McManus, L. M., Pinckard, R. N., and Harper, M. J.,** Platelet-activating factor in the rabbit uterus during early pregnancy, *J. Reprod. Fertil.,* 83, 711, 1988.

192. **Nakayama, R., Yasuda, K., and Saito, K.,** Existence of endogenous inhibitors of platelet-activating factor (PAF) with PAF in rat uterus, *J. Biol. Chem.,* 262, 13174, 1987.

193. **Yasuda, K., Satouchi, K., Nakayama, R., and Saito, K.,** Acyl type platelet-activating factor in normal rat uterus determined by gas chromatography mass spectrometry, *Biomed. Environ. Mass Spectrom.,* 16, 137, 1988.

194. **Nakayama, R. and Saito, K.,** Presence of 1-O-alk-1′-enyl-2-O-acetyl glycerophosphocholine (vinyl form of PAF) in perfused rat and guinea pig hearts, *J. Biochem. Tokyo,* 105, 494, 1989.

195. **Lynch, J. M. and Henson, P. M.,** The intracellular retention of newly synthesized platelet-activating factor, *J. Immunol.,* 137, 2653, 1986.

196. **Bratton, D. L., Harris, R. A., Clay, K. L., and Henson, P. M.,** Effects of platelet activating factor on calcium-lipid interactions and lateral phase separations in phospholipid vesicles, *Biochim. Biophys. Acta,* 943, 211, 1988.
197. **Honda, Z., Nakamura, M., Miki, I., Minami, M., Watanabe, T., Seyama, Y., Okado, H., Toh, H., Ito, K., Miyamoto, T. et al.,** Cloning by functional expression of platelet-activating factor receptor from guinea-pig lung, *Nature,* 349, 342, 1991.
198. **Wang, C.-T. and Tai, H.-H.,** Monoclonal anti-idiotypic antibodies to platelet-activating factor (PAF) and their interaction with PAF receptors, *J. Biol. Chem.,* 266, 12372, 1991.
199. **Delbridge, L. M., Harris, P. J., and Morgan, T. O.,** Characterization of single heart cell contractility by rapid imaging, *Clin. Exp. Pharmacol. Physiol.,* 16, 179, 1989.
200. **Delbridge, L. M., Harris, P. J., Pringle, J. T., Dally, L. J., and Morgan, T. O.,** A superfusion bath for single cell recording with high precision optical depth control, temperature regulation, and rapid solution switching, *Pflugers Arch.,* 416, 94, 1990.
201. **Harris, P. J., Stewart, D., Cullinan, M. C., Delbridge, L. M., Dally, L., and Grinwald, P.,** Rapid measurement of isolated cardiac muscle cell length using a line scan camera, *IEEE Trans. Biomed. Eng.,* BME-34, 463, 1987.
202. **Tomlinson, Harris, Croft, and Stewart,** unpublished observations.

Chapter 10

SIGNAL TRANSDUCTION MECHANISMS INVOLVED IN PLATELET ACTIVATING FACTOR-INDUCED PRIMARY RESPONSE GENE EXPRESSION IN A431 CELLS

Yamini B. Tripathi and Shivendra D. Shukla

TABLE OF CONTENTS

ISBN 0-8493-7299-2
© 1993 by CRC Press, Inc.

I. INTRODUCTION

Intracellular signals generated by an agonist play a key role in various cell responses. In this chapter, features of the signal transduction mechanism in relation to platelet activating factor (PAF) -induced gene expression are elaborated. Individual cells have receptors for many extracellular ligands, but the ligand-activated second messengers are limited. Many ligands activate the common second messengers. How different ligands produce their specific cell response by using common pathways is poorly understood. Regulation of gene expression is a complex phenomenon. The preexisting transcription modulators get phosphorylated/dephosphorylated and regulate the expression of some genes known as primary response genes,[1] immediate early genes,[2] cell division cycle genes,[3] or the competence genes.[4] The newly synthesized proteins from some of these genes (primary response gene products) further regulate the expression of specific genes, termed secondary response genes. The products of other primary response genes act as a receptor for a particular ligand, or mediate the intracellular signal transduction pathway.[5] These genes are induced by several agents/stimuli such as growth factors, hormones, heat shock, stress, etc.[6-8] *c-fos* and TIS-1 are the members of this family. As early as 1982, it was observed that the *fos* oncogene (*v-fos*) was responsible for the induction of osteogenic sarcomas by FBJ murine sarcoma virus.[9] It was later observed that its normal cellular homologue *c-fos* encoded a nuclear protein. This *c-fos* product is a transcriptional cofactor and in combination with the *c-jun* product, it forms a protein complex which is called activator protein-1 (AP-1) factor.[10-12] This complex binds to the AP-1 site of many genes and presumably regulates their transcription.[11] The expression of *c-fos* oncogene is transient and rapid.[13] After receptor occupancy, its induction starts as early as 5 min and peaks by 30 to 40 min. After 60 min, the *c-fos* message declines to basal level. The expression of the *c-fos* gene is autoregulated, i.e., *c-fos* protein negatively regulates its own transcription and also destabilizes the preexisting messages. Therefore, in the presence of protein synthesis inhibitor (cycloheximide) the *c-fos* message could be detected up to 2 to 3 h.[14-16]

The *c-fos* gene is conserved among vertebrates and differentially expressed during development.[17] Its product is essential for growth and differentiation of certain tissues, but its uncontrolled expression can be pathological. *c-fos* mRNA is 2.2 kb. *c-fos* protein differs from *v-fos* protein at the C terminal region.[18,19] The mechanism of *c-fos* expression is discussed later in this chapter.

TIS-1 is another primary response gene which is a member of tetradecanoyl phorbol acetate (TPA) -induced sequences (TIS). It was first reported by Lim et al. in 1987.[20] They isolated seven clones from a cDNA library constructed from TPA-induced mRNA in Swiss 3T3 cells. One of the TIS genes (TIS-28) is the *c-fos* protooncogene. Later it was observed that these TIS genes are transiently expressed in many cell lines in response to several growth factors and hormones mediating growth/differentiation.[21] The TIS-1 protein, also known as nur 77 and NGF1B, appears to be a sequence-specific transcription factor.[6] The expression of TIS-1 gene is transient and rapid. The induction starts as early as 30 min.[22] In PC-12 cells, induction of TIS-1 messages by TPA, EGF, FGF, NGF, and voltage-dependent sodium channel agonists was observed.[22,23] TIS-1 was also induced by agents that activate cAMP production in rat astrocytes.[22] It appears that TIS genes are involved in the signal transduction cascade of cell proliferation and differentiation in cells such as PC-12, astrocytes, etc.

II. CHARACTERISTICS OF PLATELET ACTIVATING FACTOR AS AN AGONIST

PAF was first discovered in the late 1960s as a factor responsible for histamine release from rabbit platelets.[24] Benveniste et al.[25] isolated it and named it "platelet activating factor".

The biochemistry and chemistry of PAF was studied in many laboratories and finally its structure was confirmed in 1979.[26]

PAF is a phospholipid. At the *sn*-1 position, it has an alkyl side chain. The chain length and degree of unsaturation significantly affect its potency. The acetate group, at the *sn*-2-position, is also necessary for its biological activity. A chain length longer than three carbons reduces the activity and its replacement by the −OH group completely inactivates it. A phosphorylcholine polar head group is found at the *sn*-3 position.[27] PAF is involved in several pathological conditions such as increased vascular permeability, atherosclerosis, allergy, inflammation, hypotension, and many others.[28,29] PAF affects the immune system as it activates neutrophils and eosinophils, induces cytokine production by macrophages and monocytes, and suppresses T lymphocyte proliferation.[28] PAF is also accumulated during ischemia or convulsions.[30] Synthesis of PAF also occurs abundantly in cells. There are two pathways for PAF synthesis: (1) remodeling[31] and (2) *de novo*.[32] The former is a phospholipase A_2 (PLA$_2$) -dependent, two-step pathway. The activation of PLA$_2$ catalyzes the hydrolysis of *sn*-2 fatty acyl residue from alkylcholine-phosphoglycerides and produces an intermediate 1-O-alkyl-*sn*-glycerol 3-phosphocholine (lyso-PAF) and free fatty acid (usually arachidonic acid). In the next step, the hydroxyl group of the *sn*-2 position is replaced by an acetate group giving rise to PAF. This step is catalyzed by a specific acetyltransferase. In the second route, 1-O-alkyl 2-acetyl glycerol is synthesized in the first step which is then converted to active PAF by CDP- choline:1-alkyl-2-acetyl-*sn*-glycerol choline phosphotransferase. PAF is not stored within the cell.

III. PLATELET ACTIVATING FACTOR AND SIGNAL TRANSDUCTION

When PAF binds to its receptor, activation of polyphosphoinositide (PPI) turnover occurs in many systems.[33] This pathway, mediated by phospholipase C (PLC), is also active, with many other agonists generating second messengers. The primary phospholipid substrate for PLC is phosphatidylinositol 4,5-bisphosphate (PIP$_2$). This pathway was first discovered by Hokin[34] and then examined in detail by Michell[35] and Berridge and Irvine.[36] The two generated products (second messengers) are inositol trisphosphate (IP$_3$) and diacylglycerol (DG). IP$_3$ mobilizes the intracellular Ca^{2+} [36] and DG activates protein kinase C (PKC).[37] Initial studies with rabbit platelets demonstrated that PAF enhanced the PPI turnover,[38] and released IP, IP$_2$, and IP$_3$.[33] It also increases free arachidonate.[39] Forskolin, or PGI$_2$, the activator of adenylate cyclase, inhibited PAF-stimulated PPI turnover;[40,41] staurosporine, a PKC inhibitor, potentiates the IP$_3$ production[42] and phorbol myristate acetate (PMA) inhibits it.[42,43] Interestingly, PAF also has an inhibitory effect on adenylate cyclase activity.[44]

Previous reports suggest the role of guanine nucleotide binding protein (G-protein) in PAF-coupled PLC activation, but the experiments with pertussis toxin (PT) have provided inconclusive results. For example, in platelets PLC activation is both PT sensitive[45] and insensitive.[46] In macrophages and neutrophils it is sensitive, whereas in U937 cells, PAF induced PLC activation is insensitive to PT.[33] Involvement of tyrosine kinases has also been proposed.[47] Dhar et al.[46] have recently reported that PAF phosphorylates 50 and 60 kDa protein in rabbit platelets, which were reactive to the monoclonal antibody to phosphotyrosine. This phosphorylation was blocked by genistein, a protein tyrosine kinase (PTK) inhibitor.[48]

IV. PLATELET ACTIVATING FACTOR AND GENE EXPRESSION

The role of PAF in gene expression is poorly investigated. Because PAF is involved in many pathological conditions and affects cell physiology, PAF might have important effects

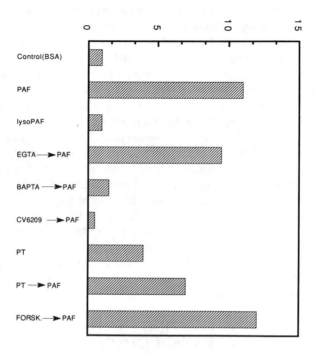

FIGURE 1. Characteristics of PAF-induced *c-fos* gene expression in A431 cells. The results from several experimental protocols are presented to emphasize the behavior of PAF-induced *c-fos* gene expression. In these experiments, A431 cells were treated with drugs/agents and then challenged with PAF (10^{-7} *M*) for 60 min. For PT treatment, cells were incubated overnight with the activated toxin (5 μg/ml) before challenge with PAF. For BAPTA experiments, cells were loaded with BAPTA (25 μ*M*) for 1 h, washed, and then challenged with PAF. The concentrations of other agents were as follows: EGTA (2 m*M*), forskolin (5 μ*M*), and lyso-PAF (1 μ*M*).

on gene expression. In order to test this hypothesis, we treated the A431 cells (human epidermoid carcinoma cells) with PAF and determined the expression of the primary response genes. It was observed that PAF induced the expression of *c-fos* and TIS-1 genes in a receptor-coupled manner.[49-51] When the A431 cells were pretreated with the PAF antagonist CV6209 for 20 min, PAF failed to induce these genes (Figure 1). CV6209 is a receptor antagonist and competes with PAF for its receptor binding site. Lyso-PAF (Figure 1), which is an inactive structural analogue of PAF, failed to induce this gene up to 10^{-6} *M* concentration, whereas PAF response was noted at 10^{-10} *M*. This result indicates the structural specificity of PAF. The dose-response profile showed that the optimum dose of PAF for *c-fos* induction in A431 cells is 10^{-7} *M*. Interestingly, PAF also induces expression of the *c-fos* gene in other cells, e.g., neuroblastoma cells,[52] human B lymphoblastoma cells,[53] and monocytes.[54]

V. KINETICS OF *c-fos* EXPRESSION

Induction of *c-fos* is rapid and transient. In the absence of cycloheximide, expression was seen as early as 15 to 20 min of PAF incubation, increased up to 40 min, and then gradually decreased. By 60 min, no detectable signal was seen. However, in the presence of cycloheximide, expression was maintained up to 4 h.[49-51] Cycloheximide is a protein synthesis inhibitor and its treatment of cells inhibits about 90% of protein synthesis. Because the expression of *c-fos* was rapid and transient, we examined whether PAF is needed for the entire time course of induction or if it relays a signal in the early stage that is responsible for the *c-fos* expression. When cells were incubated with PAF for brief periods, washed to remove the free PAF, and incubated again in fresh medium for a fixed period of time, it was observed that even 1 min of PAF incubation was enough for optimum expression of the *c-fos* gene.[51]

The induction of the *c-fos* gene could be mediated by at least two known pathways: by the involvement of adenylate cyclase and PKC. The two pathways involve different regions of the *c-fos* promoter.[6] Activation by cAMP, a product of adenylate cyclase, requires the cAMP response element (CRE), which is located at position -60 and -350 of the *c-fos* gene. On the other hand, PKC phosphorylates a protein (62 kDa) which binds to the dyad symmetry element (DSE), also known as the serum response element (SRE).[19] Further, a role for tyrosine kinase has not yet been assessed. To study the possible role of these pathways, we used several pharmacological tools which selectively inhibit or activate these pathways.

VI. INVOLVEMENT OF TYROSINE KINASE

Genistein, a putative tyrosine kinase inhibitor, inhibited the PAF-induced *c-fos* expression in a dose-dependent manner in A431 cells.[51] This suggested an involvement of protein tyrosine kinase (PTK) in the signaling pathway of PAF-induced *c-fos* expression. PTK activity is broadly divided into two groups: (1) receptor and (2) nonreceptor PTK which could be membrane bound or cytosolic.[56] The former possibility is unlikely in this case because the PAF receptor was recently cloned, and its sequence homology is different from typical tyrosine kinase receptors.[55] We also observed that genistein failed to inhibit *c-fos* expression when added 90 s after the addition of PAF. This indicates that tyrosine kinase may be involved in the very early steps of signal transduction (Figure 2). At present, it is not clear if this tyrosine kinase activity is membrane bound or cytosolic. In rabbit platelets, PAF activates the tyrosine kinase activity of pp60[c-src] and its movement from cytosol to membrane.[57] Thus, the role of the nonreceptor, cytosolic tyrosine kinase (e.g., pp60[c-src]), in this pathway would be worthy of investigation.

VII. INVOLVEMENT OF PROTEIN KINASE C

PMA pretreatment of cells down-regulates the cellular PKC activity.[58,59] PAF did not show any expression of *c-fos* in A431 cells pretreated with PMA for 20 h. Therefore, a role of PKC in the PAF-induced *c-fos* expression appears likely. When PMA and PAF were simultaneously added to these cells in optimal concentrations, no synergistic response was observed, although at lower concentrations, an additive response was seen. This further supports the role of PKC in this pathway because if two agonists are operating through a similar pathway, competition will occur and an additive induction will not be expected.

Staurosporine, a potent inhibitor of PKC,[60,61] inhibited the expression of *c-fos* induced by PAF at low concentrations. This further supports the involvement of PKC in this pathway. In order to determine the hierarchical status of PKC relative to PTK, we added staurosporine at different time points after the addition of PAF. Staurosporine inhibited *c-fos* expression when added within 4 to 5 min of PAF addition, but failed when added 10 min after the PAF addition. These data suggested that PTK is activated before PKC.

PKC has been shown to be involved in transducing signals initiated by several peptide hormone ligands.[58,62] It is a Ca^{2+}-dependent protein kinase that is directly activated by DG, a product of phospholipase C (PLC),[63] and also by tumor promoters such as TPA, PDBu,

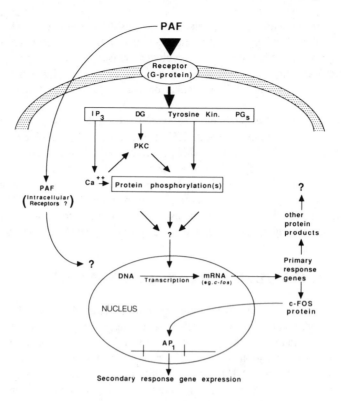

FIGURE 2. A schematic diagram depicting the relationship between PAF receptor signaling and the primary response gene expression in A-431 cells. The role of both PKC and tyrosine kinase is proposed. IP$_3$, inositol trisphosphate; DG, diacylglycerol; PGs, prostaglandins.

and mezerein. Metabolites of other phospholipases such as PLA$_2$ and PLD can also activate the PKC. More than seven isoforms of PKC have been characterized thus far.[58] The involvement of PKC in the cellular responses induced by PAF has been studied in platelets and neutrophils. It has been shown that PKC activation inhibits the PLC activity, whereas the PAF-induced homologous desensitization is not affected by PKC inhibition or down-regulation.[42,43] In relation to *c-fos* expression, it appears that this response is mediated through PKC. Thus, it is probable that PAF-induced PKC activation occurs not only through the PLC pathway, but there may be other possibilities as well. A point of considerable interest is the observation that staurosporine potentiated PAF stimulated production of IP$_3$,[42] while it inhibited the *c-fos* expression. It is therefore suggested that IP$_3$ per se is not directly involved in the *c-fos* gene expression.

PAF desensitizes its own receptor responses. When A431 cells were pretreated with PAF (in the absence of cycloheximide) for 90 min, further addition of PAF failed to induce *c-fos* genes. This desensitization was effective only up to 4 h because after that period, the addition of PAF induced the expression of the *c-fos* in A-431 cells.

Cloned PAF receptor shows homology to the G-protein-coupled receptor family. However, PT failed to completely abolish the PAF-induced *c-fos* expression in A431 cells, as only 20 to 30% inhibition was seen (Figure 1). Under similar conditions, PAF-induced IP$_3$ production was inhibited by about 50%.[68] This suggests that PAF receptors may be coupled with two types of G-proteins, PT sensitive and PT insensitive.

VIII. ROLE OF cAMP-MEDIATED PATHWAY

In A431 cells, inducible CRE is defective.[64] We have found that forskolin, an activator of adenylate cyclase, fails to induce c-fos in A431 cells, but it does elevate the cAMP level in similar conditions (unpublished). Furthermore, forskolin had no effect on PAF-induced c-fos expression (Figure 1). PAF-induced expression in this particular cell line suggests that the PKA pathway might not be involved in this signal cascade.

In neuroblastoma cells, involvement of both CRE and SRE has been proposed.[52] Taking both reports into consideration, it could be concluded that SRE alone, which is not affected by cAMP,[65] is sufficient to induce the PAF-induced c-fos expression. In those cells in which both CRE and SRE are active, however, c-fos expression may be regulated separately by both elements.

IX. ROLE OF CA²⁺

No change in the induction of c-fos was seen when A431 cells were treated with PAF in the presence of up to 2 mM EGTA. This suggests that PAF-induced c-fos expression is independent of extracellular Ca^{2+}. In rabbit platelets EGTA had no influence on PAF-induced PLC activation.[33] On the other hand, induction was completely inhibited when PAF was incubated with A431 cells preloaded with bis(-O-aminophenoxy)ethane-N,N,N',N'-tetraacetic acid (BAPTA), an intracellular Ca^{2+} chelator (Figure 1). This observation suggests that intracellular Ca^{2+} is essential for PAF-induced gene expression. Whether this Ca^{2+} is directly responsible for the activation of c-fos promoter or it participates via activating the PKC is still not clear. Because Ca^{2+} and cAMP both regulate c-fos expression through CRE,[75] which is defective in A431 cells, it is therefore most likely that Ca^{2+} is essential for the activity of PKC only.

X. EXPRESSION OF OTHER EARLY RESPONSE GENES

Besides the induction of c-fos, PAF also induces the expression of TIS-1, whose kinetics are similar to c-fos. PAF also induces the expression of c-jun in neuroblastoma cells. Thus, it seems that the product of many of these early response genes can separately or in combination activate the promoter of other genes, the secondary response genes. At present, no direct evidence exists for the identity of such genes, but its possibility cannot be ruled out.

XI. CONCLUDING REMARKS

PAF is the most potent phospholipid agonist known. Characterization of PAF receptor and its transmembrane signaling have been topics of great interest over the past several years. However, any role of PAF at the nuclear or genetic level has only recently drawn attention. It is now documented that in several different cell types, PAF stimulates the expression of primary response genes.[47] In A431 cells, genes for both c-fos and TIS-1 are induced by PAF in a PAF receptor-dependent and structurally specific manner. Of greater interest are the results that led to the suggestion that PAF receptor signaling pathways and second messengers play key roles in the induction process (Figure 2). It appears likely that in A431 cells, c-AMP and IP$_3$ have little involvement in PAF-stimulated c-fos and TIS-1 gene expression. On the other hand, PKC and tyrosine kinase both can be implicated in the gene expression. In the cascade of events initiated after PAF receptor occupancy that lead to gene expression, it appears that the tyrosine kinase step precedes that of PKC. Further, intracellular Ca^{2+} is also essential for this gene response. The exquisite sensitivity by which

PAF elicits this gene expression is remarkable because exposure as brief as 1 min was sufficient to trigger the signal leading to the primary response gene expression. As far as it can be ascertained at present, studies with PAF provide the first example of an agonist whose receptor is coupled to G-protein and stimulates *c-fos* expression via tyrosine kinase activation. This suggests involvement of a novel pathway in PAF-induced gene expression. There are several temporal and spatial issues which remain to be addressed in this phenomenon. The nature of the message and the mechanism by which it is relayed from receptor to cytosol and then into the nucleus remains unknown. Relevance of gene expression and its consequences in pathophysiological states in which endogenous levels of PAF are elevated[67] also awaits future investigation.

ACKNOWLEDGMENTS

The authors are grateful to Dr. Robert Lim for his excellent suggestions and critical reading of this chapter. Thanks are also due to Ms. Judy Richey for her expert typing of the manuscript. YBT was supported by a Biotechnology Fellowship of the Government of India and by the University of Missouri-Columbia Molecular Biology Program. SDS was supported by an NIH Research Career Development Award (RCDA) DK01782.

REFERENCES

1. **Yamamoto, K. and Alberts, B.**, Steroid receptors: elements for modulation of eukaryotic transcription, *Annu. Rev. Biochem.*, 45, 721, 1976.
2. **Lau, L. F. and Nathans, D.**, Expression of a set of growth related immediate early genes in BALB/C 3T3 cells: coordinated regulation with *c-fos* or *c-myc*, *Proc. Natl. Acad. Sci. U.S.A.*, 84, 1182, 1987.
3. **Hirschhorn, R. R., Aller, P., Yuan, Z. A., Gibson, C. W., and Baserga, R.**, Cell-cycle-specific cDNAs from mammalian cells temperature sensitive for growth, *Proc. Natl. Acad. Sci. U.S.A.*, 81, 6004, 1984.
4. **Jones, S. D., Hall, D. J., Rollins, B. J., and Stiles, C. D.**, Platelet-derived growth factor generates at least two distinct intracellular signals that modulate gene expression, *Cold Spring Harbor Symp. Quant. Biol.*, 53, 531, 1988.
5. **Cantley, L. C., Auger, K. R., Carpenter, C., Duckworth, B., Graziani, A., Kapellar, R., and Soltoff, S.**, Oncogenes and signal transduction, *Cell*, 64, 281, 1991.
6. **Herschman, H. R.**, Primary response genes induced by growth factors and tumor promoters, *Annu. Rev. Biochem.*, 60, 281, 1991.
7. **Ransone, L. J. and Verma, I. M.**, Nuclear proto-oncotenes Fos and Jun, *Annu. Rev. Cell Biol.*, 6, 539, 1990.
8. **Jahner, D. and Hunter, T.**, The stimulation of quiescent rat fibroblasts by v-src and v-fps oncogenic protein-tyrosine kinases leads to the induction of a subset of immediate early genes, *Oncogene*, 6, 1259, 1991.
9. **Curran, T., Peters, G., Van Beveren, C., Teich, N. M., and Verma, I. M.**, FBJ murine osteosarcoma virus: identification and molecular cloning of biologically active proviral DNA, *J. Virol.*, 44, 674, 1982.
10. **Chiu, R., Boyle, W. J., Meek, J., Smeal, T., Hunter, T., and Karin, M.**, The *c-fos* protein interacts with *c-jun*/AP-1 to stimulate transcription of AP-1 responsive genes, *Cell*, 54, 541, 1988.
11. **Halazonetis, T. D., Georgopoulos, K., Greenberg, M. E., and Leder, P.**, *c-jun* dimerizes with itself and with *c-fos* forming complexes of different DNA binding affinities, *Cell*, 55, 197, 1988.
12. **Rauscher, F. J., Voulalas, P. J., Franza, B. R., Jr., and Curran, T.**, Fos and Jun bind cooperatively to the AP-1 site: reconstitution *in vitro*, *Genes Devel.*, 2, 1687, 1988.
13. **Kruijer, W., Cooper, J. A., Hunter, T., and Verma, I. M.**, Platelet-derived growth factor induces rapid but transient expression of the *c-fos* gene and protein, *Nature*, 312, 711, 1984.
14. **Sassone-Corsi, P., Lamph, W. W., and Verma, I. M.**, Regulation of proto-oncogene fos: a paradigm for early response genes, *Cold Spring Harbor Symp. Quant. Biol.*, 53, 749, 1988.
15. **Cochran, B. H., Reffel, A. C., and Stiles, C. D.**, Molecular cloning of gene sequences regulated by platelet derived growth factor, *Cell*, 33, 939, 1983.

16. **Greenberg, M. E., Hermanowski, A. L., and Ziff, E. B.,** Effect of protein synthesis inhibitors on growth factor activation of *c-fos, c-myc* and actin gene transcription, *Mol. Cell. Biol.,* 6, 1050, 1986.

17. **Müller, R., Slamon, D. J., Tremblay, J. M., Cline, M. J., and Verma, I. M.,** Differential expression of cellular oncogenes during pre- and postnatal development of the mouse, *Nature,* 299, 640, 1982.

18. **Van Beveren, C., van Straaten, F., Curran, T., Muller, R., and Verma, I. M.,** Analysis of FBJ-MuSV provirus and *c-fos* (mouse) gene reveals that viral and cellular *fos* gene products have different carboxy termini, *Cell,* 32, 1241, 1983.

19. **Ransone, L. J. and Verma, I. M.,** Nuclear proto-oncogenes fos and jun, *Annu. Rev. Cell Biol.,* 6, 539, 1990.

20. **Lim, R. W., Varnum, B. C., and Herschman, H.,** Cloning of tetradecanoyl phorbol ester-induced "primary response" sequences and their expression in density-arrested Swiss 3T3 cells and a TPA nonproliferative variant, *Oncogene,* 1, 263, 1987.

21. **Herschman, H. R.,** Extracellular signals, transcriptional responses and cellular specificity, *TIBS,* 14, 455, 1989.

22. **Arenander, A. T., Lim, R. W., Varnum, B. C., Cole, R., DeVellis, J., and Herschman, H. R.,** TIS gene expression in cultured rat astrocytes: induction by mitogens and stellation agents, *J. Neurosci. Res.,* 23, 247, 1989.

23. **Kujubu, D. A., Lim, R. W., Varnum, B. C., and Herschman, H. R.,** Induction of transiently expressed genes in PC-12-pheochromocytoma cells, *Oncogene,* 1, 257, 1987.

24. **Barbaro, J. F. and Zvaifler, N. J.,** Antigen induced histamine release from platelets of rabbits producing homologous PLA antibody, *Proc. Soc. Exp. Biol. Med.,* 122, 1245, 1966.

25. **Benveniste, J., Henson, P. M., and Cochrane, C. G.,** Leukocyte-dependent histamine release from rabbit platelets. The role of IgG, basophils, and a platelet-activating factor, *J. Exp. Med.,* 136, 1356, 1972.

26. **Hanahan, D. J., Demopoulas, C. A., Liehr, J., and Pinckard, R. N.,** Identification of platelet activating factor isolated from rabbit basophils as acetyl glyceryl ether phosphorylcholine, *J. Biol. Chem.,* 255, 5514, 1980.

27. **Prescott, S. M., Zimmerman, G. A., and McIntyre, T. M.,** Platelet activating factor, *J. Biol. Chem.,* 265, 17381, 1990.

28. **Sturk, A., Cate, J. W. T., Hosford, D., Mencia-Huerta, J. M., and Braquet, P.,** The synthesis, catabolism, and pathophysiological role of platelet-activating factor, *Adv. Lipid Res.,* 23, 219, 1989.

29. **Hanahan, D. J.,** Platelet-activating factor: a biologically active phosphoglyceride, *Annu. Rev. Biochem.,* 55, 483, 1986.

30. **Kumar, R., Harvey, S. A., Kester, M., Hanahan, D. J., and Olson, M. S.,** Production and effects of platelet activating factor in the rat brain, *Biochem. Biophys. Acta,* 963, 375, 1988.

31. **Snyder, F.,** Biochemistry of platelet activating factor: a unique class of biologically active phospholipid, *Proc. Soc. Exp. Biol. Med.,* 190, 125, 1989.

32. **Lee, T.-C.,** Enzymatic control of the cellular levels of platelet activating factor, in *Platelet-Activating Factor and Related Lipid Mediators,* Snyder, F., Ed., Plenum Press, New York, 1987, 115.

33. **Shukla, S. D.,** Inositol phospholipid turnover in PAF transmembrane signalling, *Lipids,* 26, in press.

34. **Hokin, L. E.,** Receptors and phosphoinositide-generated second messengers, *Annu. Rev. Biochem.,* 54, 205, 1985.

35. **Michell, R. H.,** Inositol phospholipids and cell surface receptor function, *Biochim. Biophys. Acta,* 415, 81, 1975.

36. **Berridge, M. J. and Irvine, R. F.,** Inositol trisphosphate, a novel second messenger in cellular signal transduction, *Nature,* 312, 315, 1984.

37. **Abdel-Latif, A. A.,** Calcium-mobilizing receptors, polyphosphoinosides, and the generation of second messengers, *Pharmacol. Rev.,* 38, 227, 1986.

38. **Shukla, S. D. and Hanahan, D. J.,** AGEPC (platelet activating factor) induced stimulation of rabbit platelets: effects of phosphatidylinositol, di- and triphosphoinositides and phosphatidic acid metabolism, *Biochem. Biophys. Res. Commun.,* 106, 697, 1982.

39. **Bonventre, J. V., Weber, P. C., and Gronich, J. H.,** PAF and PDGF increase cytosolic [Ca2+] and phospholipase activity in mesangial cells, *Am. J. Physiol.,* 254, F87, 1988.

40. **Shukla, S. D.,** Platelet activating factor-stimulated formation of inositol triphosphate in platelets and its regulation by various agents, including Ca2+, indomethacin, CV-3988, and forskolin, *Arch. Biochem. Biophys.,* 240, 674, 1985.

41. **Haye, B., Aublin, J. L., Champion, S., Lambert, B., and Jacquemin, C.,** Interactions between thyreostimulin and PAF-acether on thyroid cell metabolism, *Eur. J. Pharmacol.,* 104, 125, 1984.

42. **Morrison, W. J., Dhar, A., and Shukla, S. D.,** Staurosporine potentiates platelet activating factor stimulated phospholipase C activity in rabbit platelets but does not block desensitization by platelet activating factor, *Life Sci.,* 45, 333, 1989.

43. **Morrison, W. J. and Shukla, S. D.,** Antagonism of platelet activating factor receptor binding and stimulated phosphoinositide-specific phospholipase C in rabbit platelets, *J. Pharmacol. Exp. Ther.,* 250, 831, 1989.

44. **Haslam, R. J. and Vanderwel, M.,** Inhibition of platelet adenylate cyclase by 1-O-alkyl-O-acetyl-*sn*-glyceryl-3-phosphorylcholine (platelet activating factor), *J. Biol. Chem.,* 257, 6879, 1982.

45. **Brass, L. F., Woolkalis, M. J., and Manning, D. R.,** Interactions in platelets between G proteins and the agonists that stimulate phospholipase C and inhibit adenylyl cyclase, *J. Biol. Chem.,* 263, 5348, 1988.

46. **Dhar, A., Paul, A. K., and Shukla, S. D.,** Platelet-activating factor stimulation of tyrosine kinase and its relationship to phospholipase C in rabbit platelets: studies with genistein and monoclonal antibody to phosphotyrosine, *Mol. Pharmacol.,* 37, 519, 1990.

47. **Shukla, S. D.,** Platelet activating factor receptor and signal transduction mechanisms, *FASEB J.,* in press.

48. **Akiyama, T., Ishida, J., Nakagawa, S., Ogawara, H., Watanabe, S., Itoh, N., Shibuya, M., and Fukami, Y.,** Genistein, a specific inhibitor of tyrosine-specific protein kinases, *J. Biol. Chem.,* 262, 5592, 1987.

49. **Tripathi, Y. B., Kandala, J., Guntaka, R. V., Lim, R. W., and Shukla, S. D.,** Induction of *c-fos* gene expression in A-431 cells by platelet activating factor, *FASEB J.,* 5, A-895, 1991.

50. **Tripathi, Y. B., Kandala, J. C., Guntaka, R. V., Lim, R. W., and Shukla, S. D.,** Platelet activating factor induces expression of early response genes *c-fos* and TIS-1 in human epidermoid carcinoma A-431 cells, *Life Sci.,* 49, 1761, 1991.

51. **Tripathi, Y. B., Lim, R. W., Fernandez-Gallardo, S., Kandala, J. C., Guntaka, R. V., and Shukla, S. D.,** Involvement of tyrosine kinase and protein kinase C in platelet activating factor induced *c-fos* gene expression in A-431 cells, *Biochem. J.* in press.

52. **Squinto, S. P., Block, A. L., Braquet, P., and Bazan, N. G.,** Platelet-activating factor stimulates a *fos/jun*/AP-1 transcriptional signaling system in human neuroblastoma cells, *J. Neurosci. Res.,* 24, 558, 1989.

53. **Mazer, B., Domenico, J., Sawami, H., and Gelfand, E. W.,** Platelet-activating factor induces an increase in intracellular calcium and expression of regulatory genes in human B lymphoblastoid cells, *J. Immunol.,* 146, 1914, 1991.

54. **Ho, Y. S., Lee, W. M. F., and Synderman, R.,** Chemoattractant-induced activation of *c-fos* gene expression in human monocytes, *J. Exp. Med.,* 165, 1524, 1987.

55. **Honda, Z., Nakamura, M., Miki, I., Minami, M., Watanabe, T., Seyama, Y., Okado, H., Toh, H., Ito, K., Miyamoto, T., and Shimizu, T.,** Cloning by functional expression of platelet-activating factor receptor from guinea pig lung, *Nature,* 349, 342, 1991.

56. **Hanks, S. K., Quinn, A. M., and Hunter, T.,** The protein kinase family: conserved features and deduced phylogeny of the catalytic domains, *Science,* 241, 42, 1988.

57. **Dhar, A. and Shukla, S. D.,** Involvement of pp60[c-src] in platelet-activating factor-stimulated platelets, *J. Biol. Chem.,* 266, 18797, 1991.

58. **Nishizuka, Y.,** The molecular heterogeneity of protein kinase C and its implications for cellular regulation, *Nature,* 334, 661, 1988.

59. **Spangler, R., Bailey, S. C., and Sytkowski, A. J.,** Erythropoietin increases c-myc mRNA by a protein kinase C-dependent pathway, *J. Biol. Chem.,* 266, 681, 1991.

60. **Tamaoki, T., Nomoto, H., Takahashi, I., Kato, Y., Morimoto, M., and Tomita, F.,** Staurosporine, a potent inhibitor of phospholipid/Ca^{++} dependent protein kinase, *Biochem. Biophys. Res. Commun.,* 135, 397, 1986.

61. **Powis, G.,** Signalling targets for anticancer drug development, *TIPS,* 12, 188, 1991.

62. **Nishizuka, Y.,** The role of protein kinase C in cell surface signal transduction and tumor production, *Nature,* 308, 693, 1984.

63. **Takai, Y., Kishimoto, A., Iwasa, Y., Kawahara, Y., Mori, T., and Nishizuka, Y.,** Calcium-dependent activation of a multifunctional protein kinase by membrane phospholipids, *J. Biol. Chem.,* 254, 3692, 1979.

64. **Kanei-Ishii, C. and Ishii, S.,** Dual enhancer activities of the cyclic AMP responsive element with cell type and promoter specificity, *Nucleic Acids Res.,* 17, 1521, 1989.

65. **Gilman, M. Z.,** The *c-fos* serum response element responds to protein kinase C-dependent and -independent signals but not to cyclic AMP, *Genes Devel.,* 2, 394, 1988.

66. **Sheng, M., McFadden, G., and Greenberg, M. E.,** Membrane depolarization and calcium induce *c-fos* transcription via phosphorylation of transcription factor CREB, *Neuron,* 4, 571, 1990.

67. **Koltai, M., Hasford, D., Guinot, P., Esanu, A., and Braquet, P.,** Platelet activating factor (PAF): a review of its effects, antagonists, and possible future clinical implications, *Drugs,* 42, 9, 1991.

68. **Thurston, A. and Shukla, S. D.,** unpublished data.

Chapter 11

PLATELET ACTIVATING FACTOR AND INTRACELLULAR SIGNALING PATHWAYS THAT MODULATE GENE EXPRESSION

Nicolas G. Bazan and John P. Doucet

TABLE OF CONTENTS

ISBN 0-8493-7299-2
© 1993 by CRC Press, Inc.

I. INTRODUCTION

Platelet-activating factor (PAF; 1-alkyl-2-acetyl-*sn*-glycero-3-phosphocholine) is a potent, bioactive phospholipid derived from cellular membranes following cell stimulation. PAF mediates a wide variety of biological phenomena, and this pervasiveness reflects a general role as a cellular messenger generated in response to cell stimulation. Several signal transduction pathways are affected by PAF, including promotion of Ca^{2+} influx and activation of protein kinase C (PKC) and phospholipases A_2 (PLA$_2$) and C (PLC).[1] As a consequence, PAF stimulates intracellular Ca^{2+} mobilization, inositol phosphate and diacylglycerol generation, serine/threonine and tyrosine protein phosphorylation,[2] and an increased availability of arachidonic acid for lipoxygenation.[3,4]

PAF may elicit some of its actions though intracellular pathways. One phenomenon that suggests this role is the avidity with which certain cells retain stimulus-evoked PAF. Intracellular retention of synthesized PAF occurs in several cell types in culture, including a variety of leukocytes and endothelial cells,[5] human fetal brain cells,[6] and rat cerebellar granule cells[7] and neurotransmitter-stimulated retina.[8] Intracellular PAF has been proposed as a second messenger regulating arachidonic acid release and eicosanoid generation.[9-11] The finding of high affinity PAF binding sites in purified intracellular membranes of the cerebral cortex[12] and the demonstration of selective antagonism of these sites[13] has provided an opportunity to experimentally approach specific roles for intracellular PAF, such as the regulation of gene expression.

II. INTRACELLULAR PAF AND SELECTIVE BINDING ANTAGONISTS

PAF is generated inside the cell by two pathways:[1] (1) through remodeling of membrane constituent alkyl-acylglycerophosphocholines by sequential PLA$_2$ and cholinetransferase activities or (2) through *de novo* acetate transfer, phosphate hydrolysis, and phosphocholine transfer activities upon alkyl-lysophosphatidic acids. Signal transduction through the generation of PAF may involve both pathways. The PLA$_2$-initiated pathway probably mediates the pathologic reactions in tissues.

Several studies indicate that the PLA$_2$ responsible for remodeling PAF precursor from membrane alkyl-phospholipids may be polyenoic specific with arachidonoyl esters being the preferred substrate, suggesting that *sn*-2 hydrolysis of alkyl-acylglycerophosphocholines generates both eicosanoid and PAF precursors. In brain following seizures or ischemia, PAF is generated,[14] and isolated synaptosomes from convulsing rats are the only subcellular fraction to show the accumulation of free polyenoic fatty acids (arachidonic and docosahexaenoic), suggesting that synaptic PLA$_2$ activity is enhanced under these conditions.[15] However, whether a single phospholipase releases both PAF and free fatty acids at the synapse during convulsions is not known.

Subcellular localizations of PAF generating enzymes and precursors have provided insight into the intracellular mechanism of PAF metabolism and retention.[16,17] Both acetyl- and choline-phosphotransferases (enzymes of the remodeling and *de novo* pathways, respectively) localize to the endoplasmic reticulum, whereas PAF and lyso-PAF are components of the inner leaflet of the plasma membrane. In addition, alkyl-acylglycerophosphocholine is apparently available for remodeling from both the plasma membrane and intracellular organelles. Thus, the mixed localization of PAF, PAF precursors, and PAF-synthetic enzymes suggests that (1) a high degree of efficient and rapid alkylphospholipid transport is required between membranes during PAF synthesis and that (2) newly synthesized, plasma membrane-associated PAF is accessible for intracellular usage.

Calcium ion plays an integral role in PAF metabolism.[1] PAF production through remodeling requires Ca^{2+}, but enzymes of the *de novo* pathway are each inhibited by Ca^{2+}, as are the activities of PAF deacetylation and lyso-PAF transacetylation. Therefore, calcium may drive the PAF synthetic equilibrium toward phospholipid hydrolysis and, through inhibiting its reacylation, maintain stimulated PAF levels. The protective effects of PAF antagonists in experimental epilepsy and ischemia studies suggests that elevated PAF levels are pathologic, and Ca^{2+} influx through massive neurotransmitter discharges may be responsible for initiating membrane lipid changes and the pathologic state. PAF itself induces Ca^{2+} influx, and its stimulation of PLC in turn induces intracellular Ca^{2+} ionization though polyphosphoinositide (PPI) hydrolysis.[18] Thus, PAF may act to maintain or amplify its Ca^{2+} signal intracellularly.

A second messenger role for intracellularly generated PAF is suggested by the inhibition of stimulus-induced arachidonic acid mobilization, eicosanoid production, and superoxide anion generation by structurally unrelated PAF antagonists in leukocytic and epithelial cells.[9-11] The time course of these stimulus responses parallels the intracellular generation and retention of PAF, suggesting that agonist-evoked PAF is the second messenger for these responses.

The discovery of two high affinity, Ca^{2+}-sensitive intracellular PAF binding sites[12] is consistent with an intracellular activity PAF. These sites were identified in purified microsomal membranes derived from rat cerebral cortex. In addition, a low affinity binding site exists on synaptic membranes, and binding is absent on mitochondria and myelin membranes. To minimize the contamination of microsomal membranes with plasma membranes, the postmitochondrial supernatant was first centrifuged at $43,500 \times g$ for 20 min. This pellet was enriched in plasma membranes. The supernatant was then centrifuged at $105,000 \times g$ for 60 min. Further subfractionation of this microsomal pellet by density-gradient centrifugation was performed to study the microsomal PAF binding site. The microsomal and synaptic sites seem to be different, because saturation curves in the microsomes but not in synaptic membranes fit a model compatible with multiple binding sites.

Because the intracellular sites could represent the same cell surface site undergoing intracellular recycling, a pharmacological approach has been used to further characterize these sites. A variety of PAF receptor antagonists was found to differentially bind the cell surface and the microsomal sites, supporting the notion that these sites are distinct.[12,13] The distinct nature of these sites will ultimately be characterized by molecular cloning and functional expression of the protein structures they represent. Recently, the cloning of PAF receptors possessing sequence similarity to membrane-spanning, G-protein-linked receptors such as the β_2-adrenergic receptor have been reported.[20,21] This similarity strongly suggests that the cloned PAF receptors are plasma membrane receptors and may be similar or identical to the synaptic site that has been pharmacologically identified.

III. PLATELET ACTIVATING FACTOR IS A MODULATOR OF THE PRIMARY GENOMIC RESPONSE

The primary genomic response of a cell is collectively the earliest transcriptional activity following cell stimulation and is comprised of expression of immediate-early genes. PAF stimulates immediate-early gene expression in several cells, including neuroblastoma,[21] retinoblastoma,[22] neuroglial hybrid,[23] T cells,[21] B cells,[24,25] and epidermal carcinoma cells.[26] In neuroblastoma cells,[21] exogenously added PAF exerts a rapid and transient increase both on c-*fos* and c-*jun* mRNA abundance, and a PAF antagonist inhibits this effect. *In vitro* nuclear transcription shows that PAF accomplishes the increase in immediate-early mRNA abundance by stimulating the transcription of respective genes. PAF-stimulated transcription of *c-fos* requires a cyclic AMP/calcium-response element (CRE/CaRE)[27], which agrees with the wealth of studies demonstrating PAF-stimulated Ca^{2+} influx and phosphoinositide (PI) turnover. In addition, PAF stimulates transcription of genes possessing the Fos-Jun/AP-1 responsive sequence,[21,28] indicating that the PAF stimulus evokes synthesis of functional protein following the immediate-early transcription.

c-*fos* and c-*jun* encode proteins that create a heterodimeric transcription-regulating complex through mutual leucine zipper domains.[29] PAF also stimulates transcription of the immediate-early gene *zif/268* (also called TIS-8, Egr-1, KROX 24, or NGFI-A).[23] The *zif/268* promoter, like that of *c-fos*, contains a sequence that resembles the CRE/CaRE.[30] *zif/268* encodes a Zn^{2+}-finger protein that is widely believed to be an activator of transcription. Therefore, the induced expression of two Ca^{2+}-responsive immediate-early genes, which encode two different types of transcription factor, is a component of the intracellular signal transduction of PAF.

The relevance of a PAF-transduced genomic response is substantiated by application of subnanomolar concentrations in culture, and these concentrations are considered physiological.[18] The presence of high affinity microsomal binding sites may represent an intracellular site through which PAF elicits effects on gene expression. This idea is suggested by our findings that a potent antagonist selective for the intracellular binding site will block PAF-evoked immediate-early gene expression in neuroglial hybrid cells.[21]

A role of PAF in the primary genomic response may not be restricted to transcriptional stimulation, however. PAF stimulates the activity of p34[cdc2],[31] possibly through a Ca^{2+}-mediated phosphorylation.[32] p34[cdc2] is the catalytic subunit of a histone H1 kinase that is implicated in the control of cell cycle progression.[33] The phosphorylation of histone H1 affects its activity[34] which is believed to be control of the compaction of chromatin in the nucleus and maintenance of a transcriptionally repressed state.[35] In addition, Ca^{2+} itself condenses chromatin.[32] In as much as PAF is a Ca^{2+} ionophore and a stimulator of PLC-mediated IP_3 generation, and that the nuclear envelope exhibits functional IP_3 receptors,[36,37] PAF may regulate part of the nuclear Ca^{2+} fluxes and histone H1 phosphorylation that stimulates chromatin condensation. Histone H1 kinase and Ca^{2+} regulation by PAF suggests that PAF could play a role in the availability of chromatin-bound genomic domains for transcription. In addition to histone H1, the Fos protein is a substrate of p34[cdd2].[38] Differential phosphorylation of Fos determines whether the protein will act in a dimeric complex with Jun proteins as a transcriptional stimulator or repressor.[39,40] Thus, PAF may stimulate a primary genomic response by two mechanisms: transcriptional activation of immediate-early genes and p34[cdc2]-mediated regulation of chromatin accessibility by H1 and Fos, both of which may be regulated by PAF-induced Ca^{2+} influx.

Evidence exists that other membrane metabolites may be involved in transduction of a primary genomic response, and in turn, these metabolites may be regulated by PAF. Intracellular PAF generates free arachidonic acid for subsequent generation of cyclooxygenase- and lipoxygenase-eicosanoids.[9-11] Lipoxygenase metabolites stimulate the expression of *c-fos* and *zif/268*.[41,42] Furthermore, an inhibitor of PLC will inhibit the expression of *c-fos* and inhibit phosphorylation of the serum response factor that regulates expression from the *c-fos* promoter.[43] Thus, intracellular regulation of PLA_2 and PLC by PAF may constitute a component of the PAF-induced mechanism of primary genomic response.

Injury to the cornea epithelium rapidly promotes the accumulation of PAF.[44] At the same time, *c-fos* expression is increased and PAF antagonists block this effect.[45] In the brain resting levels both of PAF and of immediate-early gene mRNA are low. However, with stimulation such as induction of seizures, PAF[14] and immediate-early genes[44,45] accumulate rapidly. A PAF antagonist selective for the intracellular binding site inhibits the *c-fos* and *zif/268* mRNA accumulation evoked by electroconvulsive shock in the hippocampus and

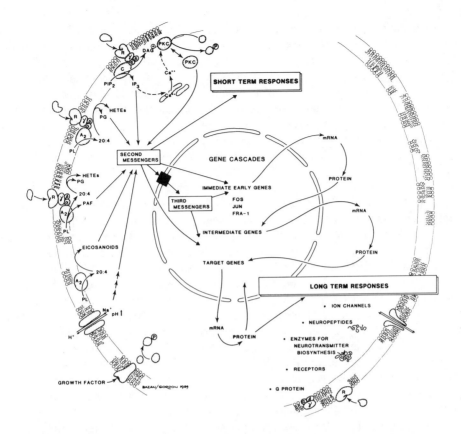

FIGURE 1. Signal transduction of acute, genomic, and long-term responses to cell stimulation. Stimulation of a cell by hormones, neurotransmitters, growth factors, or ion fluxes results in the formation of membrane phospholipid-derived second messengers (left), including inositol trisphosphate (IP$_3$), hydroxyeicosahexaenoic acids (HETEs), arachidonic acid (20:4) metabolites (eicosanoids), and PAF, through the activation of selective phospholipases. Of these, PAF, lipoxygenase eicosanoids, and the PLC metabolites have been linked to the stimulation of primary genomic responses (center). Members of the Fos, Jun, FRA (Fos-related antigens), and TIS (tetradecanoylphorbol acetate [TPA]-inducible sequences, including *zif/268*) families are transcription factors. The immediate-early expression of these transcription factors couples the generation of second messengers to long-term responses dependent upon the synthesis of new proteins. Membrane-derived second messengers accumulate as a response to injury, ischemia, convulsions, or inflammation and actively participate in the pathological process, which may include aberrant expression of long-term response genes. (From Bazan, N. G. and Bazan, H. E. P., in *New Trends in Lipid Mediators Research,* Bazan, N. G., Ed., S. Karger, Basel, 1990, 1. With permission.)

IV. PLATELET ACTIVATING FACTOR AS A SIGNAL TRANSDUCER IN ISCHEMIC AND SEIZURE RESPONSES OF THE BRAIN

One of the fundamental issues in stroke, epilepsy, and head trauma is therapeutic access to the cellular events that lead to irreversible brain damage. Similar cellular mechanisms may operate both in aging and in neurodegenerative disease, but in a time-graded fashion. These events may be the impairment of brain cell function or may link early, acute events with long-term repair processes. These early events are highlighted by the impairment of physiological neural signal transduction and may lead to abnormal concentrations of intracellular mediators. A major and early step in the biochemical progression of neurotrauma is the activation of PLA$_2$, which subsequently (1) degrades unsaturated excitable membrane phospholipids; (2) promotes the accumulation of free polyunsaturated fatty acids, biologically active eicosanoid-type metabolites, or lipid peroxidation products; and (3) leads to the generation of other bioactive lipids, such as PAF. Synaptic transmission may be impaired by (1) perturbation of Ca^{2+} fluxes and by changes in intracellular Ca^{2+} ionization, (2) release of free fatty acids and alteration of membrane-protein activities, such as inhibition of the Na^+/K^+-ATPase, and (3) generation of free radicals, which may lead to long-lasting alterations in synaptic communication. Alternatively, if the stimulus of injury is insufficient to cause irreversible damage, some of the transduction mediators accumulated may play roles as couplers to reparative processes and may initiate plasticity events.

As one of these membrane-derived mediators, PAF may play a significant role in the progression of trauma pathology. PAF accumulates during tissue injury, ischemia, inflammation, and immune reactions.[50] In the nervous system, PAF stimulates neuronal differentiation and increased cellular calcium.[51] PAF biosynthesis is stimulated by certain neurotransmitters,[8] and PAF affects the release of neuropeptides and other hormones.[52,53] PAF accumulates in the brain during seizures and during ischemia, and PAF antagonists decrease neural damage[54,55] and neurochemical changes in ischemia[55-57] and convulsions.[14,57] The increased concentration of PAF in brain under these conditions reflects early brain responses to stimulation or damage and may be related to a simultaneous or consequent PLA_2-mediated accumulation of free polyunsaturated fatty acids[58,59] and generation of their bioactive metabolites. The physiological PAF precursor, alkyl-acylglycerophosphocholine, is enriched in arachidonyl groups at sn-C_2.[50] Because the major free fatty acids accumulated in brain during ischemia are arachidonic acid and docosahexaenoic acid, PLA_2 activation is believed to be responsible for increases both in PAF precursor and in free polyunsaturated fatty acids.[58-60]

At high concentrations, PAF exhibits perturbant effects on cellular membranes,[61] and it is possible that local increases or depletions in PAF, lyso-PAF, or any partially short-chain phospholipid may be capable of altering membrane-mediated events through a nonreceptor mechanism.[5] Indeed, PAF alters membrane permeability of the blood-brain barrier.[14] During trauma, seizures, or ischemia, membrane PAF levels may attain perturbant, even lytic, concentrations. Such membrane perturbations could include alterations of ion fluxes across membranes, receptor binding and transduction, cellular transport processes, and, of course, membrane remodeling. Thus, the metabolism of PAF from cellular membranes in response to stimulation or injury may function bimodally through specific receptors or through membrane perturbations. Neuronal damage during epileptic and ischemic incidents or other injuries, and the corresponding cytoplasmic and genomic responses, may be partially accounted for by such dramatic alterations in cell membrane structure.

A rapid accumulation of PAF in brain following ischemia reperfusion is evidenced by the protective effects of PAF antagonists against cellular damage and enzymatic membrane degradation. Reperfusion is accompanied by the accumulation of components of the primary genomic response. Rats subjected to transient forebrain ischemia exhibit induction of *fos* mRNA in the cerebral cortex within 30 min of recirculation.[61] The accumulation of *fos* mRNA persists in the dentate hilus and in hippocampal area CA1 from 24 to 72 h after initiation of recirculation.[63] These findings correlate with the known time course of Ca^{2+} accumulation in CA1 following ischemia,[64,65] suggesting that accumulation of the cation is involved in *fos* induction.

Similarly, the cellular response to convulsions involves accumulation of PAF and immediate-early mRNAs in the brain. A dramatic and specific induction of *fos* in certain neuronal populations takes place in the brain of mice undergoing convulsions induced by Metrazole.[44] This surge in gene expression coincides with the increase in intracellular Ca^{2+} known to occur in neural cells during seizure.[66] In addition to *fos*, mRNAs of three other immediate-early transcription factor genes, *jun*, *jun-B*, and *zif/268*, accumulate in the hippocampus, dentate gyrus, and pyriform and cingulate cortices following Metrazole-induced seizures.[45,67]

Long-term potentiation in neural tissue is associated with establishment of altered synaptic activity and morphology. Potentiation through the perforant path in the rat selectively induces the immediate-early gene *zif/268* and inconsistently induces *fos, jun*, and *jun-B*.[68] Inhibitors of PLA[69] and a dioxolan PAF antagonist[70] inhibit the establishment of long-term potentiation. *In vitro*, PAF stimulates neurite outgrowth in neuroglial hybrid cells,[51] indicating that its availability in the environment of appropriate neurons may affect axon sprouting and subsequent synapse formation. This suggests that PLA_2 products, including PAF, may be important for the synaptic plasticity associated with synapse remodeling processes such as formation and storage of memory.

V. SUMMARY AND CONCLUSIONS

The intracellular accumulation of PAF following cell stimulation suggests an intracellular signal transduction pathway. High affinity binding sites for PAF in microsomal membranes and displacement of PAF from these sites by structurally distinct PAF antagonists suggests the existence of an intracellular receptor. Suppression of primary genomic responses by a PAF antagonist selective for the intracellular receptor suggests a cascade of events, including protein phosphorylation and generation of intracellular Ca^{2+} and arachidonic acid metabolites, linking the intracellular generation of PAF to immediate-early transcription.[68,72]

Several of the metabolites that transiently accumulate after injury may elicit beneficial effects on regenerative processes. The membrane metabolite PAF, which accumulates after seizure and ischemia, may initiate reparative processes by promoting transcriptional activation of immediate-early transcription factors. The long-term effects of these immediate-early gene transcription factors may provide a synthetic mechanism to replenish and rebuild cells following traumatic events.

ACKNOWLEDGMENT

The authors wish to acknowledge support of their research by the Jacob Javits Award NS23002.

REFERENCES

1. **Snyder, F.,** Platelet-activating factor and related acetylated lipids as potent biologically active cellular mediators, *Am. J. Physiol.*, 259, C697, 1990.
2. **Salari, H., Duronio, V., Howard, S., Demos, M., Jones, K., Reany, A., Hudson, A., and Pelch, S.,** Erbstatin blocks platelet-activating factor-induced protein-tyrosine phosphorylation, phosphoinositide hydrolysis, protein kinase C activation, serotonin secretion and aggregation of rabbit platelets, *FEBS Lett.*, 263, 104, 1990.
3. **Bazan, H., Braquet, P., Reddy, S., and Bazan, N.,** Inhibition of the alkali burn-induced lipoxygenation of arachidonic acid in the rabbit cornea *in vivo* by a platelet-activating factor antagonist, *J. Ocul. Pharmacol.*, 3, 357, 1987.
4. **Bazan, H., Reddy, S., Woodland, J., and Bazan, N.,** The accumulation of platelet-activating factor in the injured cornea may be interrelated with the synthesis of lipoxygenase products, *Biochim. Biophys. Res. Commun.*, 149, 915, 1987.
5. **Henson, P.,** Extracellular and intracellular activities of PAF, in *Platelet-Activating Factor and Related Lipid Mediators*, Snyder, F., Ed., Plenum Press, New York, 1987, chap. 10.
6. **Sogos, V., Bussolino, E., Pilia, E., Torelli, S., and Gremo, F.,** Acetylcholine-induced production of platelet-activating factor by human fetal brain cells in culture, *J. Neurosci. Res.*, 27, 706, 1990.
7. **Yue, T.-L., Lysko, P. G., and Feuerstein, G.,** Production of platelet-activating factor from rat cerebellar granule cells in culture, *J. Neurochem.*, 54, 1809, 1990.

8. **Bussolino, F., Gremo, F., Tetta, C., Pescarmona, G., and Camussi, G.,** Production of platelet-activating factor by chick retina, *J. Biol. Chem.,* 261, 16502, 1986.

9. **Stewart, A. and Phillips, W.,** Intracellular platelet-activating factor regulates eicosanoid generation in guinea-pig resident peritoneal macrophages, *Br. J. Pharmacol.,* 98, 141, 1989.

10. **Stewart, A., Dubbin, P., Harris, T., and Dusting, G.,** Evidence for an intracellular action of platelet-activating factor in bovine cultured aortic endothelial cells, *Br. J. Pharmacol.,* 96, 503, 1989.

11. **Stewart, A., Dubbin, P., Harris, T., and Dusting, G.,** Platelet-activating factor may act as a second messenger in the release of icosanoids and superoxide anions from leukocytes and endothelial cells, *Proc. Natl. Acad. Sci. U.S.A.,* 87, 3215, 1990.

12. **Marcheselli, V. L., Rossowska, M., Domingo, M. T., Braquet, P., and Bazan, N. G.,** Distinct platelet-activating factor binding sites in synaptic endings and in intracellular membranes of rat cerebral cortex, *J. Biol. Chem.,* 265, 9140, 1990.

13. **Marcheselli, V. L. and Bazan, N. G.,** A specific antagonist for intracellular platelet-activating factor (PAF) binding sites lacks activity on synaptic membranes, *Trans. Am. Soc. Neurochem.,* 22, 187, 1991.

14. **Kumar, R., Harvey, S., Kester, M., Hanahan, D., and Olson, M.,** Production and effects of platelet-activating factor in the rat brain, *Biochim. Biophys. Acta,* 963, 375, 1988.

15. **Birkle, D. L. and Bazan, N. G.,** Effect of bicuculline-induced status epilepticus on prostaglandins and hydroxyeicosatetraenoic acid in rat brain subcellular fractions, *J. Neurochem.,* 48, 1768, 1987.

16. **Record, M., Ribbes, G., Terce, F., and Chap, H.,** Subcellular localization of phospholipids and enzymes involved in PAF-acether metabolism, *J. Cell. Biochem.,* 40, 353, 1989.

17. **Vallari, D., Record, M., and Snyder, F.,** Conversion of alkylacetylglycerol to platelet-activating factor in HL-60 cells and subcellular localization of the mediator, *Arch. Biochem. Biophys.,* 276, 538, 1990.

18. **Yue, T.-L., Gleason, M., Gu, J.-L., Lysko, P. G., Hallenbeck, J., and Feuerstein, G.,** Platelet-activating factor (PAF) receptor-mediated calcium mobilization and phosphoinositiel turnover in neurohybrid NG108-15 cells: studies with BN50739, a new PAF antagonist, *J. Pharmacol. Exp. Ther.,* 257, 374, 1991.

19. **Honda, Z.-I., Nakamura, M., Miki, I., Minami, M., Watanabe, T., Seyama, Y., Okado, H., Toh, H., Ito, K., Miyamoto, T., and Shimizu, T.,** Cloning by functional expression of platelet-activating factor receptor from guinea pig lung, *Nature,* 349, 342, 1991.

20. **Nakamura, M., Honda, Z.-I., Izumi, T., Sakanaka, C., Mutoh, H., Minami, M., Bito, H., Seyama, Y., Matsumoto, T., Noma, M., and Shimizu, T.,** Molecular cloning and expression of platelet-activating factor receptor from human leukocytes, *J. Biol. Chem.,* 266, 20400, 1991.

21. **Squinto, S. P., Block, A. L., Braquet, P., and Bazan, N. G.,** Platelet-activating factor stimulates a Fos/Jun/AP-1 transcriptional signaling system in human neuroblastoma cells, *J. Neurosci. Res.,* 24, 558, 1989.

22. **Doucet, J. P. and Bazan, N. G.,** Platelet-activating factor stimulates immediate-early gene expression in proliferating human Y79 retinoblastoma cells, *FASEB J.,* 4, A1815, 1990.

23. **Doucet, J. and Bazan, N. G.,** A primary genomic response to platelet-activating factor in neurohybrid NG108-15 cells, manuscript in preparation.

24. **Mazer, B., Domenico, J., Sawami, H., and Gelfand, E. W.,** Platelet-activating factor induces an increase in intracellular calcium and expression of regulatory genes in human B lymphoblastoid cells, *J. Immunol.,* 146, 1914, 1991.

25. **Shulman, P. G., Kuruvilla, A., Putcha, G., Mangus, L., F-Johnson, J., and Shearer, W. T.,** Platelet-activating factor induces phospholipid turnover calcium flux, arachidonic acid liberation, eicosanoid generation, and oncogene expression in a human B cell line, *J. Immunol.,* 146, 1642, 1991.

26. **Tripathi, Y., Kandala, J., Guntaka, R., Lim, R., and Shukla, S.,** Platelet-activating factor induces expression of early response genes c-fos and tis-1 in human epidermoid carcinoma cells, *Life Sci.,* 49, 1761, 1991.

27. **Sheng, M., Dougan, S., McFadden, G., and Greenberg, M.,** Calcium and growth factor pathways of c-fos transcriptional activation require distinct upstream regulatory sequences, *Mol. Cell. Biol.,* 8, 2782, 1988.

28. **Squinto, S. P., Braquet, P., Block, A., and Bazan, N. G.,** Platelet-activating factor activated HIV promoter in transfected SH-SY5Y neuroblastoma cells and MOLT-4 T-lymphocytes, *J. Mol. Neurosci.,* 2, 79, 1990.

29. **Ransone, L. and Verma, I.,** Nuclear proto-oncogenes *fos* and *jun, Annu. Rev. Cell. Biol.,* 6, 539, 1990.

30. **Christy, B., Lau, L., and Nathans, D.,** A gene activated in mouse 3T3 cells by serum growth factors encodes a protein with ''zinc finger'' sequences, *Proc. Natl. Acad. Sci. U.S.A.,* 85, 7857, 1988.

31. **Samiei, M., Maleki, D.-M., Clark-Lewis, I., and Pelech, S.,** Platelet-activating factor- and thrombin-induced stimulation of p34cdc2-cyclin histone H1 kinase activity in platelets, *J. Biol. Chem.,* 266, 14889, 1991.

32. **Patel, R., Twigg, J., Crossley, I., Golsteyn, R., and Whitaker, M.,** Calcium-induced chromatin condensation and cyclin phosphorylation during chromatin condensation cycles in ammonia-activated sea urchin eggs, *J. Cell. Sci. Suppl.,* 12, 129, 189.

33. **Lewin, B.,** Driving the cell cycle: M phase kinase, HS partners and substrates, *Cell,* 61, 743, 1990.

34. **Banerjee, S., Bennion, G., Goldberg, M., and Allen, T.,** ATP-dependent histone H1 phosphorylation and nucleosome assembly in a human cell-free extract, *Nucleic Acids Res.,* 19, 5999, 1991.

35. **Zlatanov, J.,** Histone H1 and the regulation of transcription of eukaryotic genes, *TIBS,* 15, 273, 1990.

36. **Nicotera, P., McConkey, D., Jones, D., and Orrenius, S.,** ATP stimulates Ca^{2+} uptake and increases free Ca^{2+} concentration in isolated rat liver nuclei, *Proc. Natl. Acad. Sci. U.S.A.,* 86, 453, 1989.

37. **Malviya, A., Rogue, P., and Vincendon, G.,** Stereospecific inositol 1,4,5-$[^{32}P]$phosphate binding to isolated rat liver nuclei: evidence for inositol trisphosphate receptor-mediated calcium release from the nucleus, *Proc. Natl. Acad. Sci. U.S.A.,* 87, 9270, 1990.

38. **Abate, C., Marshak, D., and Curran, T.,** Fos is phosphorylated by p34^{cdc2}, cyclic AMP-dependent protein kinase and protein kinase C at multiple sites clustered within regulatory regions, *Oncogene,* 6, 2179, 1991.

39. **Ofir, R., Dwarki, V., Rashid, D., and Verma, I.,** Phosphorylation of the C-terminus of Fos protein is required for transcriptional transrepression of the *c-fos* promoter, *Nature,* 348, 80, 1990.

40. **Guis, D., Cao, X., Rauscher, F., Cohen, D., Curran, T., and Sukhatme, V.,** Transcriptional activation and repression by Fos are independent functions: the C-terminus represses immediate-early gene expression via CArG elements, *Mol. Cell. Biol.,* 10, 4243, 1990.

41. **Sellmayer, A., Uedelhoven, W., Weber, P., and Bonventre, J.,** Endogenous non-cyclooxygenase metabolites of arachidonic acid modulate growth and mRNA levels of immediate-early response genes in rat mesangial cells, *J. Biol. Chem.,* 266, 3800, 1991.

42. **Haliday, E., Ramesha, C., and Ringold, G.,** TNF induces *c-fos* via a novel pathway requiring conversion of arachidonic acid to a lipoxygenase metabolite, *EMBO J.,* 10, 10, 1991.

43. **Schalasta, G. and Doppler, C.,** Inhibition of *c-fos* transcription and phosphorylation of the serum response factor by an inhibitor of phospholipase C-type reactions, *Mol. Cell. Biol.,* 10, 5558, 1990.

44. **Bazan, H. E. P., Reddy, S. T. K., and Lin, N.,** Platelet-activating factor (PAF) accumulation correlates with injury in the cornea, *Exp. Eye Res.,* 52, 4891, 1991.

45. **Allan, G., Bazan, H. E. P., Tao, Y., and Bazan, N. G.,** Expression of the *c-fos* proto-oncogene mRNA is rapidly enhanced in the corneal epithelium following alkali burn, *Suppl. Invest. Ophthalmol. Vis. Sci.,* 31, 316, 1990.

46. **Morgan, J., Cohen, D., Hempstead, J., and Curran, T.,** Mapping patterns of c-fos in the nervous system, *Science,* 237, 192, 1987.

47. **Saffen, D., Cole, A., Worley, P., Christy, B., Ryder, K., and Baraban, J.,** Convulsant-induced increase in transcription factor messenger RNAs in rat brain, *Proc. Natl. Acad. Sci. U.S.A.,* 85, 7795, 1988.

48. **Marcheselli, V. L., Doucet, J. P., and Bazan, N. G.,** Platelet-activating factor is a mediator of *fos* expression induced by a single seizure in rat hippocampus, *Soc. Neurosci.,* 17, 349, 1991.

49. **Marcheselli, N. G. and Bazan, N. G.,** ECS-induced zif-268 in hippocampus is inhibited by a PAF antagonist, *Trans. Am. Soc. Neurochem.,* 23, 1992 (in press).

50. **Braquet, P., Touqui, L., Shen, T., and Vargaftig, B.,** Perspectives in platelet-activating factor research, *Pharmacol. Rev.,* 39, 97, 1987.

51. **Kornecki, E. and Ehrlich, Y.,** Neuroregulatory and neuropathological actions of the ether-phospholipid platelet-activating factor, *Science,* 240, 1792, 1988.

52. **Junier, M., Tiberghien, C., Rougeot, C. et al.,** Inhibitory effect of PAF on lutenizing hormone-releasing hormone and somatostatin release from rat median eminence *in vitro* correlated with characterization of specific PAF receptor sites, *Endocrinology,* 123, 72, 1988.

53. **Rougeot, C., Junier, M., Minary, P., Weidenfeld, J., Braquet, P., and Dray, F.,** Intracerebroventricular injection of platelet-activating factor induces secretion of adrenocorticotropin, beta-endorphin and corticosterone in conscious rats — a possible link between the immune and nervous systems, *Neuroendocrinology,* 51, 315, 1990.

54. **Oberpichler, H., Sauer, D., Rosberg, C., Mennel, H., and Krieglstein, J.,** PAF antagonist gingkolide-B reduces postischemic neuronal damage in the rat-brain hippocampus, *J. Cereb. Blood Flow Metab.,* 10, 133, 1990.

55. **Panetta, T., Marcheselli, V. L., Braquet, P., Spinnewyn, B., and Bazan, N. G.,** Effects of a platelet-activating factor antagonist (BN 52021) on free fatty acids, diacylglycerols, polyphosphoinositides, and blood flow in the gerbil brain: inhibition of ischemia-reperfusion-induced cerebral injury, *Biochem. Biophys. Res. Commun.,* 149, 580, 1987.

56. **Spinnewyn, B., Blavet, N., Clostre, F., Bazan, N., and Braquet, P.,** Involvement of platelet-activating factor (PAF) in cerebral post-ischemic phase in mongolian gerbils, *Prostaglandins,* 34, 337, 1987.

57. **Birkle, D., Kurian, P., Braquet, P., and Bazan, N. G.,** The platelet-activating factor antagonist BN 52021 decreases accumulation of free polyunsaturated fatty acid in mouse brain during ischemia and electroconvulsive shock, *J. Neurochem.,* 151, 88, 1988.

58. **Bazan, N.,** Effects of ischemia and electroconvulsive shock on free fatty acid pool in the brain, *Biochim. Biophys. Acta,* 218, 1, 1970.

59. **Bazan, N., Birkle, D., Tang, W., and Reddy, T.,** The accumulation of free arachidonic acid, diacylglycerols, prostaglandins, and lipoxygenase reaction products in the brain during experimental epilepsy, *Adv. Neurol.,* 44, 879, 1986.

60. **Bazan, N. and Rodriguez de Turco, E.,** Membrane lipids in the pathogenesis of brain edema: phospholipids and arachidonic acid, the earliest membrane components changed at the onset of ischemia, *Adv. Neurol.,* 28, 197, 1980.

61. **Sawyer, D. and Anderson, O.,** Platelet-activating factor is a general membrane perturbant, *Biochim. Biophys. Acta,* 987, 129, 1989.

62. **Onodera, H., Kogure, K., Ono, Y., Igarashi, K., Kiyota, Y., and Nagaoka, A.,** Protooncogene *c-fos* is transiently induced in the rat cerebral cortex after forebrain ischemia, *Neurosci. Lett.,* 98, 101, 1989.

63. **Jorgenson, M., Deckert, J., Wright, D., and Gehlert, D.,** Delayed *c-fos* proto-oncogene expression in the rat hippocampus induced by transient global cerebral ischemia: an *in situ* hybridization study, *Brain Res.,* 484, 393, 1989.

64. **Dienel, G.,** Regional accumulation of calcium in post-ischemic brain, *J. Neurochem.,* 43, 913, 1984.

65. **Siesjö, B. K. and Bengtsson, F.,** Calcium fluxes, calcium antagonists, and calcium-related pathology in brain ischemia, hypoglycemia, and spreading depression: a unifying hypothesis, *J. Cereb. Blood Flow Metab.,* 9, 127, 1989.

66. **Siesjö, B.,** Calcium in the brain under physiological and pathological conditions, *Eur. Neurol.,* 30, 3, 1990.

67. **Sukhatme, V., Cao, X., Chang, L., Tsai-Morris, C., Stamenkovich, D., Ferreira, P., Cohen, D., Edwards, S., Shows, T., Curran, T., Le Beau, M., and Adamson, E.,** A zinc finger-encoding gene coregulated with *c-fos* during growth and differentiation, and after cellular depolarization, *Cell,* 53, 37, 1988.

68. **Cole, A., Saffen, D., Baraban, J., and Worley, P.,** Rapid increase of an immediate early gene messenger RNA in hippocampal neurons by synaptic NMDA receptor activation, *Nature,* 340, 474, 1989.

69. **Linden, D., Sheu, F., Murakami, K., and Routtenberg, A.,** Enhancement of long-term potentiation by *cis*-unsaturated fatty acid. Relation to protein kinase C and phospholipase A_2, *J. Neurosci.,* 7, 3783, 1987.

70. **del Cerro, S., Arai, A., and Lynch, G.,** Inhibition of long-term potentiation by an antagonist of platelet-activating factor receptors, *Behav. Neural Biol.,* 54, 213, 1990.

71. **Bazan, N. G., Squinto, S. P., Braquet, P., Panetta, T., and Marcheselli, V. L.,** Platelet-activating factor and polyunsaturated fatty acids in cerebral ischemia or convulsions: intracellular PAF-binding sites and activation of a Fos/Jun/Ap-1 transcriptional signaling system, *Lipids,* 26, 1236, 1991.

72. **Shukla, S. D.,** Platelet-activating factor receptor and signal transduction mechanisms, *FASEB J.,* 6, 2296, 1992.

Chapter 12

PLATELET ACTIVATING FACTOR AND ARACHIDONOYL-PREFERENTIAL PHOSPHOLIPASE A_2

Shuntaro Hara, Ichiro Kudo, and Keizo Inoue

TABLE OF CONTENTS

ISBN 0-8493-7299-2
© 1993 by CRC Press, Inc.

I. INTRODUCTION

In a variety of mammalian cells, arachidonic acid can be released from membrane phospholipids in response to receptor-mediated signals and the main enzyme responsible for this process is believed to be phospholipase A_2 (PLA_2).[1,2] The arachidonic acid thus released is metabolized further to biologically active lipids, such as prostaglandins, leukotrienes, and thromboxanes.[3,4] Lysophospholipids, which include lysoPAF, a precursor for PAF biosynthesis, are the other products of the PLA_2 reaction.[5,6] However, the molecular basis of action of PLA_2 is not well understood.

To date, most of the direct studies on PLA_2 have focused on the 14-kDa PLA_2, which requires the presence of millimolar levels of Ca^{2+} for full activation.[7] In mammalian systems, two isoforms of 14-kDa PLA_2 with different primary sequences are known, which have been called types I and II enzymes.[8-12] Both of the genes that encode these isoforms carry typical secretory signals. Therefore, it has been suggested that these enzymes are secretory proteins and their activities are expressed exclusively extracellularly. Recently, a new type of PLA_2 from various sources has been identified, which, unlike the types I and II enzymes, exhibited a preference for *sn*-2-arachidonic acid-containing substrates and was activated by physiologically relevant concentrations of calcium.[13-26] These properties made it a likely candidate for involvement with receptor-mediated signal transduction. We propose that this enzyme be called type IV PLA_2, because bee venom PLA_2, the structure of which is quite different from types I and II, has been called type III PLA_2 by Dennis.[7] In this chapter, we focus on this type IV PLA_2 and its possible involvement in PAF biosynthesis and discuss its regulatory effects on PAF-induced cellular activation.

II. BIOCHEMICAL ASPECTS OF TYPE IV PHOSPHOLIPASE A_2

A. DETECTION AND PURIFICATION

The first biochemical indication of the existence of type IV PLA_2 was reported by Alonso et al.,[13] who detected an arachidonoyl-preferential hydrolyzing activity in human neutrophils. Similar such activities were detected subsequently in various cells, such as the mouse macrophage-like cell line RAW264.7,[14] mouse peritoneal macrophages,[15] the human monocytic cell line U937,[16] and human platelets.[17] In these cells, the arachidonoyl-preferential hydrolyzing activity was found predominantly in the $100,000 \times g$ soluble fraction when they were homogenized in the presence of Ca^{2+} chelators. However, when the cells were homogenized in a Ca^{2+}-containing buffer, 60 to 70% of the activity was lost from the soluble fraction and became associated with the particulate fraction,[16,18] which suggested that the intracellular distribution of type IV PLA_2 was regulated by the Ca^{2+} concentration.

In some cells, such as rabbit platelets,[19] the coexistence of other PLA_2 enzyme, such as types I and II, neither of which exhibit fatty acid selectivity, prevented us from detecting the arachidonoyl-preferential hydrolyzing activity. Therefore, experiments have been designed to eliminate the activity due to other types of PLA_2. For example, addition of dithiothreitol to the cell lysate enabled us to measure the arachidonoyl-preferential hydrolyzing activity occasionally, since dithiothreitol inhibited the activity of types I and II PLA_2, but not that of the type IV enzyme.[20] Alternatively, heparin-Sepharose affinity chromatography separated the activity of the type II from that of type IV enzyme effectively.[19]

To date, type IV PLA_2 from the mouse macrophage-like cell line RAW264.7,[14] the human monocytic cell line U937,[16,20,21] rat kidney[22] and rabbit,[23] human,[24] and bovine[25] platelets has been purified to near homogeneity. Although the apparent molecular masses of the purified enzymes obtained were diverse (ranging from 60 to 140 kDa), recent immunochemical studies[27] and/or molecular cloning experiments[28,29] revealed that their actual

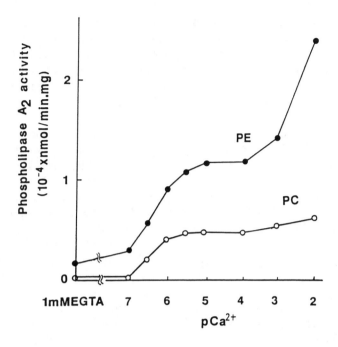

FIGURE 1. Effect of calcium ion on the purified rabbit platelet type IV PLA$_2$. PLA$_2$ activity at various concentrations of CaCl$_2$ were measured using 1-acyl-2-arachidonoylglycerophosphoethanolamine (PE) (●) and 1-acyl-2-arachidonoylglycerophosphocholine (PC) (○).

molecular masses are about 85 kDa. Specific antibodies raised against type IV PLA$_2$ isolated from rabbit platelets[27] and the human monocytic cell line U937[21] have been established, which enabled us to detect PLA$_2$ activities related to the type IV enzyme in various cells and tissues. Neutrophils, mast cells, brain, lung, and liver have been found to contain a type IV-like enzyme.[27]

B. PROPERTIES

Type IV PLA$_2$ exhibits a preference for substrates containing arachidonate at the *sn*-2 position of the glycerol backbone. For example, the human platelet-derived enzyme hydrolyzed arachidonate-containing phosphatidylcholine and phosphatidylethanolamine about ten times more effectively than the corresponding linoleate-containing phospholipids.[24] When natural membrane vesicles were used as substrates instead of synthetic phospholipid liposomes, this enzyme also hydrolyzed arachidonate-containing phospholipids selectively.[28]

In addition to PLA$_2$ activity, the type IV enzyme purified from mouse RAW264.7 cells[30] or rabbit platelets[31] exhibited lysophospholipase activity. This dual activity may represent an efficient mechanism whereby a single enzyme can function as PLA$_2$ and then degrade potentially toxic lysophospholipids rapidly.

One of the most remarkable features of type IV PLA$_2$ is its calcium dependence. Figure 1 shows the calcium dependency of the type IV enzyme, which has been purified from rabbit platelets.[23] The catalytic activity observed with either phosphatidylcholine or phosphatidylethanolamine substrates increased as the free calcium ion concentration increased from 10^{-7} to 10^{-6} M. This calcium ion concentration range is of a similar order of magnitude to the free calcium ion concentration increase induced during cell activation. This finding is consistent with the hypothesis that type IV PLA$_2$ may be involved mainly with stimulus-coupled arachidonate metabolism. The results obtained with reconstitution systems of partially purified type IV enzyme and synaptosomal membranes from rat brain[26] indicate that the type IV enzyme translocates to the membrane in a Ca^{2+}- and time-dependent manner, and appear to agree with the findings that type IV PLA_2 activity is lost from the cytosolic fraction and appears in the membrane fraction when cells are homogenized in Ca^{2+}-containing buffers.[16,18] Therefore, in addition to activating the type IV enzyme, increasing the Ca^{2+} concentration appears to induce translocation of the enzyme to the membrane.

C. STRUCTURE AND GENE CLONING

The cDNA, which encodes human type IV PLA_2, recently was cloned from the human monocytic cell line U937.[28,29] The human type IV enzyme has been demonstrated to comprise 749 amino acids and its estimated molecular mass is about 85.2 kDa. The deduced amino acid sequence of this enzyme possesses no region with high homology to the known 14-kDa types I and II PLA_2 enzymes. The corresponding murine cDNA clone also was isolated from the mouse macrophage-like cell line RAW264.7 using the human cDNA clone.[28] More than 95% of the inferred amino acid sequence of the murine type IV PLA_2 is identical to that of the human type IV enzyme. This observation, together with the results of immunochemical studies, which showed that the specific antibodies against the rabbit type IV enzyme cross-reacted with both human and rat type IV enzymes,[27] indicates that the type IV enzyme exhibits a high degree of interspecies homology.

It has been demonstrated that the amino-terminal portion of the type IV enzyme possesses a significant sequence homology with the constant region 2 (C2 region) of protein kinase C (PKC).[28,29] This domain also is homologous with the synaptic vesicle protein p65, GTPase activating protein and phospholipase C (PLC). It has been proposed that the C2 domain is the Ca^{2+}-dependent phospholipid-binding (CaLB) domain, as it is present in all PKC isoforms that translocate to membranes in response to Ca^{2+}, but is absent in those that do not.[32] The amino-terminal 138-amino acid fragment of recombinant type IV PLA_2 which possesses the CaLB domain was able to associate with membrane vesicles in response to Ca^{2+}, as was the whole type IV enzyme,[28] which supports this hypothesis.

In addition to this domain, the type IV enzyme has some potential protein kinase recognition sites (12 potential PKC phosphorylation sites: 9 serine and 3 threonine residues), and 3 potential tyrosine kinase phosphorylation sites).[29]

III. POSSIBLE INVOLVEMENT OF TYPE IV PHOSPHOLIPASE A_2 IN PLATELET ACTIVATING FACTOR BIOSYNTHESIS

The remodeling pathway of PAF biosynthesis is initiated by hydrolysis of 1-O-alkyl-2-acylglycerophosphocholine (-GPC) via an intracellular PLA_2, and the 1-O-alkyllyso-GPC (lyso-PAF) formed as a result of this reaction is then acetylated by an acetyl-CoA:lyso-PAF acetyltransferase.[5,6] It has been postulated that 1-O-alkyl-2-arachidonoyl-GPC may serve as a common precursor for arachidonic acid and lyso-PAF synthesis in the activated cells, because both arachidonate metabolites and PAF can be generated by agonistic or inflammatory stimuli.[33] Type IV PLA_2 can hydrolyze 1-O-alkyl-2-arachidonoyl-GPC and, therefore, may be involved in the remodeling pathway of PAF biosynthesis. Suga et al.[34] demonstrated that the alkylarachidonoyl molecular species was the only one of the 1-O-alkyl-2-acyl-GPC pool that decreased significantly during calcium ionophore-induced PAF formation in differentiated HL-60 cells, which indicates that arachidonoyl-preferential hydrolyzing PLA_2 activity plays an important role in PAF biosynthesis.

In human neutrophils, some lipoxygenase products, such as 5-hydroxyeicosatetraenoic acid, were demonstrated to modulate PAF biosynthesis,[35] and neutrophils and differentiated HL-60 cells both lost their capacity to form PAF when depleted of arachidonate.[34,36] When the depleted cells were supplemented with arachidonic acid, the formation of PAF by these

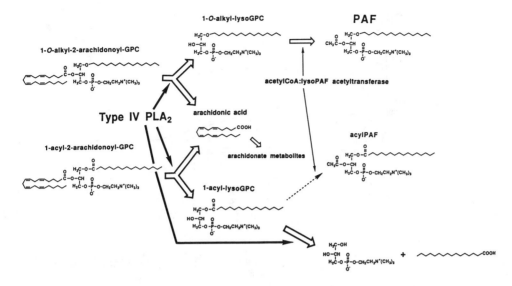

FIGURE 2. Possible role of the type IV PLA$_2$ in PAF biosynthesis.

cells was stimulated several-fold.[34] These findings indicate the probable importance of arachidonic acid and/or its metabolites in PAF biosynthesis. If it is assumed that all arachidonate substrates are provided as a result of type IV PLA$_2$ activity, the activation of this enzyme may be involved in PAF biosynthesis.

The type IV enzyme hydrolyzes both 1-*O*-alkyl-2-arachidonoyl-GPC and 1-acyl-2-arachidonoyl-GPC.[14,16] As it possesses lysophospholipase activity in addition to PLA$_2$ activity, 1-acyl-lyso-GPC would be degraded rapidly, whereas 1-*O*-alkyl-lyso-GPC would remain unchanged.[30,31] Both 1-acyl-lyso-GPC and 1-*O*-alkyl-lyso-GPC are substrates for acetyl-CoA:lysoPAF acetyltransferase.[37] Therefore, the function of the type IV enzyme may be to reduce the generation of PAF analogues with an acyl chain at the *sn*-1 position. The generation of PAF and its analogues with an alkenyl or acyl chain, induced after appropriate stimulation, was enhanced several fold with ether-linked precursor species compared to the diradyl-GPC precursors.[38] However, Sturk et al. have reported that a selective degradation system, which is phenylmethanesulfonyl fluoride (PMSF) -sensitive, regulated the ratio of the concomitantly produced PAF acyl analogues,[38] which cannot be explained by the reactivity of the type IV enzyme, as its lysophospholipase activities appeared to be insensitive to PMSF.[31]

Figure 2 shows the possible role of the type IV enzyme in PAF biosynthesis.

IV. MECHANISM OF PLATELET ACTIVATING FACTOR-INDUCED TYPE IV PHOSPHOLIPASE A$_2$ ACTIVATION

The actions of PAF are exerted via the activation of specific PAF receptors, which are found in a variety of cells and tissues.[39] The signal transduction process induced by PAF appears to be modulated by guanine nucleotide-regulatory proteins (G-proteins), which has been demonstrated by the inhibition of PAF binding by GTP in neutrophils[40] and platelets,[41] and by its stimulation of GTPase activity in platelet membranes.[41,42] Recently, Honda et al. isolated the cDNA which encodes for the PAF receptors from guinea-pig lung. Its primary structure reveals that the receptor belongs to the G-protein-coupled receptor superfamily.[43]

PAF receptors are linked to various intracellular pathways that generate second messengers by coupling with G-proteins. PAF stimulated phosphatidylinositol turnover in platelets,[44-49] polymorphonuclear leukocytes,[50] and hepatocytes,[51,52] and induced a transient el-

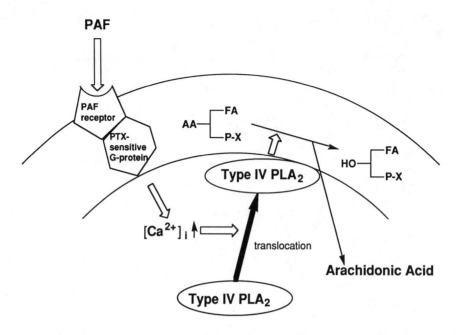

FIGURE 3.   Possible pathways for PAF-induced arachidonic acid liberation.

evation of intracellular Ca^{2+}-concentration in platelets,[53,54] neutrophils,[55,56] mononuclear leukocytes,[57] neural cells,[58] and vascular endothelial cells.[59] Release of arachidonic acid and production of arachidonate metabolites in response to PAF has been reported in various cells and tissues, including horse platelets,[44] human neutrophils,[60] guinea pig alveolar macrophages,[61] rat and human mesangial cells,[62,63] rat Kupffer cells,[64] the mouse macrophage-like cell line P388D$_1$,[65] the mouse osteoblast-like cell line MC3T3-E1,[66] and human amnion.[67] In addition, PAF was observed to stimulate the synthesis of PAF in human neutrophils,[68] where intracellular Ca^{2+}-antagonists reduced the PAF-induced liberation of arachidonic acid drastically, which indicates that Ca^{2+} is an essential factor for PLA$_2$ activation.[60] Pretreatment of human neutrophils[60] and guinea pig macrophages[61] with pertussis toxin resulted in almost complete abolition of PAF-induced arachidonic acid liberation. These data suggest that PAF potentiates the activity of Ca^{2+}-dependent PLA$_2$ via G-proteins and that type IV PLA$_2$ is one of the prime candidates to be this activated PLA$_2$. An outline of the possible involvement of the type IV enzyme in PAF-induced arachidonic acid liberation is summarized in Figure 3. Further studies must be conducted in order to ratify this scheme.

REFERENCES

1. **Van den Bosch, H.,** Intracellular phospholipases A, *Biochim. Biophys. Acta,* 604, 191, 1980.
2. **Irvine, R. F.,** How is the level of free arachidonic acid controlled in mammalian cells?, *Biochem. J.,* 204, 3, 1982.
3. **Samuelsson, B., Goldyne, M., Granström, E., Hamberg, M., Hammarström, S., and Malmsten, C.,** Prostaglandins and thromboxanes, *Annu. Rev. Biochem.,* 47, 997, 1978.
4. **Samuelsson, B., Dahlen, S. E., Lindgren, J. A., Rouzer, C. A., and Serhan, C. N.,** Leukotrienes and lipoxins: structures, biosynthesis, and biological effects, *Science,* 237, 1171, 1987.
5. **Snyder, F.,** Chemical and biochemical aspects of "platelet activating factor", a novel class of acetylated ether-linked choline phospholipids, *Med. Res. Rev.,* 5, 107, 1985.

6. **Hanahan, D. J.**, Platelet activating factor: a biologically active phosphoglyceride, *Annu. Rev. Biochem.*, 55, 483, 1986.
7. **Davidson, F. F. and Dennis, E. A.**, Evolutionary relationships and implications for the regulation of phospholipase A₂ from snake venom to human secreted forms, *J. Mol. Evol.*, 31, 228, 1990.
8. **Seilhamer, J. J., Randall, T. L., Yamanaka, M., and Johnson, L. K.**, Pancreatic phospholipase A₂: isolation of the human gene and cDNAs from porcine pancreas and human lung, *DNA*, 5, 519, 1986.
9. **Ohara, O., Tamaki, M., Nakamura, E., Tsuruta, Y., Fujii, Y., Shin, M., Teraoka, H., and Okamoto, M.**, Dog and rat pancreatic phospholipases A₂: complete amino acid sequences deduced from complementary DNAs, *J. Biochem.*, 99, 733, 1986.
10. **Seilhamer, J. J., Pruzanski, W., Vadas, P., Plant, S., Miller, J. A., Kloss, J., and Johnson, L. K.**, Cloning and recombinant expression of phospholipase A₂ present in rheumatoid arthritic synovial fluid, *J. Biol. Chem.*, 264, 5335, 1989.
11. **Kramer, R. M., Hession, C., Johansen, B., Hayes, G., McGray, P., Chow, E. P., Tizard, R., and Pepinsky, R. B.**, Structure and properties of a human non-pancreatic phospholipase A₂, *J. Biol. Chem.*, 264, 5768, 1989.
12. **Komada, M., Kudo, I., Mizushima, H., Kitamura, N., and Inoue, K.**, Structure of cDNA coding for rat platelet phospholipase A₂, *J. Biochem.*, 106, 545, 1989.
13. **Alonso, F., Henson, P. M., and Leslie, C. C.**, A cytosolic phospholipase in human neutrophils that hydrolyzes arachidonoyl-containing phosphatidylcholine, *Biochim. Biophys. Acta*, 878, 273, 1986.
14. **Leslie, C. C., Voelker, D. R., Channon, J. Y., Wall, M. M., and Zelarney, P. T.**, Properties and purification of an arachidonoyl-hydrolyzing phospholipase A₂ from a macrophage cell line, RAW264.7, *Biochim. Biophys. Acta*, 963, 476, 1988.
15. **Wijkander, J. and Sundler, R.**, A phospholipase A₂ hydrolyzing arachidonoyl-phospholipids in mouse peritoneal macrophages, *FEBS Lett.*, 244, 51, 1989.
16. **Diez, E. and Mong, S.**, Purification of a phospholipase A₂ from human monocytic leukemic U937 cells. Calcium-dependent activation and membrane association, *J. Biol. Chem.*, 265, 14654, 1990.
17. **Kim, D. K., Kudo, I., and Inoue, K.**, Detection in human platelets of phospholipase A₂ activity which preferentially hydrolyzes an arachidonoyl residue, *J. Biochem.*, 104, 492, 1988.
18. **Channon, J. Y. and Leslie, C. C.**, A calcium-dependent mechanism for associating a soluble arachidonoyl-hydrolyzing phospholipase A₂ with membrane in the macrophage cell line RAW 264.7, *J. Biol. Chem.*, 265, 5409, 1990.
19. **Kim, D. K., Kudo, I., Fujimori, Y., Mizushima, H., Masuda, M., Kikuchi, R., Ikizawa, K., and Inoue, K.**, Detection and subcellular localization of rabbit platelet phospholipase A₂ which preferentially hydrolyzes an arachidonoyl residue, *J. Biochem.*, 108, 903, 1990.
20. **Clark, J. D., Milona, N., and Knopf, J. L.**, Purification of a 110-kilodalton cytosolic phospholipase A₂ from the human monocytic cell line U937, *Proc. Natl. Acad. Sci. U.S.A.*, 87, 7708, 1990.
21. **Kramer, R. M., Roberts, E. F., Manetta, J., and Putnam, J. E.**, The Ca²⁺-sensitive cytosolic phospholipase A₂ is a 100-kDa protein in human monoblast U937 cells, *J. Biol. Chem.*, 266, 5268, 1991.
22. **Gronich, J. H., Bonventre, J. V., and Nemenoff, R. A.**, Purification of a high-molecular-mass form of phospholipase A₂ from rat kidney activated at physiological calcium concentrations, *Biochem. J.*, 271, 37, 1990.
23. **Kim, D. K., Kudo, I., and Inoue, K.**, Purification and characterization of rabbit platelet cytosolic phospholipase A₂, *Biochim. Biophys. Acta*, 1083, 80, 1991.
24. **Takayama, K., Kudo, I., Kim, D. K., Nagata, K., Nozawa, Y., and Inoue, K.**, Purification and characterization of human platelet phospholipase A₂ which preferentially hydrolyzes an arachidonoyl residue, *FEBS Lett.*, 282, 326, 1991.
25. **Kim, D. K., Suh, P. G., and Ryu, S. H.**, Purification and some properties of a phospholipase A₂ from bovine platelets, *Biochem. Biophys. Res. Commun.*, 174, 189, 1991.
26. **Yoshihara, Y. and Watanabe, Y.**, Translocation of phospholipase A₂ from cytosol to membranes in rat brain induced by calcium ions, *Biochem. Biophys. Res. Commun.*, 170, 484, 1990.
27. **Fujimori, Y., Murakami, M., Kim, D. K., Hara, S., Takayama, K., Kudo, I., and Inoue, K.**, Immunochemical detection of arachidonoyl-preferential phospholipase A₂, *J. Biochem.*, 111, 54, 1994.
28. **Clark, J. D., Lin, L.-L., Kritz, R. W., Ramesha, C. S., Sultzman, L. A., Lin, A. Y., Milona, N., and Knopf, J. L.**, A novel arachidonic acid-selective cytosolic PLA₂ contains a Ca²⁺-dependent translocation domain with homology to PKC and GAP, *Cell*, 65, 1043, 1991.
29. **Sharp, J. D., White, D. L., Chiou, X. G., Goodson, T., Gamboa, G. C., McClure, D., Burgett, S., Hoskins, J., Skatrud, P. L., Sportsman, J. R., Becker, G. W., Kang, L. H., Roberts, E. F., and Kramer, R. M.**, Molecular cloning and expression of human Ca²⁺-sensitive cytosolic phospholipase A₂, *J. Biol. Chem.*, 266, 14850, 1991.
30. **Leslie, C. C.**, Kinetic properties of a high molecular mass arachidonoyl-hydrolyzing phospholipase A₂ that exhibits lysophospholipase activity, *J. Biol. Chem.*, 266, 11366, 1991.

31. **Fujimori, Y., Kudo, I., and Inoue, K.,** unpublished data, 1992.

32. **Ohno, S., Akita, Y., Konno, Y., Imajoh, S., and Suzuki, K.,** A novel phorbol ester receptor/protein kinase, nPKC, distantly related to the protein kinase C family, *Cell,* 53, 731, 1988.

33. **Chilton, F. H., Ellis, J. M., Olson, S. C., and Wykle, R. L.,** 1-*O*-Alkyl-2-arachidonoyl-*sn*-glycero-3-phosphocholine. A common source of platelet-activating factor and arachidonate in human polymorpho-nuclear leukocytes, *J. Biol. Chem.,* 259, 12014, 1984.

34. **Suga, K., Kawasaki, T., Blank, M. L., and Snyder, F.,** An arachidonoyl(polyenoic)-specific phospho-lipase A_2 activity regulates the synthesis of platelet-activating factor in granulocytic HL-60 cells, *J. Biol. Chem.,* 265, 12363, 1990.

35. **Billah, M. M., Bryant, R. W., and Siegel, M. I.,** Lipoxygenase products of arachidonic acid modulate biosynthesis of platelet-activating factor (1-*O*-alkyl-2-acetyl-*sn*-glycero-3-phosphocholine) by human neu-trophils via phospholipase A_2, *J. Biol. Chem.,* 260, 6899, 1985.

36. **Ramesha, C. S. and Pickett, W. C.,** Platelet-activating factor and leukotriene biosynthesis is inhibited in polymorphonuclear leukocytes depleted of arachidonic acid, *J. Biol. Chem.,* 261, 7592, 1986.

37. **Wykle, R. L., Malone, B., and Snyder, F.,** Enzymatic synthesis of 1-alkyl-2-acetyl-*sn*-glycero-3-phos-phocholine, a hypotensive and platelet-aggregating lipid, *J. Biol. Chem.,* 255, 10256, 1980.

38. **Sturk, A., Schaap, M. C. L., Prins, A., Ten Cate, J. W., and Van den Bosch, H.,** Synthesis of platelet-activating factor by human blood platelets and leucocytes. Evidence against selective utilization of cellular ether-linked phospholipids, *Biochim. Biophys. Acta,* 993, 148, 1989.

39. **Hwang, S.-B.,** Specific receptors of platelet-activating factor, receptor heterogeneity, and signal transduction mechanisms, *J. Lipid Mediators,* 2, 123, 1990.

40. **Ng, D. S. and Wong, K.,** GTP regulation of platelet-activating factor binding to human neutrophil mem-branes, *Biochem. Biophys. Res. Commun.,* 141, 353, 1986.

41. **Hwang, S.-B., Lam, M.-H., and Pong, S.-S.,** Ionic and GTP regulation of binding of platelet-activating factor to receptors and platelet-activating factor-induced activation of GTPase in rabbit platelet membranes, *J. Biol. Chem.,* 261, 532, 1986.

42. **Houslay, M. D., Bojanic, D., and Wilson, A.,** Platelet activating factor and U44069 stimulate a GTPase activity in human platelets which is distinct from the guanine nucleotide regulatory proteins, N_s and N_i, *Biochem. J.,* 234, 737, 1986.

43. **Honda, Z., Nakamura, M., Miki, I., Minami, M., Watanabe, T., Seyama, Y., Okado, H., Toh, H., Ito, K., Miyamoto, T., and Shimizu, T.,** Cloning by functional expression of platelet-activating factor receptor from guinea-pig lung, *Nature,* 349, 342, 1991.

44. **Lapetina, E. G.,** Platelet-activating factor stimulates the phosphatidylinositol cycle. Appearance of phos-phatidic acid is associated with the release of serotonin in horse platelets, *J. Biol. Chem.,* 257, 7314, 1982.

45. **Billah, M. M. and Lapetina, E. G.,** Platelet-activating factor stimulates metabolism of phosphoinositides in horse platelets: possible relationship to Ca^{2+} mobilization during stimulation, *Proc. Natl. Acad. Sci. U.S.A.,* 80, 965, 1983.

46. **MacIntyre, D. E. and Pollock, W. K.,** Platelet-activating factor stimulates phosphatidylinositol turnover in human platelets, *Biochem. J.,* 212, 433, 1983.

47. **Mauco, G., Chap, H., and Douste-Blazy, L.,** Platelet activating factor (PAF-acether) promotes an early degradation of phosphatidylinositol-4,5-biophosphate in rabbit platelets, *FEBS Lett.,* 153, 361, 1983.

48. **Shukla, S. D.,** Platelet activating factor-stimulated formation of inositol triphosphate in platelets and its regulation by various agents including Ca^{2+}, indomethacin, CV-3988 and forskolin, *Arch. Biochem. Bio-phys.,* 240, 674, 1985.

49. **Morrison, W. J. and Shukla, S. D.,** Desensitization of receptor-coupled activation of phosphoinositide-specific phospholipase C in platelets: evidence for distinct mechanisms for platelet-activating factor and thrombin, *Mol. Pharmacol.,* 33, 58, 1988.

50. **Verghese, M. W., Charles, L., Jakoi, L., Dillon, S. B., and Snyderman, R.,** Role of a guanine nucleotide regulatory protein in activation of phospholipase C by different chemoattractants, *J. Immunol.,* 138, 4374, 1987.

51. **Shukla, S. D., Buxton, D. B., Olson, M. S., and Hanahan, D. J.,** Acetylglyceryl ether phosphorylcholine. A potent activator of hepatic phosphoinositide metabolism and glycogenolysis, *J. Biol. Chem.,* 258, 10212, 1983.

52. **Fisher, R. A., Shukla, S. D., Debuysere, M. S., Hanahan, D. J., and Olson, M. S.,** The effect of acetylglyceryl ether phosphorylcholine on glycogenolysis and phosphatidylinositol 4,5-bisphosphate me-tabolism in rat hepatocytes, *J. Biol. Chem.,* 259, 8685, 1984.

53. **Avdonin, P. V., Chelakov, I. B., Boogry, E. M., Svitina-Ulitina, I. V., Mazaev, A. V., and Tkachuk, V. A.,** Evidence for the receptor-operated calcium channels in human platelet plasma membranes, *Thromb. Res.,* 46, 29, 1987.

54. **Valone, F. H. and Johnson, B.,** Modulation of cytoplasmic calcium in human platelets by the phospholipid platelet-activating factor, 1-*O*-alkyl-2-acetyl-*sn*-glycero-3-phosphorylcholine, *J. Immunol.,* 134, 1120, 1985.

55. **Naccache, P. H., Molski, M. M. Volpi, M., Becker, E. L., and Sha'afi, R. I.,** Unique inhibitory profile of platelet-activating factor induced calcium mobilization, polyphosphoinositide turnover and granule enzyme secretion in rabbit neutrophils towards pertussis toxin and phorbol ester, *Biochem. Biophys. Res. Commun.,* 130, 677, 1985.

56. **Molski, T. F. P., Tao, W., Becker, E. L., and Sha'afi, R. I.,** Intracellular calcium rise produced by platelet-activating factor is deactivated by fMet-Leu-Phe and this requires uninterrupted activation sequence: role of protein kinase C, *Biochem. Biophys. Res. Commun.,* 151, 836, 1988.

57. **Ng, D. S. and Wong, K.,** Effect of platelet-activating factor (PAF) on cytosolic free calcium in human peripheral blood mononuclear leukocytes, *Res. Commun. Chem. Pathol. Pharmacol.,* 64, 351, 1989.

58. **Kornecki, E. and Ehrlich, Y. H.,** Neuroregulatory and neuropathological actions of the ether-phospholipid platelet-activating factor, *Science,* 240, 1792, 1988.

59. **Hirafuji, M., Maeyama, K., Watanabe, T., and Ogura, Y.,** Transient increase of cytosolic free calcium in cultured human vascular endothelial cells by platelet-activating factor, *Biochem. Biophys. Res. Commun.,* 154, 910, 1988.

60. **Nakashima, S., Suganuma, A., Sato, M., Tohmatsu, T., and Nozawa, Y.,** Mechanism of arachidonic acid liberation in platelet-activating factor-stimulated human polymorphonuclear neutrophils, *J. Immunol.,* 143, 1295, 1989.

61. **Kadiri, C., Cherqui, G., Masliah, J., Rybkine, T., Etienne, J., and Béréziat, G.,** Mechanism of *N*-formyl-methionyl-leucyl-phenylalanine- and platelet-activating factor-induced arachidonic acid release in guinea pig alveolar macrophages: involvement of a GTP-binding protein and role of protein kinase A and protein kinase C, *Mol. Pharmacol.,* 38, 418, 1990.

62. **Schlondorff, D., Satriano, J. A., Hagege, J., Perez, J., and Baud, L.,** Effect of platelet-activating factor and serum-treated zymosan on prostaglandin E_2 synthesis, arachidonic acid release, and contraction of cultured rat mesangial cells, *J. Clin. Invest.,* 73, 1227, 1984.

63. **Ardaillou, N., Hagege, J., Nivez, M.-P., Ardaillou, R., and Schlondorff, D.,** Vasoconstrictor-evoked prostaglandin synthesis in cultured human mesangial cells, *Am. J. Physiol.,* 248, F240, 1985.

64. **Chao, W., Liu, H., Hanahan, D. J., and Olson, M. S.,** Regulation of platelet-activating factor receptor and PAF receptor-mediated arachidonic acid release by protein kinase C activation in rat Kupffer cells, *Arch. Biochem. Biophys.,* 282, 188, 1990.

65. **Glaser, K. B., Asmis, R., and Dennis, E. A.,** Bacterial lipopolysaccharide priming of P388D$_1$ macrophage-like cells for enhanced arachidonic acid metabolism. Platelet-activating factor receptor activation and regulation of phospholipase A$_2$, *J. Biol. Chem.,* 265, 8658, 1990.

66. **Shibata, Y., Ogura, N., Moriya, Y., Abiko, Y., Izumi, H., and Takiguchi, H.,** Platelet-activating factor stimulates production of prostaglandin E_2 in murine osteoblast-like cell line MC3T3-E1, *Life Sci.,* 49, 1103, 1991.

67. **Billah, M. M., Di Renzo, G. C., Ban, C., Truong, C. T., Hoffman, D. R., Anceschi, M. M., Bleasdale, J. E., and Johnston, J. M.,** Platelet-activating factor metabolism in human amnion and the responses of this tissue to extracellular platelet-activating factor, *Prostaglandins,* 30, 841, 1985.

68. **Tessner, T. G., O'Flaherty, J. T., and Wykle, R. L.,** Stimulation of platelet-activating factor synthesis by a nonmetabolizable bioactive analog of platelet-activating factor and influence of arachidonic acid metabolites, *J. Biol. Chem.,* 264, 4794, 1989.

Chapter 13

METABOLIC FATE OF PLATELET ACTIVATING FACTOR CONTROLLED BY CELLULAR SIGNALING: STUDIES ON HEMATOPOIETIC CELL LINES

Mariano Sánchez-Crespo, Maria del Carmen García, Carolina García, Miguel Angel Gijón, Sagrario Fernández-Gallardo, and Faustino Mollinedo

TABLE OF CONTENTS

ISBN 0-8493-7299-2
© 1993 by CRC Press, Inc.

I. INTRODUCTION

The phospholipid mediator platelet-activating factor (PAF) is a potent activator of many cell types taking part in inflammatory reactions.[1-4] These cells respond to PAF because they have specific PAF receptors,[5-7] and in some cases metabolize PAF within the time required for cell activation.[8,9] Some reports have suggested that a major role of macrophages could be the modulation of the inflammatory reaction by promoting PAF catabolism,[10,11] because the intracellular concentration of PAF-acetylhydrolase, a central enzyme in PAF catabolism, increases 260-fold following differentiation of human peripheral blood monocytes into macrophages.[12] At present, a few reports exist on the role played by lymphocytes on PAF catabolism,[13,14] even though some studies indicate that PAF could play a role in the modulation of the immune response.[15,16] A host of investigations have been carried out in the HL-60 cell line,[17-19] a human promyelocytic leukemic cell line, which behaves as a differentiative bipotent cell.[20] HL-60 can be induced to differentiate along the granulocytic pathway by incubation with dimethylsulfoxide (DMSO) or with retinoic acid,[21] whereas exposure to other inducers such as 1,25-dihydroxy vitamin D_3 or phorbol myristate acetate (PMA) results in monocytic/macrophage differentiation.[22] A report by Camussi et al.[17] has related the capacity of HL-60 cells to release PAF to the expression of membrane receptors and transformation into a phagocytic cell, whereas Billah et al.[18] stressed the role of defective mechanisms regulating the activity of phospholipase A_2 (PLA_2) and acetyl-CoA:lyso-PAF acetyltransferase in uninduced cells.

The biosynthesis of PAF in polymorphonuclear leukocytes (PMN) and peripheral blood monocytes occurs mainly through the remodeling pathway. This pathway includes a PLA_2-catalyzed (EC 3.1.1.4) hydrolysis of 1-alkyl-2-acyl-*sn*-glycero-3-phosphocholine and acetylation of lyso-PAF by an acetyl-CoA:lyso-PAF acetyltransferase (EC 2.3.1.67). Because the acyl moiety released by PLA_2 is most often arachidonate, PAF metabolism is tightly coupled to the formation of eicosanoids.[23] In this chapter we have selected a number of both lymphoid and myeloid cells resembling either T and B lymphocytes or yielding either granulocytes or macrophages upon differentiation, in order to characterize the features of PAF metabolism in each cell type. Our findings indicate: (1) the ability of all the cell types so far tested to metabolize exogenous PAF by a mechanism mediated by receptors, at least in part; and (2) the restriction of PAF biosynthesis to myeloid cells.

II. MATERIALS AND METHODS

HL-60 and U937 cells were induced to differentiate toward monocytes/macrophage lineage by incubation with 32 nM PMA for 24 to 48 h. The extent of monocytic/macrophage cell differentiation was assessed by morphology, and by cell surface expression of the Mol differentiation antigen (a glycoprotein heterodimer that is involved in cellular adhesion processes and functions as the C3bi receptor in human myeloid cells).[24,25] Granulocytic differentiation of HL-60 cells was induced by adding 1.3% (v/v) DMSO for 6 d, unless mentioned otherwise. Cell suspensions were washed three times with a HEPES-buffered medium and resuspended at a concentration of 5×10^6 cells per milliliter in the same medium supplemented with 1 mM $CaCl_2$ and 0.1% bovine serum albumin (BSA). Viability of the cells was always >98%, as assessed by Trypan blue exclusion. Binding studies were carried out in a volume of 0.5 ml in Eppendorf microcentrifuge tubes at both 37° and 4°C. The concentration of [³H]PAF was 0.12 nM and different concentrations of unlabeled PAF were added. The reaction was stopped by adding cold-incubation medium and centrifugation at 8000 RPM for 30 s. The supernatants were removed and the cell pellets disrupted and mixed with a scintillation solution for aqueous samples. The binding data were subjected to Scatchard analysis using the program EDBA (Elsevier-Biosoft, Cambridge, U.K.) in a personal computer.

For preparation of a membrane fraction, the cells were washed and resuspended in the HEPES-buffered medium used for lavage and disrupted with a probe-type sonicator (three 10-s pulses). Nuclei and unbroken cells were removed by centrifugation at 27,000 $\times$ g for 15 min and the supernatant was centrifuged at 100,000 $\times$ g for 60 min. The pellet was resuspended in washing buffer in the presence of 1 mM CaCl$_2$, 1 mM MgCl$_2$, and 0.1% BSA, and binding studies were carried out in membrane fractions containing 100 μg of protein measured with the Bradford method.[26] [^{3}H]PAF was used at a concentration of 0.25 pM, and unlabeled PAF was used at concentrations up to 800 nM. The reaction was incubated for 1 h at room temperature in a volume of 0.5 ml, and stopped by the addition of 1 ml of cold medium followed by filtration in a Millipore 1225 sampling manifold, fitted with 0.22 μm fiberglass filters (Millipore Iberica, Madrid). An extraction of the filter with methanol was carried out to elute bound [^{3}H]PAF. Membrane fractions from rabbit platelets and human PMN were also studied as positive controls for comparison.

A lipid extract from cells was obtained by using the Bligh and Dyer procedure,[27] and subjected to thin-layer chromatography (TLC) on silica-gel plates using the solvent system chloroform/methanol/acetic acid/water (50:25:8:6, by vol) as developer, because this allows a good separation of PAF, lyso-PAF and 1-alkyl-2-acyl-GPC, i.e., the most predominant metabolites of PAF in the remodeling pathway. A further characterization of these products was carried out by straight-phase HPLC under the conditions described for the PAF bio-synthesis assay.

To assay PAF production, about 10^7 cells were incubated in 1 ml of a HEPES-buffered medium containing 140 mM NaCl, 3 mM KCl, 1 mM CaCl$_2$, 1 mM MgCl$_2$, 5.6 mM glucose, 0.25% BSA, and 20 μCi [^{14}C]acetate, pH 7.4. Stimulation of the cells was carried out with 10 μM ionophore A23187 for 20 min. The lipid extract was evaporated to dryness and resuspended in the mobile phase used for straight-phase HPLC. This was carried out in a Spheri-5 silica column using as a mobile phase B[96% propan-2-ol/hexane, 1/1, v/v] and A[4% water] which was linearly increased to 8% during a 15-min period.[28] The column was eluted for 60 min at 2 ml/min, and the fractions collected used for scintillation spectrometry after the addition of a scintillation cocktail for nonaqueous samples. Further characterization of the [^{14}C]acetate containing phospholipid as authentic PAF was carried out (1) by showing the loss of the label after treatment with PLA$_2$, which indicates that the [^{14}C]acetate has not been elongated; and (2) by the resistance of the label to PLA$_1$ treatment, which rules out the incorporation of [^{14}C]acetate into a moiety linked by an ester bond at the sn-1 position.

III. RESULTS

A. BINDING OF [^{3}H] PAF TO INTACT CELLS

All of the cell lines incubated in the presence of [^{3}H]PAF showed a time-dependent incorporation of [^{3}H]radioactivity into cell lipids. This is shown in Figure 1 for DMSO-differentiated HL-60 and PMA-differentiated U937 cells, whereas similar profiles obtained for Daudi and Jurkat cell lines are not shown. The accumulation of cell-associated radioactivity reached a maximum at about 60 min, was reduced when the incubation was carried out in the presence of an excess of unlabeled PAF, and was temperature dependent, as significant binding at 4°C was only observed in DMSO-differentiated HL-60 cells (data not shown). Binding of [^{3}H]PAF was accompanied by a rapid conversion into 1-alkyl-2-acyl-GPC in all of the cell lines studied (Figure 1; Table 1). When the incubation was carried out at 4°C, the incorporation of radioactivity in 1-alkyl-2-acyl-GPC was reduced by 78% to

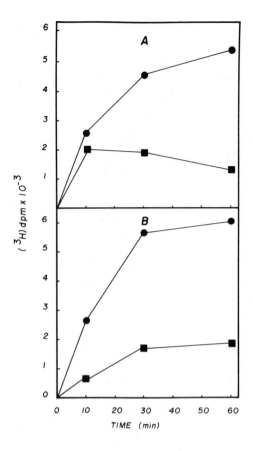

FIGURE 1.   Binding of [³H]PAF to DMSO-treated HL-60 cells (A) and to PMA-treated U937 cells (B). Cells at the concentration of 5 × 10⁶/ml were incubated at 37°C in the presence of 0.12 nM [³H]PAF. At the times indicated, cells were collected, subjected to lipid extraction, and the radioactivity incorporated in the fractions migrating as 1-[³H]alkyl-2-acyl-GPC (●) and [³H]PAF (■) in TLC quantitated. Data represent mean values of an experiment with duplicate samples. (From Garcia, M. C. et al., *Biochem. J.*, 273, 573, 1991. With permission.)

95% (Table 1). No increase of the amount of lyso-PAF associated with the cells could be detected, which is in keeping with the existence of an efficient mechanism of either reacylation or transacylation. The PAF receptor antagonist, PCA4248,[29] at a concentration of 10 μM reduced PAF conversion into 1-alkyl-2-acyl-GPC by 40% in all of the cell lines (Table 1). Scatchard analysis of [³H]PAF binding by cell lines showed a pattern consistent at first glance with the presence of receptors, but with numbers unacceptably high, i.e., above 10⁵ PAF receptors per HL-60 and U937 cell. This suggested, as already pointed out in the report by Valone,[8] that uptake and metabolism could also occur by nonreceptor-mediated mechanisms. Although these findings allow the distinction between two kinds of cell lines as regards PAF binding (i.e., myeloid cell lines, which have a larger number of high affinity binding sites, and lymphoid cells, which have a more reduced number of binding sites), further experiments were planned using membrane fraction, in order to overcome the possible influence on the quantitation of [³H]PAF binding due to endocytosis and hydrolysis by cytosolic PAF-acetylhydrolase.

B. BINDING OF [³H]PAF TO CELL MEMBRANE FRACTION

Scatchard analysis of the binding kinetics was always consistent with the existence of a single class of high affinity binding sites, irrespective of the variations detected in the

TABLE 1

Metabolism of Exogenous [³H]PAF by Different Cell Lines: Effect of Temperature and a PAF Receptor Antagonist

	1-Alkyl-2-acyl-GPC (dpm)		
Cell line	37°C[a]	37°C[b]	4°C
Uninduced HL-60	5187	2658	616
DMSO-differentiated HL-60	5432	ND	ND
PMA-differentiated HL-60	4569	3247	984
Uninduced U937	5985	2214	ND
PMA-differentiated U937	6002	4214	515
Daudi	3294	ND	276
Jurkat	3328	2234	143

Note: About 5×10^6 cells were incubated with 0.12 nM [³H]PAF (about 12,000 dpm) at 37° or at 4°C for 60 min. At the end of this period lipids were extracted and the radioactivity associated to the 1-alkyl-2-acyl-GPC fraction assessed.

[a] Indicates experiments carried out in the absence of 10 μM PCA4248.

[b] Indicates experiments carried out in the presence of 10 μM PCA4248. Cells were incubated for 6 d in the presence of DMSO to promote granulocytic differentiation. Data represent mean values of two experiments with duplicate samples.

From García, M. C. et al., *Biochem. J.*, 273, 573, 1991. With permission.

number of binding sites. Binding of [³H]PAF to membrane fractions from HL-60 and U937 cells was consistent with a number of receptors similar to that assessed in human PMN,[30] and only a significant variation of the number of receptors elicited by differentiation could be demonstrated in U937 cells after exposure to PMA. In contrast, Daudi cells showed a number of receptors reduced approximately two orders of magnitude as compared to HL-60 cells, U937, and human PMN (Table 2). Extraction of lipids from the membrane fraction used for binding showed no conversion of [³H]PAF into 1-[³H]alkyl-2-acyl-GPC, which is in keeping with the cytosolic location of PAF-acetylhydrolase, and its absence from the membrane fraction used to carry out binding studies.[31]

C. INCORPORATION OF [¹⁴C]ACETATE INTO PHOSPHOLIPIDS

Uninduced HL-60 cells incorporated the [¹⁴C]acetate label in three different lipid fractions with the retention times of neutral lipids, phosphatidylcholine (PC), and PAF, i.e., 3, 16, and 21 min, respectively (Figure 2). The incorporation of the label into the PAF fraction in control resting cells was 732 ± 215 dpm and increased to 4794 ± 915 dpm after stimulation with 10 μM ionophore A23187 for 15 min. This was enhanced to 7162 ± 1109 dpm when lyso-PAF and ionophore A23187 were used in combination (Table 3). The actual figures of incorporation of the label in DMSO-differentiated cells were lower than those detected in uninduced HL-60 cells, but showed the same tendency to increase by the addition of ionophore A23187 and 10 μM lyso-PAF (Table 3). PMA-differentiated HL-60 cells showed a reduction of the incorporation of [¹⁴C]acetate as compared to undifferentiated cells. U937 cells showed the highest rate of incorporation of [¹⁴C]acetate into neutral lipids (102,498 to

TABLE 2
Binding of [³H]PAF to Membrane Fractions

Cell line	Receptors/mg protein	K_d (M)	n
Uninduced HL-60	$1.1 \pm 0.0 \times 10^{12}$	$2.1 \pm 1.9 \times 10^{-9}$	5
PMA-differentiated HL-60[a]	0.8×10^{12}	0.5×10^{-9}	1
Uninduced U937	$6.1 \pm 2.7 \times 10^{11}$	$1.5 \pm 1.3 \times 10^{-9}$	3
PMA-differentiated U937[a]	3.4×10^{12}	1.2×10^{-9}	2
Daudi	4×10^{10}	2.1×10^{-9}	2

Note: Data obtained from the Scatchard representation are expressed as mean ± SD.

[a]   Indicates cells differentiated for 2 d in the presence of 32 n*M* PMA.

From Garcia, M. C. et al., *Biochem. J.*, 273, 573, 1991. With permission.

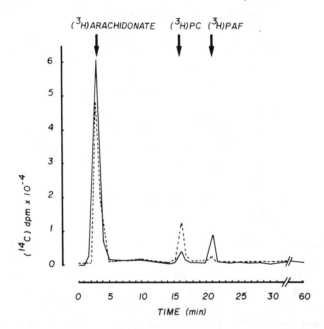

FIGURE 2.   Incorporation of [¹⁴C]acetate in lipids from uninduced HL-60 cells. Straight-phase HPLC chromatogram shows the effect of ionophore A23187 and exogenous lyso-PAF. Cells were incubated in the absence (dotted line) or presence (continuous line) of both 10 μ*M* A23187 and 10 μ*M* lyso-PAF for 15 min. At the end of this period lipids were extracted, separated by straight-phase HPLC, and the radioactivity associated to each fraction quantitated by scintillation spectrometry. The arrows indicate the retention time of the standards. (From Garcia, M. C. et al., *Biochem. J.*, 273, 573, 1991. With permission.)

152,986 dpm) and an incorporation into PC (7237 to 9891 dpm) comparable to that observed in uninduced HL-60 cells. However, the incorporation of [¹⁴C]acetate in PAF was less than that observed in HL-60 cell lines, e.g., 1169 to 1517 dpm in uninduced cells vs. 698 to 1661 dmp in PMA-differentiated cells. Daudi and Jurkat cell lines were unable to incorporate the label in [¹⁴C]PAF, and significant radioactivity only appeared associated with the neutral lipid fraction in both cell lines and to the PC fraction in Daudi cells (data not shown). Taken together, these data indicate the existence of diverse metabolic pathways for [¹⁴C]acetate. The predominant pathway seems to be either *de novo* synthesis or elongation of fatty acids, and this may explain both the incorporation of the label into the neutral lipid fraction and

TABLE 3
Incorporation of [^{14}C]Acetate in Lipid Fractions
from HL-60 Cells

Addition	PAF (dpm)	Neutral lipids (dpm)	PC (dpm)
Uninduced			
No addition	67,483 ± 21,423	14,643 ± 3,921	732 ± 215
Lyso-PAF	63,422 ± 19,486	8,428 ± 4,012	711 ± 315
A23187	69,367 ± 13,675	9,429 ± 5,102	4,794 ± 915
A23187 + lyso-PAF	48,632 ± 12,559	5,124 ± 3,006	7,762 ± 1,109
DMSO-differentiated			
No addition	20,692 ± 2,019	515 ± 84	61 ± 10
Lyso-PAF	18,221	423	57
A23187	15,083	602	1,672
A23187 + lyso-PAF	14,527 ± 4,087	963 ± 112	3,543 ± 349
PMA-differentiated			
No addition	14,650 ± 980	483 ± 16	233 ± 26
Lyso-PAF	10,884	439	261
A23187	9,548	451	824
A23187 + lyso-PAF	9,985 ± 1,507	490 ± 23	1,587 ± 263

Note: HL-60 cells were incubated in the presence of 20 μCi/ml [^{14}C]acetate and different additions. The incubation was stopped by the addition of methanol/chloroform and the lipid extract evaporated to dryness and subjected to straight-phase HPLC. To obtain granulocytic differentiation HL-60 cells were cultured for 6 d in the presence of 1.3% (v/v) DMSO. To obtain monocytic differentiation HL-60 cells were grown for 2 d in the presence of 32 nM PMA. Data represent two to four experiments with duplicate samples, and are expressed as either mean values or mean ± SD when n > 3. Background count has been subtracted.

From García, M. C. et al., *Biochem. J.*, 273, 573, 1991. With permission.

a subsequent transfer into PC, which is the most abundant phospholipid class. Because we have not observed the incorporation of [^{14}C]acetate into the PC fraction of human PMN under similar conditions of incubation and stimulation,[32] this incorporation seems to be most likely due to a high biosynthetic rate of PC in cells rapidly dividing in culture. Alternatively, our findings could reflect an enhanced turnover of PC linked to a PC cycle, as that described in a number of cells involved in immune reactions, including Jurkat and HL-60 cells.[33-35]

IV. DISCUSSION

All of the cell lines bound [^{3}H]PAF in a time-dependent manner. Binding of [^{3}H]PAF was followed by conversion of the ligand into 1-[^{3}H]alkyl-2-acyl-GPC. This raises the question as to whether this is due to binding to a membrane receptor followed by internalization and hydrolysis in the cytosol by PAF-acetylhydrolase or, in turn it is linked to another mechanism of uptake, as it has been shown for leukotriene C$_4$ in rat hepatocytes, which binds to a protein located to the cytosol rather than to a membrane receptor.[36] That we are dealing with a true membrane receptor in these cell lines stems from two main observations: blunting of both binding and catabolism by a specific antagonist of the PAF receptor at a concentration which has been able to block binding to PAF receptors on human platelets and polymorphonuclears;[29] and the occurrence of binding, but not catabolism, on a membrane fraction. Furthermore, the functional significance of the putative membrane receptors has been substantiated by showing that PAF increases free intracellular calcium in a dose-dependent manner at concentrations as low as 1 pM in P388D$_1$, U937, HL-60 and Raji cells.[13,37,38]

Another finding is the ability of HL-60 and U937 cell lines to synthesize PAF, in contrast to the absence of this property in two lymphoid cell lines studied. The capacity of HL-60 cells to generate PAF already exists in uninduced cells, and persists in differentiated cells, at least after periods in culture not longer than 6 d. These findings should be commented upon on the basis of previous knowledge about the different factors involved in the modulation of PAF biosynthesis in cells taking part in inflammatory reactions. Our data differ in part from those reported by Billah et al.,[18] who found that uninduced HL-60 cells were unable to generate PAF upon ionophore A23187 challenge, whereas DMSO-induced HL-60 cells produced PAF upon stimulation. A possible explanation for this difference could be the various procedures used to study PAF biosynthesis, as Billah et al.[18] carried out most studies using a bioassay with human platelets. Our studies, however, have been performed by measuring the incorporation of [^{14}C]acetate into [^{14}C]PAF. Because the addition of lyso-PAF at the time of ionophore A23187 challenge is an efficient mechanism that enhances PAF formation in uninduced cells, the most likely explanation is that a PLA$_2$ activity, by providing lyso-PAF, plays a central role in PAF formation. This is in keeping with our findings in human PMN, in which lyso-PAF disposal is a critical event for PAF formation.[32]

Our findings also show the incorporation of [^{14}C]acetate into lipid fractions other than PAF, and this depends on the cell line. A possible reason may be competition of acetyl-CoA:lyso-PAF acetyltransferase with a very efficient mechanism of biosynthesis/elongation of fatty acids from acetyl-CoA, as the incorporation of [^{14}C]acetate into the neutral lipid fraction of U937 cells is tenfold as high as that of PMA-differentiated HL-60 cells and even increases with induction. A report by Wakyl has stressed the absence of acetyl-CoA carboxylase in human leukocytes,[39] where acetate incorporation into fatty acids may only occur by chain elongation, but this enzyme activity is present in immature leukemia blast cells which are capable of carrying out *de novo* fatty acid synthesis.[40]

In summary, this chapter stresses the differences between different cell lines as regards PAF metabolism and suggests that cell lines with the ability to differentiate into granulocytes are the most efficient producers of PAF. Lymphoid cells could play a role in the modulation of inflammatory reactions by metabolizing PAF produced by other cell types.

ACKNOWLEDGMENTS

The study described in this chapter has been supported by DGICYT grants PM88-0010 and PM89-0003.

REFERENCES

1. **Benveniste, J., Henson, P. M., and Cochrane, C. G.,** Leukocyte-dependent histamine release from rabbit platelets. The role of IgE, basophils and a platelet-activating factor, *J. Exp. Med.,* 136, 1356, 1972.
2. **Demopoulos, C. A., Pinckard, R. N., and Hanahan, D. J.,** Platelet-activating factor. Evidence for 1-O-alkyl-2-acetyl-*sn*-glycero-3-phosphocholine as the active component (a new class of lipid chemical mediators), *J. Biol. Chem.,* 254, 9355, 1979.
3. **Blank, M. L., Snyder, F., Byers, L. W., Brooks, B., and Muirhead, E. E.,** Antihypertensive activity of an alkyl ether analogue of phosphatidylcholine, *Biochem. Biophys. Res. Commun.,* 90, 1194, 1979.
4. **Benveniste, J., Tence, M., Varenne, P., Bidault, J., and Polonski, J.,** Semi-synthese et structure proposée du facteur activant les plaquettes (P.A.F.): PAF-acether, un alkyl ether analogue de la lysophosphatidylcholine, *C. R. Hebd. Acad. Sci. D (Paris),* 289, 1037, 1979.
5. **Valone, F. H., Coles, E., Reinhold, V. R., and Goetzl, E. J.,** Specific binding of phospholipid platelet-activating factor by human platelets, *J. Immunol.,* 129, 1637, 1982.

6. **Hwang, S.-B., Lee, C.-S., Cheah, M. J., and Shen, T. Y.,** Specific receptor sites for 1-O-alkyl-2-acetyl-*sn*-glycero-3-phosphocholine (platelet activating factor) on rabbit platelet and guinea pig smooth muscle membranes, *Biochemistry,* 22, 4756, 1983.

7. **Kloprogge, E. and Akkerman, J. W. N.,** Binding kinetics of PAF-acether (1-O-alkyl-2-acetyl-*sn*-glycero-3-phosphocholine) to intact human platelets, *Biochem. J.,* 223, 901, 1984.

8. **Valone, F. H.,** Identification of platelet-activating factor receptors in P388D$_1$ murine macrophages, *J. Immunol.,* 140, 2389, 1988.

9. **Homma, H. A., Tokumura, A., and Hanahan, D. J.,** Binding and internalization of platelet-activating factor 1-O-alkyl-2-acetyl-*sn*-glycero-3-phosphocholine in washed rabbit platelets, *J. Biol. Chem.,* 262, 10582, 1987.

10. **Roubin, R., Mencia-Huerta, J. M., Landes, A., and Benveniste, J.,** Biosynthesis of platelet-activating factor (PAF-acether). IV. Impairment of acetyl-transferase activity in thioglycollate-elicited mouse macrophages, *J. Immunol.,* 129, 809, 1982.

11. **Dulioust, A., Vivier, E., Meslier, N., Roubin, R., Haye-Legrand, I., and Benveniste, J.,** Biosynthesis of paf-acether. Paf-acether but not leukotriene C$_4$ production is impaired in cultured macrophages, *Biochem. J.,* 263, 165, 1989.

12. **Elstad, M. R., Stafforini, D. M., McIntyre, T. M., Prescott, S. M., and Zimmerman, G. A.,** Platelet-activating factor acetylhydrolase increases during macrophage differentiation, *J. Biol. Chem.,* 264, 8467, 1989.

13. **Travers, J. B., Li, Q., Kniss, D. A., and Fertel, R. H.,** Identification of functional platelet-activating factor receptors in Raji lymphoblasts, *J. Immunol.,* 143, 3708, 1989.

14. **Travers, J. B., Sprecher, H., and Fertel, R. H.,** The metabolism of platelet-activating factor in human T-lymphocytes, *Biochim. Biophys. Acta,* 1042, 193, 1990.

15. **Schulam, P. G., Kuruvilla, A., Putcha, G., Mangus, L., Franklin-Johnson, J., and Shearer, W. T.,** Platelet-activating factor induces phospholipid turnover, calcium flux, arachidonic acid liberation, eicosanoid generation and oncogene expression in a human B cell line, *J. Immunol.,* 146, 1642, 1991.

16. **Rola-Pleszczynski, M., Pignol, B., Pouliot, C., and Braquet, P.,** Inhibition of human lymphocyte proliferation and interleukin 2 production by platelet-activating factor (PAF-acether): reversal by a specific antagonist, BN52021, *Biochem. Biophys. Res. Commun.,* 142, 754, 1987.

17. **Camussi, G., Bussolino, F., Ghezzo, F., and Pegoraro, L.,** Release of platelet-activating factor from HL-60 human leukemic cells following macrophage-like differentiation, *Blood,* 59, 16, 1982.

18. **Billah, M., Eckel, S., Myers, R. F., and Siegel, M. I.,** Metabolism of platelet-activating factor (1-O-alkyl-2-acetyl-*sn*-glycero-phosphocholine) by human promyelocytic leukemic HL60 cells, *J. Biol. Chem.,* 261, 5824, 1986.

19. **Vallari, D. S., Austinhirst, R., and Snyder, F.,** Development of specific functionally active receptors for platelet-activating factor in HL-60 cells following granulocytic differentiation, *J. Biol. Chem.,* 265, 4261, 1990.

20. **Collins, J. S., Gallo, R. C., and Gallagher, R. E.,** Continuous growth and differentiation of human myeloid leukemia cells in suspension culture, *Nature,* 270, 347, 1977.

21. **Collins, S. J., Ruscetti, F. W., Gallagher, R. E., and Gallo, R. C.,** Terminal differentiation of human promyelocytic leukemia cells induced by dimethyl sulfoxide and other polar compounds, *Proc. Natl. Acad. Sci. U.S.A.,* 75, 2458, 1978.

22. **Rovera, G., Santoli, D. E., and Damsky, C.,** Human promyelocytic leukemia cells differentiate into macrophage-like cells when treated with a phorbol diester, *Proc. Natl. Acad. Sci. U.S.A.,* 76, 2779, 1979.

23. **Chilton, F. H., Ellis, J. M., Olson, S. C., and Wykle, R. L.,** 1-O-alkyl-2-arachidonoyl-*sn*-glycero-3-phosphocholine. A common source of platelet-activating factor and arachidonate in human polymorphonuclear leukocytes, *J. Biol. Chem.,* 259, 12014, 1984.

24. **Miller, L. J., Schwarting, R., and Springer, T. A.,** Regulated expression of the Mac-1, LFA-1, p150,95 glycoprotein family during leukocyte differentiation, *J. Immunol.,* 137, 2891, 1986.

25. **Lacal, P., Pulido, R., Sanchez-Madrid, F., and Mollinedo, F.,** Intracellular location of T200 and M01 glycoproteins in human neutrophils, *J. Biol. Chem.,* 263, 9946, 1988.

26. **Bradford, M.,** A rapid and sensitive method for the quantitation of microgram quantities of protein using the principle of protein-dye binding, *Anal. Biochem.,* 72, 248, 1976.

27. **Bligh, E. G. and Dyer, W. J.,** A rapid method of total lipid extraction and purification, *Can. J. Biochem. Physiol.,* 37, 911, 1959.

28. **Blank, M. L. and Snyder, F.,** Improved high-performance liquid chromatographic method for the isolation of platelet-activating factor from other phospholipids, *J. Chromatogr.,* 273, 415, 1983.

29. **Ortega, M. P., García, M. C., Gijón, M. A., de Casa-Juana, M. F., Priego, J. G., Sánchez Crespo, M., and Sunkel, C.,** 1,4-Dihydropyridines, a new class of platelet-activating factor receptor antagonists: *in vitro* pharmacologic studies, *J. Pharmacol. Exp. Ther.,* 255, 28, 1990.

30. **Hwang, S.-B.,** Identification of a second putative receptor of platelet-activating factor from human polymorphonuclear leukocytes, *J. Biol. Chem.,* 263, 3225, 1988.

31. **Blank, M. L., Lee, T.-C., Fitzgerald, V., and Snyder, F.,** A specific acetylhydrolase for 1-alkyl-2-acetyl-*sn*-glycero-3-phosphocholine (a hypotensive and platelet-activating phospholipid), *J. Biol. Chem.,* 256, 175, 1981.

32. **García, M. C., Fernández-Gallardo, S., Gijón, M. A., García, C., Nieto, M. L., and Sánchez Crespo, M.,** Biosynthesis of platelet-activating factor (PAF) in human polymorphonuclear leukocytes. The role of lyso-PAF disposal and free arachidonic acid, *Biochem. J.,* 268, 91, 1990.

33. **Daniel, L. W., Waite, M., and Wykle, R. L.,** A novel mechanism of diglyceride formation. 12-O-tetradecanoylphorbol-13-acetate stimualtes the cyclic breakdown and synthesis of phosphatidylcholine, *J. Biol. Chem.,* 261, 9128, 1986.

34. **Rosoff, P. M., Savage, N., and Dinarello, C. A.,** Interleukin-1 stimulates diacylglycerol production in T lymphocytes by a novel mechanism, *Cell,* 54, 73, 1988.

35. **Pai, J.-K., Siegel, M. I., Egan, R. W., and Billah, M. M.,** Phospholipase D catalyzes phospholipid metabolism in chemotactic peptide-stimulated HL60 granulocytes, *J. Biol. Chem.,* 263, 12472, 1988.

36. **Sun, F. F., Chau, L.-W., Spur, B., Corey, E. J., and Austen, K. F.,** Identification of a high affinity leukotriene C_4-binding protein in rat liver cytosol as glutathione S-transferase, *J. Biol. Chem.,* 261, 8540, 1986.

37. **Maudsley, D. J. and Morris, A. G.,** Rapid intracellular calcium changes in U937 monocyte cell line: transient increases in responses to platelet-activating factor and chemotactic peptide but not interferon gamma or lipopolysaccharide, *Immunology,* 61, 189, 1987.

38. **Luscinskas, F. W., Brock, T. A., Wheeler, M. E., Bevilacqua, M. P., and Gimbrone, M. A.,** Biochemical and functional responses of differentiated HL-60 cells to platelet-activating factor, *Fed. Proc.,* 46, 444A, 1987.

39. **Wakyl, S. J.,** Mechanism of fatty acid synthesis, *Lipid Res.,* 2, 1, 1961.

40. **Majerus, P. W. and Lastra, R. R.,** Fatty acid biosynthesis in human leukocytes, *J. Clin. Invest.,* 46, 1596, 1967.

41. **García, M. C., García, C., Gijón, M. A., Fernández-Gallardo, S., Mollinedo, F., and Sánchez Crespo, M.,** Metabolism of platelet-activating factor in human haematopoietic cell lines. Differences between myeloid and lymphoid cells, *Biochem. J.,* 273, 573, 1991.

Chapter 14

BIOSYNTHESIS, METABOLIC FATE, AND ACTIONS OF PLATELET ACTIVATING FACTOR IN THE LOWER ANIMALS

Takayuki Sugiura, Teruo Fukuda, Tatsuya Miyamoto, Neng-neng Cheng, and Keizo Waku

TABLE OF CONTENTS

ISBN 0-8493-7299-2
© 1993 by CRC Press, Inc.

I. INTRODUCTION

Platelet-activating factor (PAF)[1] is a potent bioactive molecule, which was finally elucidated to be an alkyl ether phospholipid, 1-O-alkyl-2-acetyl-*sn*-glycero-3-phosphocholine.[2-4] It causes aggregation and degranulation of platelets and polymorphonuclear leukocytes (PMN), increased vascular permeability, smooth muscle contraction, systemic hypotension, and bronchial hyperreactivity *in vitro* or *in vivo*.[5] PAF is now considered to be an important mediator in the pathogenesis of several diseases such as endotoxin shock, anaphylactic shock, and bronchial asthma. Besides the possible involvement in various pathological reactions, PAF is now believed to be implicated in more physiological responses. Several investigators have reported the presence of PAF in various tissues and biological fluids from normal animals,[6-10] although the physiological roles of PAF are still not fully understood.

PAF was first discovered as a chemical mediator of acute hypersensitivity in mammals, and most studies have been directed toward mammalian tissues and cells. Little information is yet available concerning PAF in animals other than mammals. Recently, we presented evidence for the occurrence of high level of ether phospholipids, especially 1-O-alkyl-2-acyl(long chain)-*sn*-glycero-3-phosphocholine (GPC), which is regarded as a stored precursor form of PAF, in various types of invertebrates.[11] This characteristic is reminiscent of mammalian PMN and macrophages,[12] which are known to produce significant amounts of PAF upon stimulation. These observations prompted us to examine whether PAF is present in various types of invertebrates and whether it has physiological and pathological roles in invertebrates as well as in mammals. This chapter presents the authors' recent data on ether lipid composition as well as PAF content in these animals. Several aspects of the metabolism and actions of PAF in lower animals are also discussed.

II. ETHER PHOSPHOLIPID COMPOSITION OF VARIOUS INVERTEBRATES

It is well known that alkyl ether-containing lipids were first discovered in animals other than mammals.[13] Glyceryl ether was first isolated from the unsaponifiable fraction of lipids from sharks and rays by Tsujimoto and Toyama[14] about 70 years ago. Phospholipid containing alkyl ether residue was first isolated from chicken egg yolk by Carter and co-workers[15] in 1958. The occurrence of alkylacyl-GPC was also observed in several lower animals such as slug (*Ariolimax columbianus*; 49% of choline glycerophospholipid fraction)[16] and protozoa (*Tetrahymena pyriformis*; 62% of choline glycerophospholipid fraction).[17] The presence of alkyl ether-containing compounds in total lipid fraction and phospholipid fraction has also been pointed out for several other animals.[18-22] Thus, it has generally been assumed that lower animals may contain considerable amounts of alkyl ether phospholipids, though detailed information is not available.

Further, not much attention has been paid to alkyl ether phospholipids, as compared to alkenyl ether phospholipids (plasmalogen) in mammals, as it has long been assumed that the levels of alkylacyl-GPC in normal mammalian tissues are very low. In fact, tissues such as brain, liver, lung, heart, kidney, and erythrocytes contain only small amounts of alkylacyl-GPC in mammals.[12] The exceptions are bone marrow[23,24] and white blood cells (WBC).[25-27] These tissues and cells contain significant amounts of alkylacyl-GPC, accounting for 12 to 50% of choline glycerophospholipid (CGP) fraction.[12] After the elucidation of the structure of PAF, alkyl ether phospholipids (especially in WBC) received much more attention. Nonetheless, alkyl ether phospholipids in lower animals still remain poorly studied. Table 1 shows the data obtained for several invertebrates by us and by others. Various multi- and unicellular invertebrates — slug (*Incilaria bilineata*), water snail (*Lymnaea stagnalis*), sea anemone

TABLE 1
Alkenylacyl, Alkylacyl, and Diacyl Subclasses of Choline Glycerophospholipid Fraction from Several Species of Invertebrates

Species	Alkenylacyl (%)	Alkylacyl (%)	Diacyl (%)	Ref.
Slug	4.1	47.4	48.5	28
(*Incilaria bilineata*)				
Water snail	2.5	44.5	53.0	29
(*Lymnaea stagnalis*)				
Sea anemone	7.7	59.8	32.5	30
(*Actinia equina*)				
Sponge	9.1	79.0	11.9	30
(*Halichondria okadai*)				
Protozoa	—	83	17	31
(*Paramecium tetraurelia*)				

(*Actinia equina*), sponge (*Halichondria okadai*), protozoa (*Paramecium tetraurelia*) — all contain large amounts of alkylacyl compounds in CGP.

Recently we examined alkyl ether phospholipids in more than 25 species of multicellular invertebrates.[11] We found that alkyl ether phospholipids, especially alkylacyl-GPC, are widely distributed among various types of invertebrates, except for insects. Animals in Arthropoda other than insects also seem to contain smaller amounts of alkylacyl-GPC as compared to other lower animals. The percentages of alkylacyl-GPC in CGP fraction were 1.9% (beetle, *Allomyrina dichotoma*), 1.9% (cabbage butterfly, *Pieris rapae*), 1.8% (butterfly, *Papilio xuthus*), 1.3% (silkworm, *Bombyx mori*), 1.3% (dragonfly, *Sympetrum pedemontanum elatum*), 0.8% (grasshopper, *Oedaleus infernalis*), 1.7% (praying mantis, *Statilia maculata*), 7.0% (prawn, *Penaeus japonicus*), 17.9% (spider, *Grammostola* sp.), 8.6% (pill bug, *Armadillidium vulgare*), 45.2% (freshwater mussel, *Cristaria plicata*), 10.3% (turban shell, *Batillus cornutus*), 45.4% (sea hare, *Aplysia* sp.), 61.4% (earthworm, *Eisenia foetida*), 68.5% (earthworm, *Pheretima* sp.), 49.6% (clam worm, *Marphysa sanguinea*), 23.4% (spoon worm, *Urechis unicinctus*), 47.3% (freshwater planaria, *Dugesia japonica*), 72.6% (free-living flatworm, *Bipalium fuscatum*), 22.5% (sea squirt, *Halocynthia roretzi*), 35.4% (sea urchin, *Anthocidaris crassispina*), 64.5% (starfish, *Astropecten scoparius*), 69.7% (sea cucumber, *Stichopus japonicus*), 52.5% (jellyfish, *Aurelia aurita*), 69.8% (sea anemone, *Anthopleura japonica*), and 81.8% (sponge, *Halichondria japonica*).[11] Thus, it seems a possible common feature of invertebrates, other than insects, and especially in the lower phyla, to contain large amounts of alkylacyl-GPC.

The biological roles of alkyl ether phospholipids in these animals still remain obscure. However, the abundance of alkylacyl-GPC is of interest in relation to the possible production of PAF, since alkylacyl-GPC is regarded as a stored precursor form of PAF in mammals. We next explored the possibility of the presence of PAF in these lower animals.

III. PLATELET ACTIVATING FACTOR LEVELS IN VARIOUS INVERTEBRATES

The authors first investigated slugs[28] and found platelet-aggregating activity in their total lipid fraction. As shown in Figure 1, the activity comigrated with authentic PAF on a thin-layer chromatography (TLC) plate, suggesting that the biologically active material is PAF. This was further confirmed by the findings that the biological activity was lost after treatment

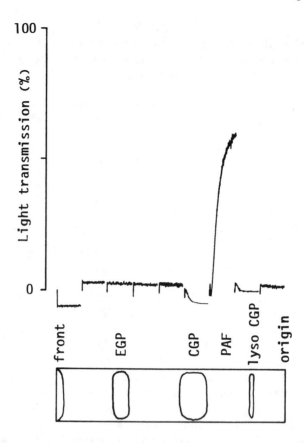

FIGURE 1. Ability of individual phospholipid fractions of the slug, *Incilaria bilineata*, to aggregate washed rabbit platelets. Total lipid fraction was subjected to TLC developed with chloroform:methanol:water (65:35:6, v/v). After the development, silica gel was zonally scraped from (2 cm width) the plate. The extracted lipid was dispersed in 0.25 % BSA-containing Tyrode's solution. An aliquot was added to platelet suspension and the changes in light transmission were recorded. (From Sugiura, T., Ojima, T., Fukuda, T., Satouchi, K., Saito, K., and Waku, K., Production of platelet-activating factor in slugs, *J. Lipid Res.*, 32, 1795, 1991. With permission.)

of the sample either with alkaline solution or with phospholipases (A$_2$ and C; PLA$_2$ and PLC) and that the aggregation of washed rabbit platelets upon the addition of the sample was completely inhibited when platelets were pretreated with a specific PAF antagonist, CV6209 (0.1 μM). The levels of PAF in the slugs, *Incilaria bilineata* and *Incilaria fruhstorferi*, were 2.1 and 1.7 pmol/g body weight, respectively.

Gas chromatography/mass spectrometric (GC/MS) analysis also provided evidence for the occurrence of PAF in *Incilaria bilineata*[28] (Figure 2). The predominant molecular species of PAF in this animal was shown to be C16:0 PAF (peak 2). A small amount of C16:0 1-acyl-PAF (peak 3) was also observed, besides C16:0 PAF. A minor peak (peak 1) was tentatively identified as C15:0 PAF based on its retention time. On the other hand, peak 4 still remains unidentified. We were not able to observe peaks of which the retention times correspond to C18:0 PAF and C18:1 PAF in slugs. The abundance of C16:0 moiety in PAF seems to be of interest, because the alkyl fatty chain at the 1-position of alkylacyl-GPC in slugs was composed mainly of C16:0 (94%) together with a small amount of C15:0 (6%).[16] It is possible, therefore, that PAF is produced from preexisting alkylacyl-GPC through a deacylation acetylation pathway in slugs, as in WBC in mammals (see Section IV).

The presence of PAF was further investigated in more than 40 species of multicellular invertebrates.[11] We found that PAF is widely distributed among these lower animals, although

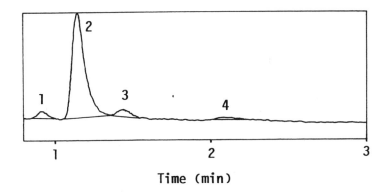

Time (min)

FIGURE 2. A trace of selected ion monitoring (m/z 117) of *t*-butyldimethylsilyl deriative of PAF from DMSO-injected slugs (*Incilaria bilineata*). The percentages of peak areas were 5.0% (peak 1), 85.9% (peak 2), 6.3% (peak 3), and 2.8% (peak 4). (From Sugiura, T., Ojima, T., Fukuda, T., Satouchi, K., Saito, K., and Waku, K., Production of platelet-activating factor in slugs, *J. Lipid Res.*, 32, 1795, 1991. With permission.)

the levels differ considerably from species to species. For instance, the estimated levels of PAF (in pmol/g body weight) were 0.2 (cricket, *Homoeogryllus japonicus*), 0.1 (grasshopper, *Oedaleus infernalis*), 0.5 (dragonfly, *Sympetrum pedemontanum elatum*), 0.1 (beetle, *Allomyrina dichotoma*), 1.3 (cabbage butterfly, *Pieris rapae*), 0.1 (silkworm, *Bombyx mori*), 0.1 (butterfly, *Papilio xuthus*), 0.1 (praying mantis, *Statilia maculata*), 0.1 (flower-fly, *Eristalomyia tenax*), 2.6 (pill bug, *Armadillidium vulgare*), 0.2 (shrimp, *Palaemon paucidens*), 0.2 (prawn, *Penaeus japonicus*), 9.2 (earthworm, *Pheretima* sp.), 3.2 (clam worm, *Perinereis nuntia brevicirris*), 3.6 (clam worm, *Marphysa sanguinea*), 5.4 *(spoon worm, Urechis unicinctus*), 0.7 (freshwater mussel, *Inversidens japanensis*), 2.3 (river snail, *Sinotaia quadratus historica*), 8.0 (Asian hard clam, *Meretrix* sp.), 2.5 (Japanese little neck clam, *Tapes philippinarum*), 0.7 (turban shell, *Batillus cornutus*), 0.3 (button shell, *Omphaliūs pfeifferi*), 0.5 (sea mussel, *Mytilus edulis*), 7.6 (freshwater planaria, *Dugesia japonica*), 0.1 (sea squirt, *Halocynthia roretzi*), 10.5 (sea cucumber, *Stichopus japonicus*), 0.1 (sea urchin, *Anthocidaris crassispina*), 0.8 (sea urchin, *Hemicentrotus pulcherrimus*), 0.1 (starfish, *Astropecten scoparius*), 0.1 (jellyfish, *Aurelia aurita*), 0.9 (sea anemone, *Anthopleura japonica*), 4.3 (sponge, *Halichondria japonica*), and 4.9 (sponge, *Halichondria okadai*).

It is clear from the above results that various types of animals contain considerable amounts of PAF. In particular, high levels of PAF are present in several species of Annelida (e.g., earthworms), Mollusca (e.g., clams), Plantherminthes (e.g., planaria) and Echinoderm (e.g., sea cucumber). Interestingly, substantial amounts of PAF were also detected in sponge, which is the lowest animal among multicellular invertebrates. As for sea cucumber (*Stichopus japonicus*), we found that PAF is not localized in particular tissues, but is distributed throughout the body.[11] This is quite different from the case of rat tissues, in which the levels of PAF are usually low except for a few tissues such as spleen and the digestive system.[11]

In contrast to these lower animals, several species contain only small amounts of PAF. The absence of PAF in various types of insects could be attributed, at least in part, to the very low levels of alkyl ether phospholipids in these animals. Several other animals such as sea squirt, sea urchin, and starfish were also shown to include only small amounts of PAF, though these animals contain large amounts of alkyl ether phospholipids. It is obvious, therefore, that the amounts of PAF are not directly proportional to the levels of alkylacyl-GPC observed in animals. The absence of PAF, however, does not necessarily imply the impairment of the ability to produce PAF. It is possible that these animals, including insects, produce considerable amounts of PAF when stimulated. In fact, we found that the levels of

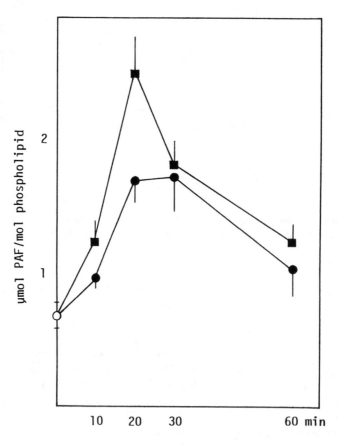

FIGURE 3. Effect of cutting on the levels of PAF in earthworms (*Eisenia foetida*). Earthworms were cut into small pieces (ca. 2 mm) in physiologically balanced salt solution in the presence (■) or absence (●) of A23187 (10 μ*M*). PAF levels were estimated by bioassay using washed rabbit platelets. Values are means ± from four determinations. (From Cheng, N.-N., Sugiura, T., Fukuda, T., and Waku, K., unpublished data, 1991.)

PAF in several types of lower animals were increased when the animals underwent physical or chemical treatments. Figure 3 shows the changes in PAF levels in earthworms, *Eisenia foetida*. The amount of PAF was transiently elevated after the cutting of the body (Figure 3) or after pricking with needles.[32] We also found that the levels of PAF in slugs were markedly increased after the injection of organic solvents such as dimethylsulfoxide (DMSO) and ethanol (Figure 4).[28] Such increases were also observed after several physical stimuli that induce lethal damage (Figure 4).[28] Thus, it appeared that the levels of PAF in various types of invertebrates vary depending on the condition of the animals, although the exact physiological meanings of the changes in PAF levels in stimulated animals are as yet unknown.

PAF is present not only in multicellular but also in unicellular invertebrates. Tsoukatos and co-workers[33] demonstrated the presence of PAF in protozoa (*Tetrahymena pyriformis*) cells. They reported that these cells contain PAF at the level of 4.2 ng/10^7 cells and that only 1 to 3% of PAF was released into the culture medium. Interestingly, the amounts of PAF were not altered when the cells were treated either with calcium ionophore A23187 or with zymosan particles, which is different than the case of WBC in mammals. PAF may be produced continuously in a stimulus-independent manner in these protozoan cells. We also found that the injection or addition of A23187 causes only slight acceleration of PAF production over the control (treated with vehicle alone) in slugs and earthworms (Figures 3

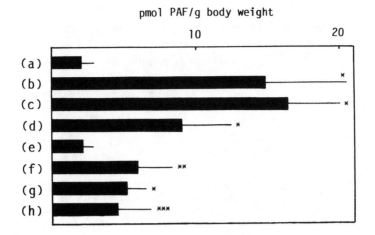

FIGURE 4. Effects of various treatments on the PAF levels in slugs (*Incilaria bileneata*): (a) control; (b) injected with DMSO (50 μl/g body weight); (c) injected with 2 m*M* A23187 in DMSO (50 μl/g body weight); (d) injected with ethanol (50 μl/g body weight); (e) injected with distilled water (50 μl/g body weight); (f) injected with zymosan water solution (4 mg/ml; 50 μl/g body weight); (g) given an electric shock; (h) cut into two. After 15 min, slugs were killed and total lipids were extracted. PAF contents were estimated by bioassay using washed rabbit platelets. Values are means ± SD from six to seven determinations. *p <0.001 vs. (a). **p <0.01 vs. (a). ***p <0.5 vs. (a). (From Sugiura, T., Ojima, T., Fukuda, T., Satouchi, K., Saito, K., and Waku, K., Production of platelet-activating factor in slugs, *J. Lipid Res.*, 32, 1795, 1991. With permission.)

and 4). However, it is evident in these multicellular animals that several other stimuli such as cutting, pricking with needles, and the injection of organic solvents are able to trigger PAF formation through unknown mechanisms.

IV. ENZYME ACTIVITIES INVOLVED IN PLATELET ACTIVATING FACTOR METABOLISM IN INVERTEBRATES

In mammals, PAF is known to be produced via two different biosynthetic routes.[34] One involves the hydrolysis of preexisting alkylacyl-GPC by PLA_2 followed by the acetylation of 1-alkyl-GPC through the action of 1-alkyl-GPC:acetyl-CoA acetyltransferase (remodeling pathway), and the other involves the transfer of phosphocholine from CDP-choline to 1-alkyl-2-acetyl-*sn*-glycerol catalyzed by alkylacetylglycerol:CDP-choline cholinephosphotransferase (*de novo* pathway). We first studied enzyme activities implicated in the biosynthesis of PAF in slugs and earthworms. We found that acetyltransferase activity catalyzing the formation of PAF from 1-alkyl-GPC (lyso-PAF) is present in microsomal fractions (105,000 × *g* pellet fraction) of slugs (Table 2)[28] and earthworms.[32] The specific activity of this enzyme reaction was about one half that of 1-alkyl-GPC:acyl(long chain)-CoA acyltransferase activity observed in the same fraction.[28] On the other hand, the cytosolic fraction (105,000 × *g* supernatant fraction) did not contain acetyltransferase activity, although substantial activity was detected in the mitochondrial fraction (7000 × *g* pellet fraction) as well (Table 2).

Interestingly, several properties of acetyltransferase in slugs and in earthworms were shown to be different than those of mammalian tissues such as spleen. For instance, the addition of EDTA or EGTA to the assay mixture inhibited the enzyme activity of acetyltransferase in microsomal fraction of mammalian tissues,[34] while the presence of these chelators did not influence the enzyme activity in microsomal fraction obtained from slugs.[28] Furthermore, acetyltransferase activity in earthworms was more resistant to increasing concentrations of substrate, 1-alkyl-GPC, than that in mammalian tissues such as rabbit spleen.[32]

TABLE 2
Subcellular Distribution of the Enzyme Activities of
Acetyltransferase and Acetylhydrolase in the Slug,
Incilaria bilineata

Fraction	Acetyltransferase (pmol/min/mg protein)	Acetylhydrolase (pmol/min/mg protein)
7,000 × *g* pellet	34 ± 5	16 ± 6
105,000 × *g* pellet	47 ± 4	31 ± 11
105,000 × *g* supernatant	1 ± 1	105 ± 10

Note: Acetyltransferase activity was estimated using [^{14}C]acetyl-CoA (100 μ*M*) and lyso-PAF (20 μ*M*) as substrates. Acetylhydrolase activity was estimated using [^{3}H]PAF (20 μ*M*) as a substrate. Enzyme activities were measured at 25°C. Values are means ± SD from three to four determinations.[28]

In addition, the activity of acetyltransferase in earthworms was not affected by cutting of the body, which is a stimulus capable of inducing PAF formation in earthworms.[32] The regulation of the enzymes involved in PAF metabolism in lower animals may be somewhat different than that in mammalian tissues.

Microsomal fractions of slugs[28] and earthworms[32] also contain the enzyme activity for the *de novo* synthesis of PAF, alkylacetylglycerol:CDP-choline cholinephosphotransferase. This enzyme activity could produce a considerable amount of PAF if a sufficient amount of the substrate, alkylacetylglycerol, is available. We found that high levels of 1-alkyl-GPC (the substrate for the remodeling pathway) are present in various types of invertebrates.[11] On the other hand, no information is thus far available concerning the levels of alkylacetylglycerol (the substrate for the *de novo* pathway) in lower animals. Therefore, the question remains unsolved whether the *de novo* pathway is physiologically relevant to the biosynthesis of PAF in these lower animals.

As for the degradation of PAF, we found that acetylhydrolase activity is mainly distributed in the cytosloic fraction (105,000 × *g* supernatant fraction) of slugs (Table 2)[28] and earthworms.[32] Lambremont et al.[35] also reported that acetylhydrolase activity is present in cytosolic fraction of corn earworm (*Heliothis zea* Boddie). Such a distribution of acetylhydrolase is similar to that observed in mammalian tissues. Acetylhydrolase activity found in slugs[28] and earthworms[32] appeared to be different than PLA$_2$, which hydrolyzes long-chain fatty acid-containing diradyl phospholipids; the former reaction is Ca^{2+} independent, whereas the latter reaction is Ca^{2+} dependent.[28] The presence of a specific hydrolyzing enzyme strongly suggests that the levels of PAF are highly controlled so that excess amounts of PAF may not exert deleterious effects.

V. METABOLIC FATE OF PLATELET ACTIVATING FACTOR

Protozoan (*Tetrahymena pyriformis*) cells rapidly take up and metabolize exogenously added PAF.[36] When *T. pyriformis* cells (2.5 × 10^6 cells) were incubated with [^{3}H]PAF (10^{-6} *M*), PAF was rapidly converted to alkylacyl(long chain)-GPC: 42 and 82% of PAF was metabolized to alkylacyl(long chain)-GPC during 5 and 30 min of incubation, respectively. Lyso-PAF was also detected as a metabolite (1 to 9%), especially during the first few minutes of the incubation, suggesting that the deacetylation of PAF is an intermediate step in the reaction. Such a rapid conversion of PAF to alkylacyl(long chain)-GPC through a deacetylation-reacylation reaction closely resembles that observed for various mammalian tissues and cells.

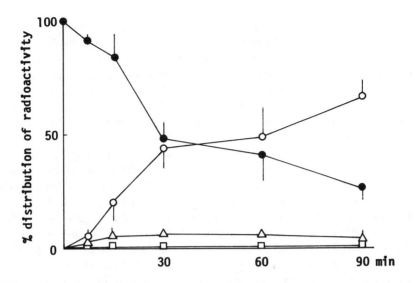

FIGURE 5. Metabolic fate of PAF in slugs (*Incilaria bilineata*). [³H]PAF was dissolved in 0.25% BSA (1 μCi(2 nmol)/ml) and dorsally injected into slugs (0.05 μCi(100 pmol)/g body weight). After the indicated periods, slugs were killed and total lipids were extracted. Individual phospholipids were separated by TLC and their radioactivities were estimated. (●) PAF; (△) lyso-PAF; (○) alkylacyl-GPC; (□) neutral lipids. Values are means ± SD from four determinations. (From Sugiura, T., Miyamoto, T., Fukuda, T., and Waku, K., unpublished data, 1991.)

We also observed that isolated sponge cells metabolize PAF.[37] Exogenously added [³H]PAF (10^{-7} M) was first metabolized to lyso-PAF: 11, 17, and 27% of the radioactivity appeared in the lyso-PAF fraction after 15, 30, and 60 min of incubation, respectively. The radioactivity in alkylacyl(long chain)-GPC also gradually increased with time, accounting for 3% (15 min), 8% (30 min), and 20% (60 min) of total radioactivity. In several types of mammalian cells, such as rabbit alveolar macrophages, the acylation of lyso-PAF is believed to proceed mainly via a cofactor-independent transacylation system.[38,39] We detected only weak activity of cofactor-independent transacylase in the membrane fraction of sponge cells.[37] This may account, at least in part, for the relatively low rate of acylation of lyso-PAF observed in intact cells. We found that cofactor-independent transacylation activity is almost absent in slugs[28] and earthworms.[32] Nevertheless, [³H]PAF was gradually metabolized to [³H]alkylacyl(long chain)-GPC in slugs (Figure 5). It is conceivable, therefore, that acylation systems other than cofactor-independent transacylase are responsible for the acylation of lyso-PAF in these animals.

VI. ACTIONS OF PLATELET ACTIVATING FACTOR ON CELLS

The physiological meaning of the presence of PAF in lower animals is not yet clear. Only limited information on this matter is currently available. Tsoukatos and co-workers[40] suggested the presence of some specific binding sites or areas for PAF in *Tetrahymena pyriformis* cells. These sites are saturable with PAF; saturation of the uptake was obtained for concentrations ranging from 5.7 to 7.8 × 10^9 molecules per cell. They also demonstrated that the administration of PAF (10^{-8} to 10^{-6} M) to *T. pyriformis* cells induces Ca^{2+} influx into the cells.[41] The intracellular levels of Ca^{2+} were elevated time and dose dependently. In contrast, lyso-PAF, even at the dose of 10^{-5} M, failed to stimulate Ca^{2+} influx. The effect of PAF occurred in two phases; one involves the early response, and the other involves the lasting response. They concluded that the rapid increase of intracellular Ca^{2+} was mainly accounted for by the increase of intracellular free Ca^{2+}. This rapid increase of intracellular free Ca^{2+}, as well as the slight increase in control cells, was completely inhibited by the treatment of cells with a Ca^{2+} channel blocker, verapamil. These results suggested that the overall effect of the alterations induced by PAF is the opening of Ca^{2+} channels. They also reported that PAF causes a slow increase of intracellular Na^+, which is possibly the result of a Ca^{2+}/Na^+ exchange mechanism.[41] On the other hand, neither the intracellular level of K^+ nor the cell volume was found to be affected by PAF.

Concerning the biological effect of PAF, they demonstrated that PAF induces glycogenolysis in *T. pyriformis* cells.[42] The concentration of PAF required for such a response (2.6×10^8 molecules per cell) was, however, considerably high compared with the native PAF level (5×10^5 molecules per cell). The level of native PAF was also fairly low compared to that observed at saturation of uptake (5.7 to 7.8×10^9 molecules per cell). On the other hand, *T. pyriformis* cells do not show any microscopic alterations in mobility, shape, or size, even when exposed to a relatively high concentration of PAF (10^{-4} M or 2.6×10^{10} molecules per cell). Thus, the biological role of PAF in these cells remains enigmatic. We also observed that PAF stimulates phospholipid metabolism in isolated sponge cells,[37] the effect being not so prominent as compared to the case of stimulated mammalian tissues. The biological meaning of such an effect is also as yet uncertain. In any event, the biological and biochemical changes induced by PAF in lower animal cells need to be much more extensively investigated. It will be of interest to know whether the mode of actions as well as the physiological meanings of PAF in lower animals are the same as those in mammalian tissues and cells.

VII. CONCLUDING REMARKS

PAF is a unique bioactive phospholipid having an alkyl ether residue at the 1-position of the glycerol backbone. A PAF analogue that contains an acyl moiety at the 1-position (1-acyl-PAF) is also present with PAF in mammalian tissues, though this compound does not possess potent biological activities. Thus, the presence of an alkyl ether residue in the PAF molecule is crucially important for binding to specific receptor(s) and/or the subsequent signal transduction mechanism(s) in mammals. It is noteworthy, however, that alkyl ether phospholipids are not abundantly present in various mammalian tissues, except for several cell types such as WBC. The ratio of alkylacyl(long chain)-GPC to diacyl(long chain)-GPC is usually <0.05.[12] We also found that several species of insects, which are regarded as rather advanced animals, are not enriched in alkylacyl-GPC. On the other hand, various other types of invertebrates, especially in the lower phyla, contain large amounts of alkylacyl-GPC, suggesting that alkyl ether phospholipids came to be produced as a major component of biomembranes at the earliest stage of the evolution of animals. It can be emphasized, therefore, alkyl ether phospholipids are important lipid molecules, particularly for lower invertebrates. The observation that significant amounts of PAF are present in various types of lower animals also suggests that PAF has been conserved through long periods on an evolutional time scale, and it is likely to play important roles in these lower animals under physiological conditions. Studies on PAF in lower animals should provide valuable information for the better understanding of the metabolic control, modes of action, and physiological as well as pathological roles of PAF in advanced higher animals.

REFERENCES

1. **Benveniste, J., Henson, P. M., and Cochrane, C. G.,** Leukocyte-dependent histamine release from rabbit platelets: the role of IgE, basophils, and a platelet-activating factor, *J. Exp. Med.,* 136, 1356, 1972.

2. **Demopoulos, C. A., Pinckard, R. N., and Hanahan, D. J.,** Platelet-activating factor. Evidence for 1-O-alkyl-2-acetyl-sn-glyceryl-3-phosphorylcholine as the active component (a new class of lipid chemical mediators), *J. Biol. Chem.,* 254, 9355, 1979.

3. **Blank, M. L., Snyder, F., Byers, L. W., Brooks, B., and Muirhead, E. E.,** Antihypertensive activity of an alkyl ether analog of phosphatidylcholine, *Biochem. Biophys. Res. Commun.,* 90, 1194, 1979.

4. **Benveniste, J., Tence, M., Varenne, P., Bidault, J., Boullet, C., and Polonsky, J.,** Semi-synthesis and proposed structure of platelet-activating factor (PAF): PAF-acether, an alkyl ether analog of lysophosphatidylcholine, *C. R. Acad. Sci.,* 289D, 1037, 1979.

5. **Braquet, P., Touqui, L., Shen, T. Y., and Vargaftig, B. B.,** Perspectives in platelet-activating factor research, *Pharmacol. Rev.,* 39, 97, 1987.

6. **Yasuda, K., Satouchi, K., and Saito, K.,** Platelet-activating factor in normal rat uterus, *Biochem. Biophys. Res. Commun.,* 138, 1231, 1986.

7. **Sugatani, J., Fujimura, K., Miwa, M., Mizuno, T., Sameshima, Y., and Saito, K.,** Occurrence of platelet-activating factor (PAF) in normal rat stomach and alteration of PAF level by water immersion stress, *FASEB J.,* 3, 65, 1989.

8. **Saito, K., Nakayama, R., Yasuda, K., Satouchi, K., and Sugatani, J.,** PAF analogues in normal rat tissues, in *Biological Mass Spectrometry,* Burlingame, A. L. and McCloskey, J. A., Eds., Elsevier, Amsterdam, 1990, 527.

9. **Johnston, J. M., Bleasdale, J. E., and Hoffman, D. R.,** Functions of PAF in reproduction and development: involvement of PAF in fetal lung maturation and parturition, in *Platelet-Activating Factor and Related Lipid Mediators,* Synder, F., Ed., Plenum Press, New York, 1987, 375.

10. **Tokumura, A., Kamiyasu, K., Takauchi, K., and Tsukatani, H.,** Evidence for existence of various homologues and analogues of platelet-activating factor in a lipid extract of bovine brain, *Biochem. Biophys. Res. Commun.,* 145, 415, 1987.

11. **Sugiura, T., Fukuda, T., Miyamoto, T., and Waku, K.,** Distribution of alkyl and alkenyl ether-linked phospholipids and platelet-activating factor-like lipid in various species of invertebrates, *Biochim. Biophys. Acta,* in press, 1991.

12. **Sugiura, T. and Waku, K.,** Composition of alkyl ether-linked phospholipids in mammalian tissues, in *Platelet-Activating Factor and Related Lipid Mediators,* Synder, F., Ed., Plenum Press, New York, 1987, 55.

13. **Debuch, H. and Seng, P.,** The history of ether-linked lipids through 1960, in *Ether Lipids, Chemistry and Biology,* Snyder, F., Ed., Academic Press, New York, 1972, 1.

14. **Tsujimoto, M. and Toyama, Y.,** *Chem. Umsch. Geb. Fette, Olele, Wachse Harze,* 29, 27, 1922.

15. **Carter, H. E., Smith, D. B., and Jones, D. N.,** A new ethanol amine-containing lipid from egg yolk, *J. Biol. Chem.,* 232, 681, 1958.

16. **Thompson, G. A., Jr. and Hanahan, D. J.,** Identification of α-glyceryl ether phospholipids as major lipid constituents in two species of terrestrial slug, *J. Biol. Chem.,* 238, 2628, 1963.

17. **Thompson, G. A., Jr.,** Studies of membrane formation in *Tetrahymena pyriformis.* I. Rates of phospholipid biosynthesis, *Biochemistry,* 6, 2015, 1967.

18. **Malins, D. C. and Varanasi, U.,** The ether bond in marine lipids, in *Ether Lipids, Chemistry and Biology,* Snyder, F., Ed., Academic Press, New York, 1972, 297.

19. **Thompson, G. A., Jr.,** Ether-linked lipids in molluscs, in *Ether Lipids, Chemistry and Biology,* Snyder, F., Ed., Academic Press, New York, 1972, 313.

20. **Thompson, G. A., Jr.,** Ether-linked lipids in protozoa, in *Ether Lipids, Chemistry and Biology,* Snyder, F., Ed., Academic Press, New York, 1972, 321.

21. **Horrocks, L. A. and Sharma, M.,** Plasmalogens and O-alkyl glycerophospholipids, in *Phospholipids,* Hawthorne, J. N. and Ansell, G. B., Eds., Elsevier, Amsterdam, 1982, 51.

22. **Isay, S. V., Makarchenko, M. A., and Vaskovsky, V. E.,** A study of glyceryl ethers. I. Content of α-glyceryl ethers in marine invertebrates from the Sea of Japan and tropical regions of the Pacific Ocean, *Comp. Biochem. Physiol.,* 55B, 301, 1976.

23. **Pietruszko, R.,** Lipids of red bone marrow from pig epiphyses, *Biochim. Biophys. Acta,* 64, 562, 1962.

24. **Thompson, G. A., Jr. and Hanahan, D. J.,** Studies on the nature and formation of α-glyceryl ether lipids in bovine bone marrow, *Biochemistry,* 2, 641, 1963.

25. **Sugiura, T., Onuma, Y., Sekiguchi, N., and Waku, K.,** Ether phosphiolipids in guinea pig polymorphonuclear leukocytes and macrophages: occurrence of high levels of 1-O-alkyl-2-acyl-sn-glycero-3-phosphocholine, *Biochim. Biophys. Acta,* 712, 515, 1982.

26. **Mueller, H. W., O'Flaherty, J. T., and Wykle, R. L.,** Ether lipid content and fatty acid distribution in rabbit polymorphonuclear neutrophil phospholipids, *Lipids,* 17, 72, 1982.
27. **Sugiura, T., Nakajima, M., Sekiguchi, N., Nakagawa, Y., and Waku, K.,** Different fatty chain compositions of alkenylacyl, alkylacyl and diacyl phospholipids in rabbit alveolar macrophages: high amounts of arachidonic acid in ether phospholipids, *Lipids,* 18, 125, 1983.
28. **Sugiura, T., Ojima, T., Fukuda, T., Satouchi, K., Saito, K., and Waku, K.,** Production of platelet-activating factor in slugs, *J. Lipid Res.,* 32, 1795, 1991.
29. **Liang, C.-R. and Strickland, K. P.,** Phospholipid metabolism in the molluscs. I. Distribution of phospholipids in the water snail *Lymnaea stagnalis, Can. J. Biochem.,* 47, 85, 1969.
30. **Sugiura, T.,** unpublished data, 1991.
31. **Kaneshiro, E. S.,** Positional distribution of fatty acids in the major glycerophospholipids of *Paramecium tetraurelia, J. Lipid Res.,* 21, 559, 1980.
32. **Cheng, N.-N., Sugiura, T., Fukuda, T., and Waku, K.,** unpublished data, 1991.
33. **Lekka, M., Tselepis, A. D., and Tsoukatos, D.,** 1-*O*-alkyl-2-acetyl-*sn*-glyceryl-3-phosphorylcholine (PAF) is a minor lipid component in the *Tetrahymena pyriformis* cells, *FEBS Lett.,* 208, 52, 1986.
34. **Lee, T.-C.,** Enzymatic control of the cellular levels of platelet-activating factor, in *Platelet-Activating Factor and Related Lipid Mediators,* Snyder, F., Ed., Plenum Press, New York, 1987, 115.
35. **Lambremont, E. N., Malone, B., and Snyder, F.,** Platelet-activating factor-acetylhydrolase in insects: identification and partial characterization of a 1-alkyl-2-acetyl-*sn*-glycero-3-phosphocholine acetylhydrolase in a cell-free system of *Heliothis, Arch. Insect Biochem. Physiol.,* 7, 37, 1988.
36. **Lekka, M. E., Tsoukatos, D., and Kapoulas, V. M.,** *In vivo* metabolism of platelet-activating factor (1-*O*-alkyl-2-acetyl-*sn*-glycero-3-phosphocholine) by the protozoan *Tetrahymena pyriformis, Biochim. Biophys. Acta,* 1042, 217, 1990.
37. **Sugiura, T., Miyamoto, T., Fukuda, T., and Waku, K.,** unpublished data, 1991.
38. **Sugiura, T. and Waku, K.,** CoA-independent transfer of arachidonic acid from 1,2-diacyl-*sn*-glycero-3-phosphocholine to 1-*O*-alkyl-*sn*-glycero-3-phosphocholine (lyso platelet-activating factor) by macrophage microsomes, *Biochem. Biophys. Res. Commun.,* 127, 384, 1985.
39. **Robinson, M., Blank, M. L., and Synder, F.,** Acylation of lysophospholipids by rabbit alveolar macrophages. Specificities of CoA-dependent and CoA-independent reactions, *J. Biol. Chem.,* 260, 7889, 1985.
40. **Lekka, M. E., Tsoukatos, D., and Kapoulas, V. M.,** Uptake of platelet-activating factor (1-*O*-alkyl-2-acetyl-(l-o-alkyl-2-acetyl-sn-)*sn*-glycero-3-phosphocholine) by *Tetrahymena pyriformis, Comp. Biochem. Physiol.,* 93B, 113, 1989.
41. **Tselepis, A., Tsoukatos, D., Demopoulos, C. A., and Kapoulas, V. M.,** Effects of AGEPC on the intracellular levels of ions in *Tetrahymena pyriformis, Biochem. Int.,* 13, 999, 1986.
42. **Tsangaris, T., Demopoulos, C. A., Tsoukatos, D., Tournis, S., and Kapoulas, V. M.,** Stimulation of glycogenolysis by AGEPC in *Tetrahymena pyriformis,* in *Abstr. 2nd Int. Conf. Platelet-Activating Factor and Structurally Related Alkyl Ether Lipids,* TN, October 26 to 29, 1986, 133.

INDEX

MERCK RESEARCH LABORATORIES
LITERATURE RESOURCES, RAHWAY